Shifting Gears

Shifting Gears:

The 1,000-Mile Ride That Changed My Mindset on Type 1 Diabetes

Dr. Ian Lake

WB
WELLNESS BOOKS

Copyright

Published in the United Kingdom by Wellness Books
www.wellnessbooks.co.uk

Cover design by Iain Hill of 1981D

ISBN: 978-1-0684581-4-9
First published 2026
Printed in the United Kingdom

Dedicated To

People living with type 1 diabetes, who face the challenge of managing it every day. You are heroes.

Disclaimer

This book reflects a personal journey of someone living with type1 diabetes through the science and practice of type 1 diabetes. It is intended for educational and general informational purposes only and should be read with that in mind. The content is not a substitute for professional medical advice, diagnosis, or treatment, and it should never replace consultation with your diabetes specialist or healthcare team. It is not intended that you compare your own diabetes numbers with the ones presented here. Everyone has different challenges in type 1 diabetes, and this book is published to support the case for a rethink.

The goal of this book is to offer a framework of understanding that can enhance collaboration with your healthcare providers in managing type 1 diabetes. If you live with type 1 diabetes and also experience complications or have other medical conditions, please consult your doctor or medical practitioner before making any adjustments. Please also refer to the appendix at the end of the book, where additional guidance is provided on safely optimising insulin therapy.

In most cases, an optimised insulin strategy is beneficial and safe; however, everybody is different. Some might decide it is not for them. Sometimes, adopting a slower, more gradual approach is the wisest path, allowing your system the time it needs to adjust. Sudden, significant changes – especially in the presence of advanced complications – can temporarily stress the body, so patience and careful pacing are strongly encouraged.

Table of Contents

Foreword

When I first began working in medicine, diabetes was taught to us in neat diagrams and tidy algorithms. Glucose went up, insulin brought it down, and success was measured by numbers on a page. Over time – through years of clinical practice, research, and conversations with people living with diabetes – I learned that real life is far less predictable. Patients do the same things on different days and get completely different results. They follow the rules and still feel that something doesn't quite add up. That tension between theory and lived experience is what drew me immediately to *Shifting Gears*.

Dr Lake writes not only as a physician but as someone who has lived inside the daily reality of type 1 diabetes for decades. That dual perspective gives this book a rare authenticity. It is one thing to understand insulin physiology from the outside; it is another to feel its effects hour by hour, mile by mile, decision by decision. His willingness to question assumptions – while remaining grounded in science – is both refreshing and necessary. In many ways, this work carries forward the spirit and books of Dr. Richard Bernstein and Dr. Keith Runyan, whose pioneering efforts challenged conventional thinking and empowered individuals with diabetes to better understand their own physiology.

Throughout my career, I have come to see insulin as far more than a glucose-lowering medication. It is a master metabolic hormone that influences energy, fat metabolism, appetite, and the broader rhythms of human physiology. Yet traditional teaching has often narrowed the conversation to carbohydrates and dosing strategies alone. What Dr Lake offers in these pages is not a rejection of established care but an expansion of it, encouraging deeper metabolic thinking while remaining practical and grounded in lived experience. He invites readers to look at the wider context – the interaction between nutrition, movement, sleep, stress, environment, and circadian rhythm – and to consider how these factors shape insulin sensitivity and day-to-day stability.

The journey at the heart of this book – a 1,000-mile cycling expedition – is more than a physical challenge. It becomes a framework for exploration: of endurance, adaptation, and the evolving relationship between insulin and lifestyle. As I read, I was reminded of many patients who discovered that meaningful change often begins not with a new device or a new prescription, but with a new understanding of how their bodies respond to the world around them.

What I appreciate most is the tone of humility that runs through these pages. Dr Lake does not present a rigid set of instructions. Instead, he offers a way of thinking – an invitation to observe patterns, ask better questions, and approach type 1 diabetes with curiosity rather than frustration. That approach resonates deeply with my own experience in metabolic medicine, where progress often comes from stepping back and reconsidering assumptions that have long gone unquestioned.

For clinicians, *Shifting Gears* provides a reminder that physiology is dynamic and deeply influenced by lifestyle inputs that extend far beyond the plate. For individuals living with type 1 diabetes, it offers validation – that the variability they experience is not a personal failure, but a reflection of a complex metabolic system responding to countless signals.

Books like this matter because they bridge worlds that are too often separated: the clinical and the personal, the scientific and the experiential. By sharing his story with clarity and openness, Dr Lake contributes to a broader conversation about how we understand insulin, metabolism, and the lived reality of type 1 diabetes – very much in the tradition of those who have challenged us to think differently about insulin and metabolic health.

It is my hope that readers approach these pages with an open mind and a spirit of exploration. Whether you are a clinician, a researcher, or someone navigating type 1 diabetes yourself, you may find – as I did – that this journey encourages you to rethink familiar ideas and see metabolism through a wider lens.

Eric C. Westman, MD, MHS
Duke University Health System
Durham, North Carolina USA

Introduction

Silencing the Chainsaw and Hearing the Birds Sing

The morning I cracked three eggs into a pan of melted butter, I did not know I was beginning a revolution. I was not planning one. I was not trying to break rules or challenge a system, I just wanted a peaceful morning. I wanted to avoid another hypo by 10 am. I wanted, if I am honest, a break from the constant firefighting of my glucose levels.

That omelette turned out to be the first moment of clarity I had had in over two decades of living with type 1 diabetes. For the first time, I ate a meal without needing to react. I did not crash or spike. I just... stayed steady. The chainsaw of diabetes – the relentless mental noise, corrections, recalculations, corrections of corrections – finally fell quiet. And when I silenced the chainsaw, I could hear the birds sing. I began to tune into my body.

And so began the shift. Not just a change in diet or insulin strategy, but a complete rethinking of what it means to live with type 1 diabetes: a paradigm shift. A rebellion, gentle but grounded in science and lived experience. I was a doctor; I was also a patient. I had followed the guidelines for years – and I had been getting sicker.

This book is the story of how I found another way, one that is simpler, saner, and more sustainable. One that replaces chaos with calm. One that does more than manage blood sugar – it transforms lives.

From Guidelines to Guesswork

I was diagnosed in 1995. Like most of us, I followed the medical advice of the time: eat complex carbs, keep fat low, match insulin accordingly, and exercise as much as you can. I did all of it. I cycled to work, counted carbs, carried glucose tablets, and chased my numbers with good intentions – and a growing sense of frustration.

The blood test for long-term glucose control, HbA1c, is less than 42 mmol/mol (6%) for those without the condition. The guideline-accepted target for good type 1 control is 48 mmol/mol (6.5%). Back when I was diagnosed, the number was 58 mmol/mol (7.5%). HbA1c is a predictor of the likelihood of diabetes complications. The higher it is, the higher the risk of complications.

My numbers hovered in the high 50s mmol/mol (7.5%) for years. Sometimes they were close to that, sometimes much worse. I was told, and believed, that this was acceptable, I was doing okay; after all, at the time, it was the guideline target. But it was way off normal. I can get to normal nowadays but back then, it seemed impossible. No one went for normal.

Every Monday was a reset as I tried to do better. Porridge for breakfast, then a cycle ride to work. I was aiming for stability. But by 10:30 am, I was treating a hypo. By lunch, I was spiking. Then crashing again. This repeated until… burnout! Yet I never questioned it; I was part of the system delivering it. I was always told that type 1 diabetes was a tough condition, and so I thought this was as good as it got.

When the Student Becomes the Rebel

The turning point came when I stumbled upon Dr Richard Bernstein, an American physician and pioneer in diabetes management. His story mirrored mine: someone living with type 1 diabetes who became fed up with the chaos of trying to manage it. He found stability through a low-carb diet and minimal insulin. His logic was sound and his results compelling. But it ran counter to everything I had been taught, and everything I was teaching others. At first, I dismissed it; it did not fit my paradigm. I was not ready.

But when early complications began to appear – when brain fog became my default state, when my HbA1c drifted into the 80's (9%) – I gave Bernstein's method a try. The result was immediate and dramatic. My glucose stabilised. My insulin use dropped. The fog lifted. Aches vanished. My mood improved. My sleep deepened. I had not realised how unwell I had been until I started feeling well.

Optimised Insulin, Not Just Normalised Glucose

The breakthrough was not just cutting carbs; it was understanding insulin itself.

In medical school, we are taught that insulin is just a glucose-lowering drug, but it is more than that. It is a master hormone of energy balance, inflammation, fat storage and ageing. Excess insulin, even in the presence of normal glucose, can harm the body. The goal is not just to lower glucose; it is to use insulin wisely as well.

What I needed was not more insulin, it was less – better timed, more in sync with how my body would naturally release it. This was the beginning of what I call "optimised insulin".

A Broader Framework for the Foundations of Health

As I refined my insulin strategy, I began noticing how other aspects of life affected my control of diabetes. I grouped them into what I now call the five foundations of health:

1. **Nutrition** – A diet based on real food, prioritising protein and fat whilst restricting carbohydrate. It transformed my need for insulin and my glucose control.
2. **Activity** – Exercise became a tool to support insulin sensitivity, not to compensate for poor control or be feared.
3. **Mindset** – The psychological burden lifted. With fewer hypos and less chaos, I felt human again.
4. **Environment** – Light exposure, temperature and stress altered my glucose. I learned to work with these forces.
5. **Circadian rhythms** – Understanding how my body clock regulates hormones helped me align insulin dosing more precisely.

This became my new model of care: optimised insulin, rooted in biology, but personalised by lived experience.

A 1,000-Mile Journey of Proof

To test this model in real life, I set off on a three-week cycle ride from my home in the southwest of England to a medical conference in St Moritz, Switzerland, a journey of 1,000 miles (1,600km). I was not aiming for superhuman activity levels but rather to explore how accessible this lifestyle is to everyone; I was going to take my time and enjoy the view. This was not the challenge of a "man of a certain age", or a Lycra-fest. It was not a race. It was an experiment. My bike was my office chair, and my office was the cycle route across South England, along the River Rhine and over the Swiss Alps. My goal was to cover a modest, achievable daily distance and arrive on time in St Moritz.

Along the way, I tracked glucose, ketones, insulin, heart rate, food and distance. Could optimised insulin carry me over the Alps? Could the five foundations of health keep me steady, fuelled and well? Spoiler: yes, they could!

I felt strong. I slept soundly. My glucose stayed in range. My mind was clear. My body – flexible and pain-free – kept going without fuss. I did not chase perfection. In reality, I could not; I had no pump to finesse the numbers, and I am not painstakingly diligent by nature. However, I did chase consistency, based on knowledge of how to optimise insulin.

Technology: A Tool, Not the Solution

Modern tools like continuous glucose meters (CGMs) and pumps are remarkable advances, and can be very helpful – but they can easily dazzle us with their technological prowess, and we can forget the fundamental question: how much insulin are we using, and why?

We are told that a flat glucose line is the gold standard. But if that flatline is driven by excess insulin with no regard for volume, it may be doing more harm than good. Optimised insulin uses smaller doses, less often, with more impact. It will augment technology, not replace it. It respects Dr. Bernstein's "law of small numbers":

Smaller mealtime carbohydrates + smaller insulin doses = smaller margins of error.

The Science Is Clear, The Culture Isn't

The very-low-carb, or ketogenic, approach is backed by strong evidence: lower HbA1c, reduced hypoglycaemia, improved lipid profiles, mental clarity and better mood. And yet, it remains marginalised. Why? Partly because medical education still teaches outdated dietary advice.

There is, in fact, not a single piece of research that shows the superiority of the current high-carb guideline diet recommended for type 1 diabetes. We were bolted onto guidelines designed to prevent second heart attacks in people without diabetes, because it was felt that, well, we have a higher risk of heart disease anyway, so let's recommend a "heart-healthy" diet. No one, it seems, thought about the effect a high-carb diet would have on the insulin demands of the body. Partly because change is hard; new paradigms require giving up past habits. And partly because, as clinicians, we are slow to question what we ourselves were taught. New knowledge is hard to teach when almost all textbooks preach old ideas, repeated until they start to look like fact.

But science moves forward still. Paradigms shift. And I believe we are on the brink of such a shift.

A Doctor-Patient's Dilemma

My journey to Switzerland was also an identity-reckoning. I had been both prescriber and recipient of the same failed advice. Changing my mind meant confronting my professional pride. It meant standing apart. It meant admitting I had been wrong. But it also meant finding freedom – and once I experienced the power of optimised insulin, I could not go back. Not ethically, not personally.

I began teaching this method to others. And I watched them thrive.

This Is a Call to Change

If you are living with type 1 diabetes or treating someone who is, this book is an invitation – not to abandon science, but to deepen it. Not to reject tools, but to use them more wisely. Not to strive for perfection, but for peace. This is not rebellion for the sake of it; it is a quiet revolution grounded in science, experience, and a desire to do no harm. I am not promoting a fringe theory, I am living the results – and I have seen what happens when others do the same: better control, less insulin.

This approach will not cure your diabetes. But it can silence the chainsaw. It can replace firefighting with foresight, panic with pattern, and guesswork with understanding. It can help you – or those you care for – hear the birdsong again.

What This Book Offers

This is not a diet book. It is not a how-to-manage-diabetes manual. I know what it is like to be on both sides of type 1 diabetes, and so I have written this primarily for my fellow T1s. I have put all of my learning about type 1 diabetes into this book. It contains a wealth of information that should also be useful to clinicians – they are very welcome to read it, and I think it will provide some valuable insights into the optimised insulin approach.

By the end of this book, you should have a deep understanding of how optimised insulin can work with your unique type 1 diabetes and feel confident in its management. You should be knowledgeable enough to feel empowered to collaborate with your clinician about your care. This is a condition that has to be managed 24 hours a day. You will be lucky indeed to find a diabetologist available at three in the morning; often the only person in charge is the person with the condition.

This is a story of paradigm shift – a lived experiment in healing and hope. It weaves personal experience with clinical insight. It is grounded in data but told with heart. And above all, it is optimistic – because I have seen what is possible. I have lived it.

Shifting Gears is two books in one. Firstly, it is an account of my cycling journey to Switzerland; it is a daily diary of the three-week adventure, with details of how I managed my type 1 diabetes with optimised insulin. Alternating with this travel adventure are chapters that will take you through how the body metabolises insulin, what insulin is, and how insulin impacts many aspects of our daily life. It explores the foundations of health: nutrition, activity, mindset, our environment, sleep, and circadian rhythms. The diary chapters begin with a cycle symbol, and the detail chapters begin with the target symbol.

The book can be read solely as a travel diary which will give a lot of information about the daily management of type 1 diabetes. At the end of these chapters is a map of the day's route and a QR code linking you to a series of images taken on that day.

It can equally be read as a textbook. I hope that by alternating chapters, you will build up your knowledge and enjoy learning along the journey. You do not need a medical background to understand the medical details, though some sections may require a second read. There are references at the end of the book that you can explore, to dive deeper into the concepts that interest you.

I hope it will become clear that type 1 diabetes need not be complex to manage if you adopt the principles of optimised insulin. I hope also that by the end of the book, you are an expert, and feel confident through knowledge that your chosen path is the result of an informed choice – whatever path you choose. I think you will be surprised how straightforward it really is.

As doctors, we give ourselves an impossible task by prescribing the wrong diet. The metabolic mayhem that follows adds unnecessary complexity. This book follows an approach based on the latest findings in the science of nutrition, metabolism and biochemistry. Hopefully, by the end, you will feel more in control. When the realisation dawns as you go through the book, I challenge you not to say, *"Why wasn't I told this years ago?"* It is the most common reaction I get.

Chapter 1
Breakfast Rebellion

"We all have big changes in our lives that are more or less a second chance."
– Harrison Ford

Welcome to my world: type 1 diabetes visited me without warning in 1995 when I was in my mid-thirties. It will be with me for the rest of my life. I have to learn to live with it and give it my best shot – no pun intended.

Type 1 diabetes is a tough condition to manage; it is unpredictable, often frustrating, and never quite plays by the rules. For me, there were times when things would unexpectedly improve, those rare stretches of good glucose control that seemed to come out of nowhere. But just as often, I would experience inexplicable runs of poor control. I could do exactly the same thing two days in a row and end up with completely different results. It always felt random and deeply perplexing. It reminded me of the line often attributed to Einstein: "Insanity is doing the same thing over and over again and expecting different results." Except with type 1 diabetes, doing the same thing and getting different outcomes is practically the rule, not the exception. That is what makes it so maddening: you can be careful, disciplined and consistent, and still be punished by variability you did not see coming.

Over time, since diagnosis, I developed a pragmatic strategy. I obviously wanted normal glucose, but aimed to 'stay safe' by keeping it slightly high: between 7 and 10 mmol/L (126–180 mg/dL). High glucose levels can lead to long-term complications, and although I was not managing my blood glucose very well, I believed I could offset some of the risk. I focused on physical activity. Type 1 diabetes comes with a higher risk of cardiovascular disease, and exercise reduces that risk – so, I cycled, I ran, I moved as much as I could. I told myself that my active lifestyle could offset less-than-ideal glucose levels.

That was how I lived for years – doing the best I could. I ate what I wanted, because it was considered normal practice, and injected insulin to match. It was what I now refer to as "hedonistic management". I did not give much thought to insulin dosing beyond knowing that large doses tended to cause large hypos; I followed the guidance of the time – guidance that remains the standard even today. I hope that will change, and the early signs are there.

Living with type 1 diabetes is more than a physical challenge, it is an emotional rollercoaster. The constant vigilance, the unpredictability, the daily mental calculations. It wears you down. Just when you think you have found balance, something shifts. A minor illness, a moment of stress, a meal that digests differently, and suddenly everything is off. The condition can feel like it is in control of you, not the other way around. It can be very stressful having to manage type 1 diabetes in addition to the normal life challenges we all face. In those early years, I struggled with this mindset.

In my clinical practice, I watched complications unfold in my patients, some slowly, others suddenly. It reinforced a grim belief: no matter how well you manage your blood sugar, the condition will catch up with you. I came to believe that complications were inevitable, and the best I could do was delay them. I still remember the moment of diagnosis, when the urine test strip changed from blue to brown. I realised then that I had type 1 diabetes. And with that realisation came the silent expectation that things would only get worse – that decline was inevitable. That sense of resignation stayed with me for a long time. It shaped how I approached diabetes:

conservatively, reactively, with a kind of quiet dread in the background. But all of that would eventually change.

The framework I had been taught seemed logical and practical enough. Carbohydrates raise blood sugar more than any other variable. Insulin lowers it. People with type 1 diabetes do not produce insulin, so they have to inject it. The theory was straightforward: calculate the carbohydrates, match the insulin, and time both so that the insulin peaks just as the glucose from digestion enters the bloodstream. The two were supposed to meet like dance partners, arriving together, moving in sync, and gracefully lowering glucose levels. To this, you added a background dose of long-acting basal insulin to cover everything else, including those variables that complicate glucose control – overnight liver glucose output, hormonal fluctuations, activity fluctuations and stress. That was the model, and it sounded tidy on paper.

Some people made it look easy. I saw them occasionally in the clinic: patients with impeccable records, with HbA1c levels much lower than mine, logging their readings with discipline and precision. I assumed they were simply better organised than I was; I could never get to those levels of control. And many more were complication-free, despite having a conventional diet. Meanwhile, I was hovering around an average HbA1c of 58 mmol/mol (7.5%) for majority of the first two decades. Not terrible, not great – except for a brief spell in the honeymoon phase where, for reasons not fully understood, the body's remaining insulin-producing cells keep working. My control briefly mimicked someone without diabetes, but my diabetes did not respond like theirs.

In the years before I made any significant changes, my HbA1c crept up to 80 mmol/mol (9.5%), life got busy, priorities shifted and I lost focus. I assumed the fault was mine: my habits, my mindset, my discipline. I felt like a failure, and as a doctor it stung more. I was not walking the talk; I was not even managing to walk in a straight line. In effect, I was not a 'good' diabetic. We tend to sense the judgment when we attend a diabetes clinic – well, I do.

I remember when I was at medical school, a consultant showed us a woman who had been complication-free for 60 years, who was quite rightly looking happy and confident. He then showed us a man who had been wheeled up from the dialysis unit. This man was an amputee who had had a stroke and was wrapped in a standard-issue white, waffle-knit hospital blanket. One of the corners was dragging on the floor, collecting the dirt, and he looked beaten. After the patients had left, the consultant said, referring to the woman, "This is what happens when you manage your diabetes well…" and then, referring to the man, "this is what happens when you don't." Cruel judgment, and ignorant, as we know – but that is how I learned about type 1. I know that a lot of people living with type 1 also blame themselves for their poor HbA1c; I am not alone. So, if I am not a 'good' diabetic, what am I?

Indeed, I tried to hide my condition. It became a guilty secret. I was afraid of being judged because my numbers were not that great. How would that reflect on the rest of my clinical practice? *"If this doctor can't manage type 1 diabetes, what else can't he manage?"* I never saw other people in that way at all, so it said a lot about me that I judged myself by different standards. I had a lot of growing up to do, clearly.

Things I took for granted were reassessed in the light of my diagnosis of type 1 diabetes. I would be constantly "on call" for low and high glucose. I could not just eat when I wanted; I had to plan. My right to drive would now be medically assessed every three years, and I would be subjected to lifelong monitoring and surveillance through the NHS. I would likely die a decade earlier and possibly deteriorate with complications a decade before that; I had seen it all unravel in others. I had friends who were uneasy about driving with me. I learned that families with children living with type 1 found it difficult to let their children stay overnight at their friends' houses because their friends' parents were uneasy with the responsibility.

I reacted by staying silent about my condition. I was not helping by keeping it to myself, but acceptance takes time. They say that the final part of a doctor's training is when they get ill themselves. They are right, it is the most challenging module in my curriculum. I could accept my diabetes diagnosis but I could not take the fact that I was unable to control it. All the clichés about health and wealth come to mind. I am a team player, and this hurt a lot. When I finally managed to get control, the relief was indescribable.

It took 20 years for me to realise that I was not the problem. It did not matter how carefully I matched insulin to carbs; if I did not sleep well, if I exercised too late, if I was stressed, or even if the weather changed, my blood glucose could spiral out of control. I know now that the problem was the method I was using to manage my type 1. Diabetes education had all the veneer of science, but it was not sensitive enough to account for the chaos of real life. In fact, when I finally began to challenge "group-think", I realised that the science was not being followed at all. This was not about any lack of personal willpower; this was about poor-quality science in the management model we were being told to follow.

Dr Richard Bernstein's findings that very low-carb diets improved type1 diabetes control were revolutionary at the time, and the response from the medical establishment was rejection. The American Diabetes Association dismissed his work. At the time, he was an engineer in a medical laboratory; he trained to become a doctor so he could advocate for it himself. Bernstein lived with type 1 diabetes for over 75 years and still practised medicine in his 80s. His work has influenced tens of thousands of people living with type 1 diabetes, including me, offering them not just hope but practical, measurable results. And yet, shockingly, almost no one in my professional circles has heard of him.

For me, embracing his approach would mean tearing up everything I had been taught. Back then, I was telling patients to avoid fat and eat more carbohydrates, and to be consistent, I was following that advice myself. Bernstein was telling me to do the exact opposite. Someone had to be wrong. At the time, I found it difficult to practise against the consensus. The National Institute for Health and Care Excellence (NICE) guidelines, crafted by panels of respected experts, were clear: they reinforced the carbohydrate-heavy model. I took reassurance from the authority of it all. I continued to give that advice to my patients, and to follow the same advice myself. I was not ready to flip my thinking – not then.

I put Dr Bernstein's book back on the shelf, but not for long. The seed had been planted. And once you have seen a glimmer of truth, something that explains the chaos and promises stability, you can't unsee it. The question kept growing in the back of my mind: could it be that we have been managing it wrong all along?

I started to believe that I needed to unlearn everything I had been taught about type 1 diabetes. Was everyone else driving on the wrong side of the road, or was I? It was not easy. As a doctor, I am trained to believe in the system. I am tested on the guidelines. I am rewarded for staying inside the lines. The exams do not ask if the guidelines are right; they ask if you can recite them. I remember a colleague who failed a finals examination module for suggesting in an exam that a low-carb, high-fat diet might be a better next-step intervention in type 2 diabetes than insulin. "How to initiate insulin" was the required answer. He gave the "wrong" answer, even though it made metabolic sense and was backed up by science. He passed the resit by providing the standard and "right" response – start insulin – and went on to join the Royal College of General Practitioners as a primary care physician.

That moment stuck with me because it showed me how dogmatic our professional narratives can be, and how threatened they become when challenged by experience. Recalibrating your thinking, especially when it conflicts with professional orthodoxy, is deeply uncomfortable, and that discomfort can easily turn into defensiveness. It is easier to call someone "non-compliant" than to admit the guidance may not work. It is easier to blame the patient than to question the dogma. I had to work through some of those conflicts myself.

Additionally, type 1 diabetes is not the one-size-fits-all we are taught to obey. What works for one person might fail for another; we are all individuals. That is why fewer than 10% of people with type 1 reach the so-called "good control" benchmark of 48 mmol/mol

(6.5%) in a rigid model of management. We all need to find our way, based on quality information.

Eventually, healthwise, I arrived at a point of no return. The warning signs were there: early complications, nagging symptoms, poor sleep, brain fog, fatigue. My first letter informing me of background retinopathy was the kick I needed. I won't say I panicked, but I remember, even today, exactly where I was when I read the letter. My body was waving a flag, telling me it was time to change. If there were signs in my eyes, I could be certain that the problem was everywhere: in the brain, the heart, the joints, etc. I had seen every complication of type 1 diabetes throughout my career and I did not want to go there – so, I permitted myself to try something radical. I would try Bernstein's methods for a while, "just to see", I told myself. I would experiment – nothing permanent. If it did not work, I could always go back to the NICE guidelines and the high-carb, high-insulin roller-coaster.

To be honest, I, too, was an advocate of the "low-fat: good, high-fat: bad" belief, and it was difficult to tear myself free from this notion. I believed it – and I had more reason than most to do the opposite, having read that there was another way. My disease was catching up with me; I had to call my own bluff. My training told me it would not work. However, it *did* work – and it shocked me how immediate it was.

That first low-carb, high-fat meal – three eggs, butter, nothing else – felt almost reckless at the time. All that fat? It went against everything I had been taught. But the outcome was undeniable: my glucose graph barely moved. And it stayed flat – no post-meal correction. No hypo two hours later. No recovery snack. Just smoothness. And with that smoothness came clarity: I was in control. The next meal was the same, and the one after that. I felt a calmness I had not known in years. Within a few weeks, my confidence grew. Within months, I could reliably predict my glucose levels after most meals. That had never happened before. There was no trick, just stability. My insulin doses have been halved. My glucose variability dropped. My energy rose. And I started to believe that this was not just an anomaly, it was how the body was supposed to feel. It was the first step to freedom.

I am now as sure as I can be that this strategy actually works. I question myself every single day: "What if I am wrong?" However, the evidence that it works and is safe is accumulating daily. A growing number of healthcare professionals are reaching the same conclusions as I am. I am becoming increasingly confident that this is the best and most scientific approach to type 1 diabetes.

Good blood glucose control was just the beginning; within days, my brain fog lifted. When you have brain fog, you do not know it is there until it is gone. I had functioned well with brain fog but once it lifted, my clarity of thought and speed of thinking improved – my vision seemed clearer. Those muscle aches every morning that took an hour or so to clear, they were gone, too. I no longer had joint pains after running, and regular calf muscle strains became a thing of the past. My mindset definitely improved, my brain felt calmer, and I was less prone to negativity. At night, I slept through, having previously needed to visit the bathroom at least once. I lost a small amount of weight, though I did not need to. Within months, my HbA1c dropped from 83 mmol/mol (9.7%) to 55 mmol/mol (7.2%), then to 44 mmol/mol (6.2%), and it has gone lower than that, even reaching the 30s (5%) on occasion. A lot of people I know regularly maintain levels in the high 30s and have experienced the same benefits as I have.

I now happily live alongside my type 1 diabetes. Being in control has been freeing. One door closes, another opens: I had to give up my pilot's licence – the first thought I had when I was diagnosed – but I still do air sports and have found freedom in paragliding. I am a much sharper driver now my brain fog has gone. I do not worry every day about my glucose, as I know it will be okay. For me, this change has been positive. Of course, there are things I miss but the new positives of life far outweigh the negatives.

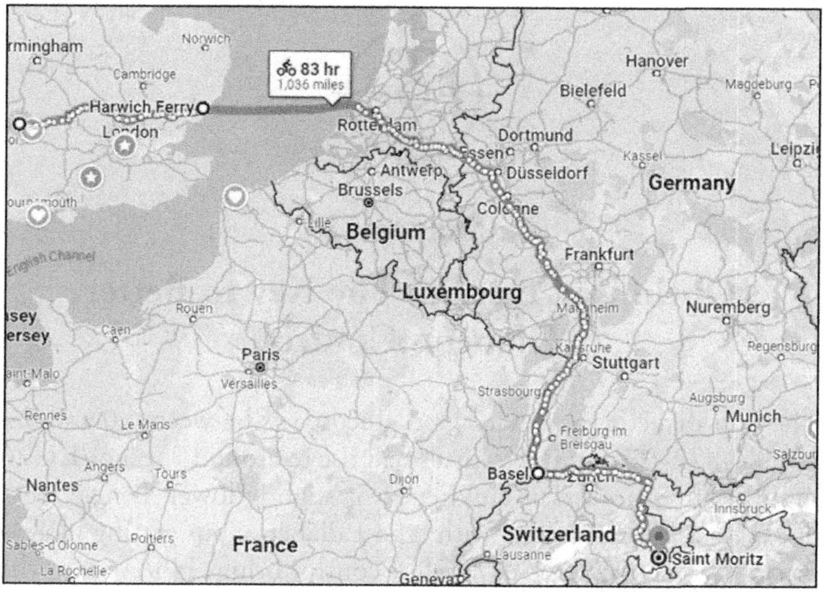
Norwich
Cambridge
83 hr
1,036 miles
Harwich Ferry
Hanover
Bielefeld
Magdeburg
Dortmund
Kassel
Düsseldorf
Germany
Antwerp
Brussels
Belgium
English Channel
Frankfurt
Luxembourg
Nuremberg
Rouen
Caen
Paris
Versailles
Stuttgart
Regensburg
Strasbourg
Augsburg
Munich
Rennes
Le Mans
Freiburg im Breisgau
Angers
Tours
Nantes
Dijon
Basel
Innsbruck
Switzerland
Lausanne
Poitiers
France
Saint Moritz
La Rochelle

Chapter 2

Optimised Insulin: The Key to Better Diabetes Control

The non-diabetic range for blood glucose sits between 4.0 and 5.4 mmol/L (72–97 mg/dL), with a small rise to around 7 mmol/L (126 mg/dL) after meals. For children, it is slightly lower. It may seem like a big ask for someone with type 1 diabetes, but getting there – or close – is possible. That level of control brings HbA1c into the normal range, somewhere around 40 mmol/mol (about 6%). It is not a competition, and some people will have an expression of diabetes that is genuinely harder to manage than others. For them, these numbers might be unrealistic or simply too stressful to maintain. But what I am suggesting is this: we should see normal glucose as something achievable, and not have to accept high numbers just because we have type 1 diabetes. There are very few markers of health where we accept being outside the normal range; we simply would not tolerate it in thyroid function, blood pressure, cholesterol, electrolytes, anaemia – the list goes on.

It might be difficult, especially given the current high-carbohydrate dietary recommendations, but there is evidence that a low-carb diet has advantages. One study found that 95% of people with type 1 diabetes following a ketogenic diet – without even factoring in other foundations of health – achieved an HbA1c of 48 mmol/mol (6.5%) or better. That compares with just 8% under "usual care". So, if lower numbers are achievable, why not aspire to them?

In my view, to achieve this requires understanding insulin and how to use it well – not simply as a tool to respond to dietary carbohydrates. If you get the insulin right, you will get the glucose right, too. And when that happens, your numbers improve naturally.

The benefits of smoother glucose control with less insulin include:

- Fewer hypoglycaemic and hyperglycaemic episodes
- Reduced risk of diabetic ketoacidosis (DKA)
- Potential for weight normalisation (although weight loss is not the primary goal)
- No need for calorie restriction
- Improved long-term glucose management

Experts increasingly agree that minimising glucose fluctuations benefits overall health and diabetes management.

Newer measures like the Coefficient of Variation (CV) and Time in Range (TIR) are more accurate indicators of diabetes control. These require a Continuous Glucose Monitor (CGM) for precise tracking. The goal of optimised insulin is to dose as precisely as possible, mimicking the natural action of insulin in someone without type 1 diabetes. This is a challenge; the more insulin we use, the harder it becomes to maintain stable glucose levels – a principle known as the Law of Small Numbers. For example, on a conventional diet, you might need eight units of rapid-acting insulin, whereas on a low-carb diet, you might only need one unit. If one unit lowers glucose by 2.5 mmol/L (45 mg/dL), the potential for overshooting and inducing a hypo is significantly reduced with smaller doses.

While diet is crucial, other aspects of health also significantly affect insulin sensitivity and glucose control. These include:

- Physical activity
- Environmental factors, such as illness, temperature or travel
- Mindset and stress management
- Circadian rhythms, which regulate hormonal function

To address these factors, we set a basal rate on our insulin pumps, or inject a basal dose. For food-related glucose fluctuations, we use rapid-acting insulin – the so-called basal-bolus approach.

Understanding how basal insulin truly works is essential, and it starts with setting your basal rate correctly.

Setting the Basal Rate: A Practical Approach

Basal adjustments follow a consistent process for adults, and similarly for children – although daily variation may require more frequent tweaks. There are only three steps to basal rate optimisation. If your HbA1c remains higher than ideal – which is the case for around 95% of people with type 1 diabetes on conventional treatment – it is worth revisiting these steps, even if you are already following a ketogenic diet.

This method is the same one taught at diagnosis when insulin is used for the first time; it may be familiar, but a quick revision might be useful.

Step 1: Ensuring Your Basal Insulin Dose Is Accurate

Basal insulin (pens or pumps) is given independently of meals to counter background glucose production. To test basal accuracy:

1. Start in the morning, skip breakfast and monitor glucose hourly.
2. Keep your usual basal rate – do not change it during the test.
3. Many people using pens settle on two basal injections per day, but to begin with, stick with what you usually do. Repeat the fasting period in the afternoon on another day, to cover a 24-hour period. Or take three fasted sessions that cover a 24-hour period over a few days. The aim is to assess how glucose fluctuates with basal insulin.

   The basal dose will then usually be close to optimal. It will need refinement from time to time; people often become more insulin-sensitive in the first few months of starting a ketogenic diet, so it is necessary to be aware that the basal dose might need reducing.

4. Indicators of accuracy:
    - If glucose stays steady (4–6 mmol/L), your dose is likely correct.
    - If glucose drops, your basal insulin may be too high.
    - If glucose rises, the dose may be too low.

Early morning rises in glucose due to growth hormone (GH), adrenaline or cortisol – known as the "dawn phenomenon" – can complicate matters. A small bolus of rapid insulin is better than altering basal.

Basal needs vary depending on how other factors influence insulin sensitivity:

- Menstruation: many women notice increased basal needs pre-menstruation.
- Sleep: poor sleep often increases insulin requirements.
- Physical activity: regular exercise may reduce basal insulin needs.

Step 2: Revising Carbohydrate Counting and Label Reading

Learning how to read food labels properly is essential. Manufacturers often use misleading front-of-pack labelling (FOPL), designed for marketing and pressure selling, not for accurate insulin dosing; it is especially deceptive for type 1, as it separates carbohydrates and added sugar. For people with type 1, we need to allow for both. On the back-of-pack label (BOPL), these come under the category of carbohydrates. The full label on the back enables calculation of total carbohydrates and protein. This gets easier with practice and is a fundamental skill for effective insulin dosing.

Count the total carbohydrates per 100g of food, including those that come from protein. Carbohydrates can be listed as total or net; net means that the insoluble fibre has been removed from the carbohydrate total. In practice, this distinction is minor for people on a very low-carb diet, as the proportion of fibre is small and has little impact on insulin estimation.

Step 3: Rapid-Acting Insulin for Meals

Inject rapid-acting insulin for meals based on carbohydrate and protein counting. The method is the same as when you were first diagnosed, but on a low-carb diet, doses are smaller, making control more predictable and safer. Over time, learning to include protein in your calculations becomes important. This will be covered later, but as a guide, protein can be estimated using around half of your insulin-to-carbohydrate ratio. For example, if you use one unit of insulin for 10g of carbohydrates, you should estimate one unit of insulin for 20g of protein.

By adopting a very low-carb diet, many people achieve stable control for the first time since diagnosis. Once the swings from high-carb meals are gone, the more subtle effects of protein become apparent.

A ketogenic diet is a very low-carb diet and is not at all about cutting calories; it is about cutting carbs and replacing the calories with protein and healthy fats. Many people can reduce their total daily insulin use by around half. Whether you transition gradually or make an immediate switch, the key is to learn from your meals and adapt. With practice, control becomes intuitive.

The main food groups in a ketogenic diet are leafy green vegetables, fish, meat, nuts, dairy, eggs, and berry fruits. For those who have a sweet tooth, some sweeteners can replace sugar, and for those who like chocolate and alcohol, there are very low-carb options. The ketogenic diet does not need to be boring or repetitive, and there are thousands of recipes available online.

Insulin optimisation is about understanding how this diet and the five foundations of health – diet, activity, environment, mindset and circadian rhythms – work together to improve diabetes control. Initially, this might seem daunting, but it is really straightforward and like all things, with repetition, the method becomes second nature in no time at all. Whether you use pens or pumps, insulin can be optimised and better glucose control will follow. When that happens, type 1 diabetes becomes something *you* manage, and not something that manages *you*. And to me, that's a win-win.

Chapter 3
My Wheels for the Ride

As with diabetes management, choosing the best bike setup is about compromise. A heavier weight is a favourable quality of a bike when cycling *with* gravity, lightness when riding *against* it; a strong, heavy frame is less likely to break than a light one. And new is likely to be more reliable than old. And so on.

Function Over Fashion

I was lucky to have two bikes to choose from. The logical choice would have been the one I used 10 years ago on a 3,500-mile tour around the North Sea. I bought it specifically for that journey: a Dawes Super Galaxy, a classic, steel-framed touring bike. Fully loaded, the bike and kit weighed 38 kg. Heavy, yes, but once moving, it had unstoppable momentum.

Steel bikes have their own personality. They are the heaviest of the lot, but they have a unique quality: a built-in flexibility in the steel that acts like suspension. You can feel it, especially on corners when fully loaded with bags: lean into a bend, and the frame seems to respond in slow motion, the front end leading and the rear gently following. I exaggerate, of course, but only slightly; it is something you only understand when you have ridden one fully loaded. Without luggage, the bike is stiff and unforgiving. With luggage, it comes alive. Over the course of that journey a decade ago, it had held up admirably. The only issue was a cracked rear rim, which, remarkably, still got me home; otherwise, the bike was solid. And steel has another perk: if it breaks, it is repairable just about anywhere.

However, my lighter road bike seemed an attractive option for this trip. In 2007, *Cycling Weekly* ran an article listing every road bike available that year – nearly 500 models in total, ranging from a few hundred euros to more than €7,000. Mine ranked 474th cheapest on the list; I bought it new from my local shop for £565 and I still use it. With care, a good bike should last a lifetime, and this had been a faithful workhorse. I used it for several years on my daily eight-mile round trip to work. The open frame meant I did not need to crouch over, and the combination of aluminium frame and carbon fibre forks gave it a slick, lightweight feel. But aluminium is not so forgiving; the ride can be harsh, especially on high-pressure tyres, and if the frame breaks, it is more specialised to repair. This road bike has gentle curves in the rear frame, which adds a little flex. I had also fitted some new, slightly wider, treadless tyres – a real find – which added just a touch of suspension, and were supposed to be puncture-resistant.

I have never been part of the branding or performance "arms race" that is promoted in the enthusiasts' magazines; I just wanted something comfortable and reliable. Over the years, I have replaced quite a few parts. At one point, the spokes began failing regularly, and I picked up a second-hand black rear wheel with high-spec, flat-profile spokes that made the bike feel just a little more "pro". Later, when the front wheel gave out, I sourced the same brand and model again, second-hand, this time in silver. The colour mismatch did not bother me in the slightest; the function was all that mattered. One of the combined gear/brake levers eventually wore out – I upgraded it. And a whole new chainset went on when the cogs finally wore down. I have been through several sets of brake pads, too. Most recently, I had to replace the cracked plastic saddle, and just before this trip, the main pedal crank bearing failed spectacularly, with only a few warning creaks, necessitating a walk home. I replaced it with just three weeks to go, thankful that it failed before I set off. This bike brings to mind the character Trigger, a council road sweeper from the British TV hit of the 1980s, *Only Fools and Horses.* He proudly told people he had the oldest broom in the council, even though it had 17 heads and 12 handles over many years. That's how

I think of my road bike: a true "Trigger's broom". And I love the concept – a well-used, well-maintained bike is the very embodiment of sustainability.

I really could not decide which bike to take until just a few weeks before setting off. The road bike felt more comfortable and while the touring bike was solid, I always felt like I was wrestling with its weight. I did a half-dozen, timed 15-mile rides on both. The road bike won every time by five minutes. That is not much per ride, but over three weeks, that is an entire day gained. So, my ageing, recycled bike was the one I decided to take; it had been well-maintained and should serve me just fine. The only question was whether the fragile-looking road frame would handle the gravel and kerbs, with the added burden of luggage it was not designed for. I did not know, but I went with optimism.

So, the black Giant SCR 2.0 from 2007 would be my companion. My chosen bike was seventeen years old but as I prepared to make new memories on it, I could only reflect that my body had not aged as quickly as the bike. Optimised insulin, as I have been doing for the past decade, has improved my fitness, in my view. Only time would tell.

Chapter 4
What Causes Type 1 Diabetes? What We Know (and What We Don't Yet)

There are several medical conditions that require insulin. For example, people with type 2 diabetes can experience failure of the insulin-producing cells in the pancreas. And people who have had their pancreas surgically removed also require insulin. For any condition requiring supplemental insulin, the principles outlined in this book will be useful information.

Type 1 diabetes is characterised by the presence of autoantibodies, which are proteins produced by your immune system that attack your body's own cells. At the present time, this can't be cured and requires insulin. It begins when the immune system, meant to defend us, mistakenly turns on the insulin-producing cells of the pancreas. Our own immune system attacks these cells as if they were foreign.

This is called **autoimmunity**, and the exact causes of many autoimmune diseases are not yet known. Once these cells are destroyed, insulin must be delivered from outside the body as an injection. Without insulin, blood sugar climbs too high and energy can't be properly managed. That is why people with type 1 rely on daily insulin therapy to stay alive.

Autoimmune diseases affect a broad range of tissues, with collagen in rheumatoid arthritis and nerve tissue in multiple sclerosis being just two examples.

No Clear Cause, Just Clues

We still do not have one clear cause for T1 diabetes. What we do have is a tangle of clues: genes that raise the risk, and environmental triggers that seem to set the process in motion. You might inherit the tendency, but something in your surroundings – such as a viral infection, a vitamin D deficiency, or even certain foods – may trigger the process. Because there is no single 'villain', scientists are focusing less on removing the cause, and more on calming or retraining the immune system.

A Condition on the Rise

Across the world, type 1 diabetes is becoming more common – although not everywhere at the same rate. Between 1989 and 2003, studies across Europe showed a steady rise of nearly 4% each year. Sweden still reports increases, though slower than before. In China, the numbers have shot up from about 1.5 cases per 100,000 people in the late 1990s to over 5 per 100,000 just 10 years later. Something is shifting; our genes have not changed that fast – but our environment has.

Genes: The Loaded Dice

There is a genetic side to the story. The human leukocyte antigen (HLA) system helps the immune system tell "self" from "foreign". Three genes in particular – DQA1, DQB1 and DRB1 on chromosome 6 – are the major risk markers. Together, the HLA genes explain around 40–50% of the inherited risk for type 1 diabetes. But even with these genes, nothing is certain; they load the dice, but they do not fix the outcome.

This is clear when you look at families. If a father has type 1, a child's lifetime risk is roughly 5%; if it is the mother, it is only about 2%. Identical twins – who share all the same DNA – show only about a 27% match within seven years, and just 4% for non-identical twins over two decades. That gap tells us that something outside genetics must tip the balance.

Autoantibodies: The Immune System's Fingerprints

Before type 1 diabetes shows up, the body often gives off signals called autoantibodies. These are antibodies that mistake your own cells for invaders. They can appear years before symptoms, gradually chipping away at insulin production.

The main ones are:

- Islet Cell Autoantibodies (ICA)
- Insulin Autoantibodies (IAA)
- Glutamic Acid Decarboxylase Autoantibodies (GAD65)
- Protein Tyrosine Phosphatase Autoantibodies (IA-2 or ICA-512)
- Zinc Transporter 8 Autoantibodies (ZnT8A)

The more types of autoantibodies you have, the higher your risk of developing full type 1 diabetes; however, it is not a guarantee – some people with several antibodies never progress, while a few people with no detectable antibodies still develop the disease. Those unexplained cases are called "idiopathic type 1 diabetes". ("Idiopathic" is a posh word for "we don't have a clue!")

Scientists have even noticed that antibodies can appear in a specific order; for example, IAA and GAD65 often appear first. Yet, even that order can change between countries. Children in Sweden and Lithuania, for instance, tend to show different patterns of which antibodies come first and how many appear at once. It is another reminder that type 1 has regional "accents", even within Europe.

Our Immune System's Fine Line

Tiny changes in DNA called single-nucleotide polymorphisms (SNPs) add extra variation. Everyone has millions of them, and most do not matter. But some influence how the immune system behaves. One gene, PTPN22, is often linked with type 1 diabetes, lupus, and Graves' disease. Curiously, the same change that increases those risks actually lowers the chance of Crohn's disease, showing that our immune system walks a fine line between too active and too quiet.

Geography: The Map of Risk

Type 1 diabetes does not strike evenly; around the world, rates can differ more than 350-fold. Finland leads the chart, with one of the highest rates anywhere, followed closely by Sardinia. That is surprising – Sardinia gets far more sunlight than Finland, which should mean higher vitamin D levels and lower risk. Yet it is the opposite. Sardinia's people also have relatively low frequencies of the risky PTPN22 gene. So, something else must be at play – perhaps unique infections, early diet differences, or historical genetic mixing.

Even within nearby countries, contrasts are sharp. Italy, right next door to Sardinia, reports only about one-fifth as many cases. The pattern repeats across Europe: northern areas such as Finland and Sweden show much higher rates than southern ones like Spain and Greece.

Migration studies add another clue. Families who move from one country to another usually carry their original risk – until the next generation. Children born in the new country take on that country's risk level: environment again, not just DNA.

There is also a seasonal rhythm. Diagnoses tend to rise in winter and dip in summer. It may relate to viral infections or vitamin D. Still, not every country follows this rule – Sardinia, for example.

Diet, Milk, and the Gut

Food is one of the most debated triggers. Several studies have found a loose link between cow's milk consumption and type 1 diabetes, especially in northern countries. Finland, for example, has both one of the highest type 1 rates and very high milk intake. Children who drink more than three glasses a day seem to face a slightly higher risk, if they already have genetic susceptibility.

But Iceland breaks the rule: its people drink even more milk than the Finns, yet their type 1 rate is much lower. That hints it might not be the *amount* of milk, but the *type*. Most European cows make A1 casein, a milk protein, which can break into BCM-7, a fragment that may trigger immune reactions. Cows in parts of Asia and Africa produce A2 casein, which does not create BCM-7. Animal studies have shown more diabetes in those fed A1 milk, though human data remains uncertain.

Sardinia again stands out: high milk consumption, sunny weather, very high type 1 rates, but relatively low vitamin D levels: an odd mix that does not neatly fit any single theory.

Another angle involves gluten. People with type 1 are more likely to have coeliac disease. Some research found that women who ate the most gluten during pregnancy had roughly double the risk of their children later developing type 1. Other studies did not find clear effects. What *is* clear is that the gut – and microbiome – play a role in immune training.

Stress: The Wild Card

Some stories link the start of type 1 to major stress or trauma. Science is thin here, but the idea fits: stress hormones can stir up the immune system and push a fragile balance over the edge. Still, stress alone does not cause the disease – it may simply accelerate what was already underway.

Where That Leaves Us

Right now, type 1 diabetes is a lifelong condition; you can live well with it, but you can't yet make it go away. The hopeful part is how fast the field is moving. New immune-modifying drugs have already shown they can delay the onset of type 1 in people at high risk – sometimes by several years. That is the first real sign we can slow the process, not just treat the result of a destroyed insulin production system.

So, for the moment, the best we can do is live well with what we know: manage blood sugar, support research, and stay ready for what is next. The more we learn about genes, diet, sunlight, and the immune system, the closer we get to turning "incurable" into "preventable".

Chapter 5
77 Miles

Day 1: Stroud to Thame
The Big Day!
Monday, 20 May 2024

"You are off to great places! Today is your day! Your mountain is waiting, so get on your way!"
– Dr. Seuss

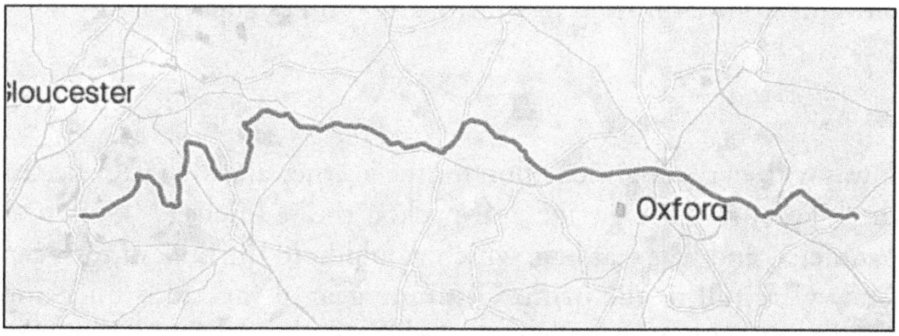

There is no stopping me now – this is it! A good night's sleep followed by my usual, spontaneous wake-up at 6 am. A quick peek through the curtains reveals a nice day; it is a good start. With patchy and prolonged rain forecast for the rest of the week, I am grateful for a sunny day today.

It is a slightly nippy morning, and clothing choices are on my mind. Years of outdoor experience tell me it is going to be a couple of hours wearing a cycling top over a long-sleeved underlayer, paired with shorts and my summer gloves. These fingerless, retro-style crocheted string gloves are ideal – you only really need protection on your palms if you fall; the string offers just enough texture to save your skin in an awkward tumble, while also wicking away sweat. The Alps might be a different story: just four degrees Celsius is predicted in St Moritz today, and I will be pedalling there in about three weeks. So, I have packed a pair of regular gloves for when that time comes. It is just a month before the summer solstice, but there has been no real summer weather yet in my corner of the southwest of England. Today's forecast suggests an easterly breeze, which means Day One begins with a headwind.

I am starting by heading vaguely north, before veering east toward Oxford, and on to the town of Thame. I will loosely follow the River Thames for the English leg of the trip, and head for Harwich. I plan to take the ferry to Hook of Holland and pick up the River Rhine cycle route, which I will follow south to Basel, then turn east to Lake Constance, and finally head south again to cross the Alps and onwards, to the finish in St Moritz 1,000 miles later.

~ ~ ~ ~ ~

It was with nervous anticipation for the journey ahead that I wheeled the bike out of the garage and packed the saddlebags (known as panniers), and rear seat bag, which would hold the bulk of my gear. They were full to the brim. Camping gear always adds bulk and weight, but without it, it does not feel like a proper trip. The weather was not looking great for it; still, I was not planning to camp in England.

I realised I need to get a move on. I had only booked two nights of accommodation so far, and needed to be at the ferry on night three; missing the overnight voyage would mean wasting time on a daytime crossing when I could be pedalling instead.

Those first three days demanded a 200-mile ride to the village of Harwich, in Essex. I had not covered that kind of distance with full luggage in a while. A few days back, I had done a ten-mile, fully packed rehearsal to see if I could manage the first hill; it is a steep one I usually avoid when riding locally – a proper first-gear, out-of-the-saddle kind of climb, which takes 15 minutes at most.

I brewed up a black coffee and wandered outside again to size up the whole bike-and-luggage situation. I was itching to get started, but had arranged to meet a friend at 8 am for the 'official' send-off. There was still an hour to go, so I leaned against the wall and ran through a mental checklist. The bike felt heavy; I wondered if the frame would hold. There were no external signs of corrosion, but water has a way of sneaking in. If it was an issue, it would reveal itself eventually – no use worrying now. Out came the scales: 32 kg; less than my North Sea Cycle Route trip, at 38 kg all-in.

It was finally time to go. I rinsed the coffee cup, fed Mitz the cat, and scribbled "Thanks, Fiona!" on the blackboard by the back door, for my lodger. She had agreed to feed Mitz while I was away. Shoes on, and I was out the door by 7:50 am to meet my good friend John Meadley in Stroud town centre. He had kindly offered to take a few pictures and wave me off.

Whilst this was a big trip, it was not some massive challenge in the traditional sense. There would be physical effort, sure, and maybe even injury, but I had planned manageable daily distances and had long-distance experience; I just needed to arrive in St Moritz by 9 June. And I had built in a three-day buffer for anything unexpected. In a worst-case scenario, I could take the train.

I saddled up, and rolled out and down the gentle half-mile slope into the town – past the hill I would tackle later. I gave it a friendly nod. On, through familiar streets: past the police station, the health food shop, along an alleyway, past a pub into the main street, and finally to the square in front of the Stroud Subscription Rooms – a large building which holds events locally known as the "Sub Rooms" and is the town's cultural heart. It was funded through public subscription.

John arrived bang on time. He is a great friend; we reminisced about our days campaigning for social prescribing in the Stroud Valleys when I was a local GP. This area really led the way. One forward-thinking GP created Art Lift, a programme that prescribed creative arts for people feeling isolated or depressed. From that grew all sorts of initiatives: gardening, dance, and, yes, even cycling. In fact, John and I spearheaded "cycling on prescription". The idea was simple: support adults who already knew how to ride but had lost confidence. Trained helpers would ease them back into the saddle.

John is a man of many hats – co-founder and honorary president of Pasture for Life.org, for one. This group of farmers champions the restorative power of grazing animals on pasture, with a focus on animal welfare and soil health. Their cattle roam outside, eating a natural diet from a biodiverse smorgasbord of plants that build an underground ecosystem teeming with life: bacteria, fungi and lichens. Those with deep roots help the pasture withstand drought, whilst lucerne, sainfoin and clovers can take nitrogen out of the atmosphere through their symbiotic relationship with bacteria in their roots, meaning chemical fertilisers are not needed. Cow pats become a natural fertiliser where dung beetles and biodiversity thrive. It is a beautiful concept – a natural, closed loop, just letting nature do its thing. Vet bills drop because the animals are not stressed and they can self-medicate by eating plants with beneficial properties in pasture and hedgerows.

There is growing evidence that this kind of farming sequesters carbon into the soil. John has worked worldwide with rural communities, and I believe his time has come. He is riding the wave of a true paradigm shift in farming.

I believe the same goes for medicine: real health comes from how we eat and live. That is how we reduce our dependence on drugs to mask chronic illness. But it will take time to convince a new generation of doctors to hold on to their curiosity – the spark that got them into medicine in the first place. Protocols and symptom-focused silos of thinking have eroded that spark.

Yet so many chronic conditions share a root cause: metabolic dysfunction, mostly from excessive carbohydrate intake. With type 2 diabetes, we treat the high blood sugar, but the real fix lies in the food. If you fix the diet, you fix the insulin and everything else falls into place – blood pressure, cholesterol, even cardiovascular risk. What is good for John's cows is good for humans: an ancestral diet grounded in real food. Of course, having type 1 diabetes adds complexity. That is what this trip is all about – exploring.

John took the mandatory departure photos and waved me off. And just like that, I had started. All the anticipation and planning, condensed into a single moment. Anyone who has ever set off on something big knows the feeling: excitement mixed with anticlimax. The destination – Thame. Off I went, past the sports shop, through the gap between the baker's and the trinket shop, up the high street and on, to the climb up the Cotswold escarpment. Funnily enough, Day One would include some of the biggest climbs of the entire trip, aside from the final days in the Alps; but it makes sense when you think about it. The River Rhine route to Lake Constance would be mostly flat, but the Cotswolds? Their beauty lies in the hills.

Stroud sits in the heart of five valleys where tributaries converge into the River Frome. The landscape here is 200-million-year-old Jurassic limestone shaped by glaciers and rivers over millennia. This limestone spine runs in an arc from Dorset and Devon in the south, and on up to North Yorkshire. And, yes, it is as pretty as you might imagine. The town is at the southern end of the Cotswolds. Its industrial rise came from waterpower, which powered wool mills. But the price for all that flowing water? An undulating, never-flat terrain. The Cotswold ridges naturally run north, which is great if you are going that way, but I am headed east – meaning I would be crossing each of those valleys, up and down, again and again; it was going to be breathtaking in every sense. And right now, it was "up": a low-gear, steady sort of grunt. Not a desperate pant, but still a workout, standing on the pedals, arms pulling on the bars – but I had trained for this. I had practised the first 20 miles several times, so nothing came as a surprise.

After climbing the steep limestone escarpment for a quarter of an hour, I was rewarded with glorious, far-reaching views. To the south, the shimmering River Severn estuary; to the west, the rugged silhouettes of the Welsh mountains; and to the northwest, the rolling, whaleback form of the Malvern Hills. On a bright, sunny morning like today, it was nothing short of spectacular.

I had the Bikemap satnav app running today, and it proved to be a little whimsical in this area; the app's voice prompts seemed overly eager to route me in unnecessary loops. That is the problem with satnavs that offer too many options, they start getting creative. Around here, minor roads were abundant – and on these minor roads, Bikemap really liked a loop. During my preparation rides around here, it once sent me three-quarters of the way around a rectangle when one straight line would have done the trick; it seemed convinced that the narrower the road, the better – assuming "quiet for traffic" meant "perfect for cycling". I was not so sure, especially when 'quiet' meant a rough track down into a valley, only to climb back up again minutes later – great for fitness, but not for pacing or making good time on Day One.

After a brief coffee stop, I finally glanced at the continuous glucose meter (CGM). It relayed a reading of blood glucose from a small disc stuck on my arm to a mobile phone app every five minutes. It was the first look since leaving Stroud an hour earlier. I had not yet taken my rapid-acting insulin, and had taken less than my usual Tresiba dose. It is still nonsensical to me – taking a drug with a 33-hour half-life twice a day – but that is a habit left over from my days of long-acting Lantus-brand basal insulin, otherwise known as "insulin glargine". Despite the marketing, I never found that it lasted 24 hours – and many people who contacted me through my website said the same. They were amazed at the difference when switching to twice-daily injections. So that is what I have stuck with. These days, I usually take 16 to 20 units total: 8–10 units twice daily; not a huge amount, but I always keep in mind Dr Richard Bernstein's principle that larger volumes can lead to erratic absorption. It is all about surface area-to-volume ratio – smaller injections spread over a greater surface are better absorbed, so twice daily makes sense.

Insulin sensitivity improves with physical activity, and today, my body was starting to adapt. I knew that once I got into the rhythm of riding every day, my glucose handling would improve and my insulin needs would drop. The question was, when, and by how much? I was already reasonably well trained, but recent weeks had been more sedentary than I would have liked. Now, firing up the muscles for several hours each day was going to shift things.

That morning, I had injected six units of Tresiba with my coffee, skipping breakfast and rapid insulin. That was less than my usual dose of 8–10 units, and depending on how my glucose behaved first thing, I might normally add two units of rapid insulin for the dawn effect.

The first couple of days of this ride needed a bit of trial and error. I thought back to my five-day, fasted run a few years ago – 100 miles, fully fasted, water and electrolytes only, no food. It was a huge experiment to show that deep ketosis in type 1 diabetes can be safe with the right knowledge. I used less than half my usual insulin back then. But this trip was different; I would be eating, albeit meals that were almost devoid of carbohydrates.

Although I had a good level of fitness, I had never done a series of daily long rides. My routine had been more like an hour or two of cycling three times a week, mixed with short running sessions; no need to adjust insulin for those. But this? This was a whole different game. Thirty years of injecting insulin has taught me a lot about my own responses, but everyone is different. Right now, I am using about 24 units a day; back in my high-carb days, it was double that. I know people who use twice what I do now, and others who get by on single digits. It all depends on your body, your experience, how long you have had type 1, how aggressive your autoimmunity is, and more.

After what felt like an age of up-and-down riding, and a few too many stops to double-check the route, I found myself in the Cotswold town of Northleach. This was familiar and fairly local territory. I had done around 35 miles, and yet Thame still felt miles away. The problem was, I had blindly followed the satnav, and it had not served me well. Three sides of a square – a needless detour, and precious time and energy spent. It was a classic case of over-trusting the tech. Tech is a tool to be used for a purpose, and understood – it is never a good idea to use tech without understanding its benefits and limitations. That applies to type 1 as well; if I ever use a pump, it will be on my terms, not the algorithms'.

Today was now looking like a very long day. I just hoped I had not overdone it too early – a common error when the excitement of Day One takes over. Northleach, though, was lovely: a rough-edged central square, surrounded by stone cottages and a few small shops. At least I was now up on the flatter part of the Cotswolds – the hills would be gentler from now on. I grabbed what I call "plastic food" from a local shop – a phrase that, unfortunately, would become familiar on this trip. Keto-friendly food was not always easy to find in the smaller towns, not without a bit of hunting. Today, I needed to keep moving. I sat on a sunny bench and let the world pass by. Salami, cheese, nuts – that would do. I logged it into the Cronometer macronutrient app. Then, a quick café stop for another coffee and back on the bike to head for the next stop, Oxford.

By the time I reached the outskirts of Northleach, 35 miles from where I had started, my glucose had nudged up to 9 mmol/L (162 mg/dL). It was likely the protein from lunch kicking in, or perhaps a spike from stress hormones, triggered by the hard climbs. I should have waited a little longer to see which way it would trend, but impatience got the better of me; I added one unit of rapid-acting insulin, thinking it would gently nudge the glucose level down by two, to 4 mmol/L.

An hour later, I was in Oxford. It was busy and nearing rush hour. Thankfully, it is a bike-friendly city with good cycle infrastructure, so I did not have to share the road with too many cars. But cyclists, scooters, and pedestrians… well, that is another matter; I swear, some cyclists ride like anarchists! I had to use every known skill of body language to hold my line and stop people from cutting me up.

By this point, I could feel it: that unmistakable drain of a serious hypo. In hindsight, the early stages were likely the reason I had been getting worked up with fellow road users a bit earlier. Just a slight loss of rapid reflexes and cognitive sharpness – but enough to affect judgement. I now experienced weakness, foggy concentration and plummeting energy levels; I had overshot with the insulin correction for the earlier high. I had overestimated the effect of exercise, and underestimated how insulin-sensitive I had already become. Plus, my basal insulin was still active in the background, dragging my glucose down further.

I had to stop. My vision was spotting, and my head was spinning – not dangerous, but not comfortable either. I estimated that three glucose tablets would bring me back to normal. It would typically be two in this situation, but my insulin was very potent – I was far more sensitive than usual at this stage in the ride. I had calculated I was around three times more sensitive than normal, based on the glucose drop. The frustrating part was that my CGM was right there on the handlebars and just a tap away; I could easily have checked it. But I had not – I figured I was in the clear. I was wrong. I had overmanaged my rapid insulin, and underestimated my increasing insulin sensitivity.

The glucose tablets kicked in quickly and I felt lucid again, but it would be 15 minutes before I could get moving. I still felt weak, which is how it is for me. Hypos mess with your logic. I have spoken to so many people who say the same. Your brain tells you to eat more. So, even though I knew I needed three tablets, based on my insulin-to-carb ratio and current sensitivity, I still wanted to devour the whole pack. It is tempting to take more, thinking it will work faster. It does not; it just sends your glucose rocketing back up.

I saw someone on X (formerly Twitter) describe it perfectly:

"It started calm, and by the end, the fridge looked like a smash-and-grab."

We have all been there.

That is the thing about experimenting. Sometimes you get it wrong. For the rest of the day, the glucose graph looked like a bouncing ball – hypos followed in waves, and I took glucose tablets to correct the lows. I never had to stop riding again that day, but I felt frustrated. This was not my finest hour; not the best advert for someone trying to demonstrate how well keto and insulin optimisation can work. A few overcorrections. A misstep or two. But the good news? This was only one of two hypos on the entire trip that forced me to stop. The second came the next day; after that, I worked out my doses and the rest of the journey had no more such incidents. There were other hurdles, of course, but more about those later.

As for today, the final 15 miles into Thame passed in calm and sunshine. The terrain flattened out, but I was tired. My planned 60 miles had become 77, and I had spent eight hours in the saddle – but I felt okay. No aches. No injuries. Just that satisfying fatigue you earn with effort.

Thame, in South Oxfordshire, was lovely; an old market town with a lively buzz for a Monday. There was no Cotswold stone here, but plenty of enchanting Tudor brickwork. I checked into a charming pub with unexpectedly plush décor: polished wooden floors, a grand bed, and a touch of Art Deco – all at a modest price. Better still, they let me keep the bike in the room.

After a shower and a well-earned medium-rare sirloin steak, I settled in for the night. I opted to cover the protein in the steak with two units of Novorapid, but left out the long-acting Tresiba. I was asymptomatic but still running low on blood glucose. I would see how it went. It was a good choice; the steak raised the glucose to 5 mmol/L (90 mg/dL), and it stayed there all night, with a slight downward drift due to the Tresiba from the morning before. It really is a long-acting drug! And my insulin sensitivity was increasing.

And with that, Day One was done. I had a lot to reflect on. It was a solid start, and five per cent of the route was completed. Plenty was learned, and there was plenty more to explore – especially around insulin, exertion, and what it really means to dial things in.

Tomorrow, onwards!

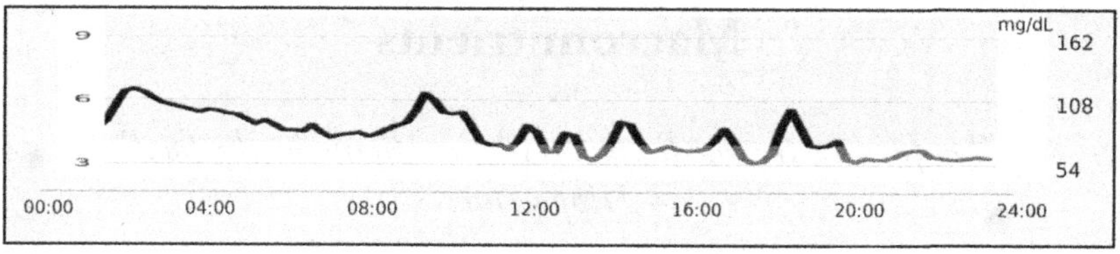

Chapter 6
Macronutrients

"Let food be thy medicine and let medicine be thy food"
– Hippocrates

How Can We Live Long and Live Well?

We all want both – to add life to years and years to life. By truly understanding insulin and how it affects our metabolism, we can achieve both; it is not a choice between the two. With knowledge and attention, we gain control of our health. There is a lot to learn, but it is worth it. Let's start with the basics, metabolism.

Metabolism

Metabolism is how the body balances the building and breaking down of materials to stay alive. It has two main sides:

- **Anabolism** – which builds tissue and stores energy.
- **Catabolism** – which breaks down tissue and releases energy.

These two processes are always running. Over time, the balance between them shapes our weight, strength and overall health. If we build more than we break down, we gain; if we break down more than we build, we lose. This is true whatever macronutrient we are talking about.

Insulin is an anabolic hormone – it helps store fuel and build tissue. It moves glucose into cells, stores excess carbohydrate as glycogen or fat, and supports growth and repair.

Energy comes from food, and from the food we store in our bodies, mainly as fat and sugar. The body is incredibly adaptable and can convert one nutrient into another as needed: protein into glucose, fat into glucose, or sugar into fat. Enzymes, which are specialised proteins produced by cells, speed up these reactions, keeping metabolism smooth and efficient.

Every cell plays its part. The brain and hormones coordinate the system, enabling the body to work as one. The primary nutrients – protein, fat and carbohydrates – provide fuel and building blocks. Vitamins and minerals (micronutrients) support these processes. Since most of our body is made up of water, protein and fat, we need enough of each to stay healthy. Sugar does not provide body structure but can be stored as energy, and some sugars act as signalling molecules.

Protein

Protein is essential for life. It comes from foods such as meat, eggs, dairy, legumes, tofu and nuts. Proteins are made of amino acids – 20 different ones – the body's building blocks. Some can be made in the body, but nine essential amino acids must come from food. The liver and kidneys constantly recycle amino acids from tissue turnover, keeping a ready supply of amino acids for repair and growth.

Unlike fat or carbohydrate, the body cannot store protein, unless you think of muscle as a protein store. There is no "protein depot", like body fat or glycogen. Instead, amino acids are constantly reused or broken down. During fasting or illness, the body first uses circulating amino acids; only in prolonged starvation does the body break down significant muscle to meet its protein and energy needs.

Insulin itself is a protein – built from a specific chain of 51 amino acids folded into a precise 3D shape. Scientists have learned to manipulate this sequence to create different types of insulin: fast-acting and long-acting versions that behave predictably in the body.

Protein's role goes far beyond muscle. It forms enzymes, hormones, neurotransmitters and cell receptors encoded by our DNA, all of which help regulate metabolism. Because we cannot store protein, we must consume it regularly. The general recommendation is about 1–2 grams per kilogram of ideal body weight per day, with more needed for activity, growth or ageing.

Adequate protein intake is essential for health. Some foods contain all essential amino acids and are known as complete proteins, while others contain fewer, meaning a variety of foods is needed to obtain the full range. This complete profile of essential amino acids supports strength, repair and healthy metabolism. Like carbohydrates, protein also provides energy, supplying 4 calories per gram.

Fat

Fat has been misunderstood for years, but it is vital for health. It is not just a source of energy but also supports brain function, hormone balance, and is an essential component of cell membranes. Fat and protein together make up roughly one-third of our body weight; water makes up most of the rest. About 60% of the brain is made of fat.

The type of fat we eat matters. Natural fats from meat, fish, eggs, nuts, seeds, avocados and dairy are good sources. In contrast, highly processed seed oils like canola or sunflower are less stable and can form harmful, inflammatory compounds when heated. Cold-pressed oils like olive or avocado oil are healthier and more stable. The fatty acid makeup of our food influences the health of our cells, the flexibility of our membranes, and even our mood and brain function.

Our fat stores are vast: tens of thousands of calories, even in lean individuals. Fat is stored mainly as triglycerides, which contain three fatty acids and a sugar-type (glycerol) backbone. When we burn fat, the glycerol can be turned into glucose, while the fatty acids provide energy directly. Fat gives 9 calories per gram – more than double the energy of protein or carbohydrates.

Fatty Acids Vary by Structure

There are many ways of describing fats. Fats like to form into chains – repetitive sequences of carbon and hydrogen molecules. The degree of saturation and chain length are two of the most common ways to describe them.

Saturation means simply the reactivity of the fats based upon the number of higher energy-containing bonds or joins between the carbon molecules that make up the fat. These chemical bonds not only define the reactivity of a fat (the opposite, of course, being stability), but also the shape of the fat molecule. Double bonds induce "kinks" in fat chains and these are thought to be instrumental in the interactions of the fat with surrounding molecules.

- **Saturated fats** have no double bonds and are stable. Double bonds are susceptible to breakdown and are less stable. Saturated fats are stored in body fat cells and can be readily mobilised to provide energy under appropriate conditions.

  Because fat stores are large and energy-dense, they serve as the body's long-term fuel reserve. Dietary saturated fats have been discouraged for the past 50 years because of the supposed association with heart disease; in reality, the picture is far more nuanced, and recent clinical reviews do not clearly support a straightforward link.

- **Monounsaturated fats** (like those in olive oil) have one double bond and can react with other molecules. Monosaturated fats are more fluid than saturated fats, and are found in adipose tissues alongside saturated fats as they maintain fluidity of the fat. They are also considered metabolically more neutral, whereas saturated fats are considered proinflammatory.

  An enzyme found in fat cells converts saturated fat into monounsaturated fat. It is called SCD1. So, carbohydrates that are converted to fat in the liver are "detoxified" in the fat cell. It is a necessary step to prevent "toxic spillover of fat". Human fat, like most animal fats, is roughly 50% saturated and 50% unsaturated.

- **Polyunsaturated fats** (like fish oil) have two or more double bonds and are delicate – easily damaged by heat or oxygen. The multiple double bonds in these fats alter their shape, and this is an integral part of their function. They play important roles in cell signalling and membrane structure, in addition to serving as an energy source.

Fats can also be described in terms of the length of the carbon chain – giving us short-, medium-, and long-chain fatty acids. Most fatty acids are medium- to long-chain. For example, a common storage fat, palmitic acid, is a long-chain, 16-carbon saturated fat. The very long-chain polyunsaturated fatty acids found in essential omega fats play a greater role in structure and hormone signalling than in providing energy.

So, fats are not just stored energy – they are part of every cell membrane. This makes them essential for cellular communication and the overall function of the body.

Carbohydrates

Carbohydrates are the body's quick fuel. They include sugars and starches in our food, which are digested and converted mainly into glucose and another sugar called fructose. Glucose is essential for energy; some tissues rely on it exclusively, such as red blood cells, but it is not required in the diet.

The body can synthesise glucose from protein and fat through a metabolic process called gluconeogenesis (the synthesis of new glucose). Glucose, when fully metabolised, yields 4 calories per gram of carbohydrate, the same as protein, but less than half that of fat. But pure calories are only part of the story; in later chapters, it will become clear that the speed of energy generation might be more important than the final amount produced. This is especially important in anaerobic reactions, where glucose is the only fuel available because the body can't use oxygen temporarily, for example, when sprinting. Everything in biology is conditional and nuanced.

The body stores carbohydrate as glycogen, a readily available form of glucose found principally in the liver and muscles. These stores hold roughly 2,000 calories of energy. Muscle glycogen powers muscle activity; liver glycogen helps maintain blood glucose levels between meals.

Only about one teaspoon of glucose circulates in the blood at any time. In someone without type 1 diabetes, insulin lowers glucose when it rises, while glucagon, adrenaline and cortisol raise it when needed. This delicate balance maintains a constant energy supply for the brain and muscles.

Carbohydrates come in three forms:

- **Monosaccharides** – simple sugars, like glucose and fructose
- **Disaccharides** – two-unit sugars, such as lactose and sucrose
- **Polysaccharides** – complex chains, like starch and glycogen

Nutrition guidelines often suggest obtaining 50–60% of calories from carbohydrates. However, for individuals with insulin-dependent diabetes, reducing carbohydrate intake results in more stable glucose levels and lower insulin doses. If carbohydrates are removed from the diet, protein and fat then provide sustainable, balanced energy, with glucose being made "in-house" as required.

Beyond the Numbers

Modern tools – like glucose sensors and insulin pumps – have changed diabetes care, but numbers alone do not tell the full story. True health depends on how we eat, move, rest, and manage stress – not just on insulin doses to match carbohydrates.

By understanding metabolism, we can make better choices. When insulin, diet and activity work together, we do not just manage disease – we support vitality, strength and longevity. That is how we add life to years, and years to life.

Chapter 7
Total Miles: 143

Day 2 – Thame to Matching Tye, 66 Miles

"When you set sail for Ithaca, wish for the road to be long, full of adventures, full of knowledge."
– C.P. Cavafy

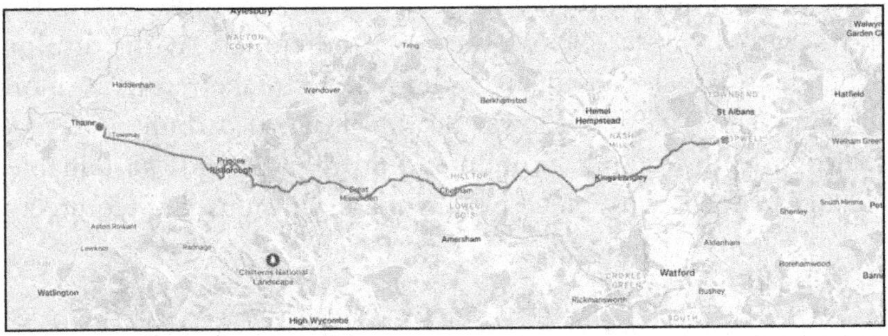

I do not need an alarm; I wake naturally around 6 am and prepare for the day ahead. I went through the morning routine that would soon become a habit. First, I checked my glucose, then the weather. To check the weather properly, a trip outside was required. What is the temperature like? The wind? It is always cooler in the mornings, even in summer, but getting a feel for the temperature helped me decide how many layers to wear; nothing is more annoying than stopping after about 10 minutes as the muscles reach operating temperature, because the body is overheating. I popped out of the patio doors onto the communal lawn. Yesterday's clothes had been drying on a wooden bench outside, but they were still damp. A damp set of clothes is a bit of a setback; they do not do well if packed damp.

Another advantage of going out into the natural light within a few hours of rising is that it helps me reset my body clock. It is a necessary action, to synchronise my circadian rhythms with the day-night cycle, but I can't do this indoors as I need ultraviolet light, which is blocked by glass. I will explore this as I travel along the Rhine, but for now I knew I was synchronised for the day.

A glance at the weather forecast showed rain was due in the afternoon and into the evening. In a hopeful but desperate attempt to get better news, I scrolled through a couple more weather apps and looked at the satellite image. It was not looking good; I would probably be riding in the rain for half of the day – but one positive was that it was forecast to be warm. I decided to have some breakfast, and then changed into the damp clothes before I set off; if I used my dry clothes on this wet day, then the next day, I might have no dry clothes at all.

I checked my ketone levels on the Sibio continuous ketone meter on my arm and compared them to the "gold standard" finger-prick test with the Keto Mojo device. I did the same calibration for blood glucose on two finger-prick devices, and photographed the results for future reference.

Then, I checked the route on the two cycle satnavs I had installed, Google and Bikemap. They were pretty much in agreement. The route was relatively flat, save for a steepish climb into the Chiltern Hills, but then it was flat or slightly downhill to my overnight stop at a pub in a village called Matching Tye, in Essex. The pub was bang on the route, give or take a mile or so, and was only just over 60 miles away. I double-checked Bikemap to ensure there were no wild detours along what the mapping software thought might be a good route, and chose that app for the day.

My routine also included filling the two 500 ml water bottles, putting on my heart-rate monitor, checking I had enough glucose tablets, and using my insulin pens to inject the estimated insulin.

Breakfast depended on whether or not it was available. That day it was, so I decided to break my fast earlier than usual. I recorded everything on a food app called Cronometer. I also brought some scales with me, but found them largely impractical. They were occasionally useful; they also helped me weigh coffee. My Jetboil stove and AeroPress coffee maker combination were my luxury items, and, when combined with a hand coffee-bean grinder and some expensive beans, they enhanced the trip no end. Freeze-dried granules in thin sachets were a poor substitute, and when I woke up early, I liked a coffee to sip outside whilst planning the day and synchronising my body clock.

It was time I headed for breakfast. It was usually eggs and bacon plus or minus mushrooms in the UK, or cold meats, cheese and eggs in mainland Europe. That day it was the full deal: bacon, eggs and mushrooms. There were no carbs in this meal, but there was protein. I needed to decide whether to inject rapid-acting insulin for the protein in this meal; yesterday's insulin had been way too much. Of course, that was looking back – as we know with type 1, predicting the future is far trickier than analysing and criticising the past.

That morning's glucose was 4 mmol/L (72 mg/dL). Outside of this adventure, I usually take two units of rapid-acting insulin in the morning to cover the effects of waking, coffee and any food, then 8–10 – sometimes six – units of long-acting Tresiba insulin to cover the many background factors that influence insulin needs. This amount of insulin usually works for my ketogenic diet, two meals a day, and 45 minutes to an hour of dedicated physical activity. Other people have a different way. The rest of my typical day away from this adventure is spent either pottering about or mostly sitting at a desk, looking at a screen.

The first thing that was blindingly obvious that day was the amount of physical activity I was doing; the other factors were roughly the same. There was no correct answer to this one. I had had type 1 for 30 years and had some insulin sensitivity, but likely far less than someone who had had it for less than a decade. I had a family history of type 2 diabetes, so I had about a one-in-four chance of having the genetic profile that made me less likely to handle carbohydrates efficiently as I aged. That was irrelevant in some ways, but it might have a bearing on how I could become resistant to insulin later in life. On the other hand, I did not have any of the other autoimmune conditions which commonly accompany type 1 diabetes, such as thyroid or coeliac disease, so I was lucky in that respect.

So, my decision was based on how my own "type" of type 1 expressed itself. I hoped to avoid any hypos. Trial and error were part of a type 1 day when we did something different. I finally decided to ignore the rapid that morning and take six units of Tresiba, and possibly six that night. Or a different dose. It would depend on how the day went. I could have justified covering the glucose-raising effects of waking, the coffee, and the protein in the bacon and eggs with a rapid insulin bolus; I might even have reflected later in the day that I should, in fact, have taken some rapid insulin, but my sensitivity to this type of insulin the previous day had made me cautious.

This was a significant deviation from orthodox practice seen in diabetes clinics. Typically, we only count carbs and adjust for the dawn effect. Here, I was thinking about protein and the stimulant effect of caffeine. I would discover further into the journey the other factors of daily living that affect our insulin, which go right to the heart of how I think we should be managing type 1 diabetes. I would begin addressing all of the root causes of health, to give me more finesse. I have never been told to realign my body clock, for instance, or to consider the insulin requirements of circadian biology.

I do think it matters how much insulin I use. What if I had perfect glucose but needed 1,000 units of insulin? Was that good? I would have got a clap from my diabetes department for my normal HbA1c, but I might have been stacking up consequences of continually higher-than-optimal insulin – and there were plenty of conditions in those without diabetes that were related to higher-than-normal insulin, especially neurological diseases, which I will explore later.

So, I figured I needed to look at how I might use the least insulin by studying the five foundations of health: diet, activity, mindset, movement and circadian rhythms. I needed to mimic the life practices of a healthy person without type 1, who would almost certainly make less insulin than I inject. Insulin in people with type 1 diabetes, whether through a pen or pump, does not behave in the same way as in someone with a functioning pancreatic hormonal metabolism – but I can try to get close.

I reflected on the change in my diabetes management since diagnosis and how radically different it was that day; it was almost the complete opposite of my dietary choices a decade earlier. I had been on the North Sea Cycle trip 10 years before and had not had protein and fat for breakfast. Carbohydrates were the primary food source, with lean protein included and fat minimised. Going through my diary of that North Sea Cycle Route trip, I came across this entry:

Sundebru to Grimstad, Saturday, 23 August 2014

"Stacked up with carbs. Breakfast not particularly imaginative – cereal, rolls, packet meat, and jam with fresh coffee. But I made the most of it."

On that day, I had stopped over in a guest house in Norway, on a rare departure from camping. It had been raining for two days, and my clothes had been wet. I could not bear another night of camping in the damp, so I bailed out to a place where I could dry my stuff, charge up all of the electronics, and have a comfortable bed. This place also served breakfast. It had been a cold table offering, but the fresh coffee had been a welcome bonus. I had had type 1 diabetes for around 20 years back then, and carbohydrates had been my staple; after all, I had been about to spend a day hauling a fully laden touring bike up and down hills. I needed energy. And what was the best source of energy? Well, carbohydrates, naturally! Or so I had thought at the time. Fizzy drinks companies will tell you that sugar is good for athletic performance, and popular breakfast cereal companies will tell you that breakfast – preferably a cereal that they manufacture – is the most important meal of the day. You can't entirely negate those arguments because there is nuance, and these companies know it.

Back then, continuous glucose monitors were not widely available, and pumps were not commonly used. I had insulin pens containing Lantus and Novorapid, as well as a finger-prick glucose meter. It had been a case of avoiding hypos and keeping a lid on high glucose. All of that exercise had stabilised control most of the time; however, after three months on the road back then, my HbA1c had hardly moved. Now, with a ketogenic diet and optimised insulin, everything had changed. The key has been to challenge outdated thinking and focus on what truly optimises health and insulin management.

Before I changed my diet, I frequently had palpitations, background joint pains and postural hypotension – extreme light-headedness when standing from sitting. Most of the time, I had to stand still to gather myself and, more often than not, put my head down to get the blood flowing to my brain. Imagine being a patient and watching your doctor almost faint as they got up to examine you.

This is a side-effect called autonomic neuropathy – damage to the autonomic nervous system. The autonomic nervous system consists of the nerves that control all of the background functions we need to stay alive but do not need to remember to do consciously. Imagine having to remember to blink, breathe, and control your heart rate and blood pressure, not to mention all digestive functions. These are all handled by the autonomic nervous system, and the nerve that coordinates them is the vagus nerve. It is the longest nerve in the body. It is well named; "vagus" comes from the Latin word for "wanderer", which fits perfectly, as this nerve supplies the organs of the thorax and abdomen.

If the vagus nerve succumbs to the relentless effects of high glucose – and nerve tissue is highly vulnerable to it – we can experience side effects. Many would know about the unpredictable and often delayed stomach response to food, as the vagus nerve supplying it is affected. It is called gastroparesis – slow stomach emptying – which can affect glucose control as food absorption becomes unreliable. At the other end is the horribly named diabetic diarrhoea. So, it is beneficial to have a fully functioning autonomic nervous system.

The autonomic nervous system also plays a role in regulating blood glucose levels by modulating the vagus nerve's action on pancreatic islet cells that release insulin. We have to take control of that function manually if we have type 1 diabetes; we can't produce insulin, let alone worry about how it is released. We need to mimic both the beta cells and the vagal control of the pancreas. We have to inject our insulin before we eat, well before the vagus nerve would typically send a signal to our pancreas if we had no type 1 diabetes. We then have to hope that the glucose rise from the food and the insulin dose coincide. And even if it does, we have to hope that the many other functions of the vagus nerve are intact to help us balance our insulin with other hormones that work with it. Someone has likened it to driving a car and having to anticipate a bend by turning the steering wheel 30 minutes ahead of it. We were heroes.

I set off at a good pace to try to get some miles under my belt before the rain set in. The cloud was building as I approached Kings Langley, a small town on the southeast edge of the Chiltern Hills. The road through it took me past the Grand Union Canal. I paused there, leaning my bike against the iron bridge railings where the canal went under the road. I looked up and down the canal, then had a brief jog along the towpath, up to and over some lock gates. There were no boats on the canal that day and just a handful of people walking the towpath. I was feeling nostalgic; just over a year earlier, I had passed that very spot when on a long-distance, 145-mile run along the length of the Grand Union Canal from Brentford in London to Gas Street Basin in Birmingham.

I checked my CGM. I had felt okay all morning and was curious to see whether my insulin calculation had been accurate. It had been perfect so far. There had been a slight rise from 4 to 5.5 mmol/L (72 to 99 mg/dL), but all was good; I just hoped that the Tresiba dose had not been too high.

I got back on my bike and set off with a short sprint downhill and into the drizzle, then a steady rain. There were some well-tended cycle tracks there, and I followed them to the garden city of St Albans, its cathedral just visible through the heavy mist and rain. I never got very close because I was on a set of cycle paths that staggered, literally, around the city's suburbs – every road junction at right angles to the cycle path, often with railings meant to protect the cyclist, the occasional bollard adding to the slow progress.

Cycling through the rain brought the first problem of the adventure. It got into my phone's charging port, so now I had no way of navigating, nor a way of measuring glucose. My hands were wet, and manual glucose testing would have been a chore. I had a backup phone, which was unfortunately out of charge. I had been so careless – and that day, I needed diabetes monitoring more than ever, after the previous day's excitement with hypos.

The task right then was to find a hairdryer. I hoped to find a hairdresser, but passed a veterinary clinic on a suburban road out of town; I figured they might have had one to dry off small animals. They did not, but the receptionist told me there was a hand dryer in the toilet. Why had not I thought of that? After 10 minutes of drying, I was back online. At about that time, there was a knock on the door and I was booted out; there was, by then, a queue for the loo.

After the excellent start to the day with normal glucose levels, the afternoon deteriorated into one of managing hypos; not bad ones, and easily managed with chomping on 6–9 grams of glucose tablets as I rode along. I did have to stop once, though, on a hill. I just literally ran out of energy – like a clockwork motor winding down, I ground to a halt. I felt it coming on at the bottom of the hill, and took the necessary correction of glucose tablets. However, they did not cut in on time. It was annoying – but part of the life of someone with type 1.

Hypos on a ketogenic diet sneak in ever so gently, with no drama – not like the bad old days when high insulin volumes, poorly estimated with the meal, would send the glucose into a near-vertical dive and it was all drama. Those days were over, thank goodness. I was grateful, though, to have hypo awareness; it can't be easy without that. In those days, alarms were mandatory.

The hypo was doubly annoying because I knew people who attempt to raise glucose by putting in an intense bout of riding to boost stress hormones. I was doing all that, yet it did not work for me; I rarely had the extra capacity to put in an anaerobic shift on a hill, anyway. But that hypo, that day, was the last significant hypo I experienced in the next three weeks of cycling.

Onward to Hertford: it was thoroughly wet, so choosing not to fit mudguards to the bike I now realised was an error. I needed a break. I had not eaten, and was getting demoralised and cold. I parked up near a supermarket and discovered some Sainsbury's zip-close sandwich bags, and thoroughly recommend them as effective waterproof phone covers; the screen was even operable through the polythene covering. I was back to full function.

I sat on the railings near the shopping trolleys and ate my meal – some cheese and cooked bacon. A motorcycle courier was sheltering under the same canopy, sitting on a yellow road-salt box, sheltering from the rain and scrolling away on his phone. I briefly chatted with a passing outdoorsy couple who turned out to be avid touring cyclists. They pointed out the cycle path in the corner of the car park as a shortcut to the main cycleway – I would never have found that one without their help.

The path was a mud-fest, and I came out of it with dirt-splattered legs and shoes. With 17 miles to go, I dug in to tick them off. Soon, there were ten to go – and a great, smooth, minor road to indulge myself on. The plus side of the rain was that the mud washed off in the spray from the front wheel; I sought out the puddles to get a jet wash. Of course, one of the more stupid things about riding in puddles is that you do not know if they are hiding a pothole. As the road was freshly metalled, I took the chance. It was all good.

In that final hour, I flew along feeling full of energy. The rain was still pouring down, and I noticed that the morning's east wind had become a westerly tailwind as a weather front approached. I freewheeled with a backwind into the sartorially named village of Matching Tye, with its pub called The Fox on the village green. I was allowed to put my bike in the cellar. I took a nice, warm shower, threw my cycling gear in there, too – stamping on it to give it the washing-machine effect – hung it out to dry, and headed for supper. The bar had a local vibe – rough plaster, dark wooden beams, velour upholstery, and a cosy glow from the wall lights. I was happy there while it poured down outside. It was early evening, but the low cloud made it seem like late evening on an autumn night.

A second night in a restaurant brought an opportunity to indulge. Liver and bacon were on the menu; it was a no-brainer – minus the mashed potato, of course. We should eat more offal; lightly cooked liver is sweet and succulent – although overdone, it becomes rubber in texture and dull in taste, losing its sweetness. I also had some broccoli to accompany it, along with a starter of cooked goat's cheese. I also, against my better judgment, had a glass of red wine. I guessed I was celebrating the success of the often-tough second day. It might have interfered with my sleep, and I tried to avoid it when I could. I needed to find alternative ways of celebrating small wins.

The meal was calculated as 800 calories. It was protein-heavy, but the carb count was only 14 grams. For the 70 grams of protein and carbs, I used four units of insulin: one for the carbs and three for the protein. I continued with six units of Tresiba. I used an insulin-to-carb ratio of one unit of insulin per 10 g of carbs, and for protein, one unit per 20 g.

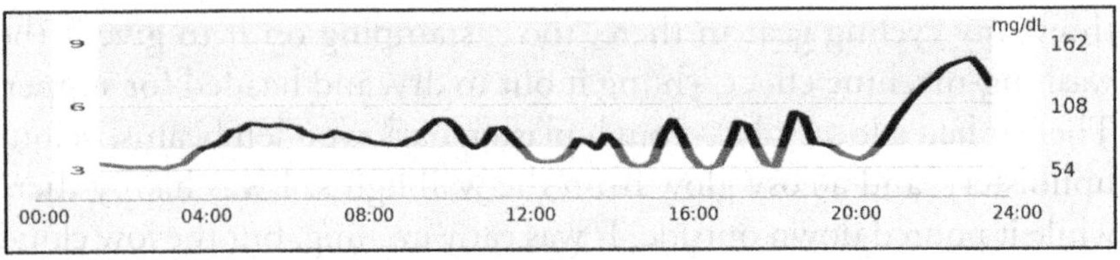
mg/dL
9
6
3
162
108
54
00:00
04:00
08:00
12:00
16:00
20:00
24:00

Chapter 8
Hypoglycaemia

On the first day of this trip, I became susceptible to even a tiny amount of rapid-acting insulin. I usually expect around a 2.5 mmol/L (45 mg/dL) drop in glucose per unit, but this time I got two to three times that. So naturally, I was very cautious about using rapid insulin in the context of exercise. I could have approached it differently, perhaps by reducing my basal insulin and using small, carefully titrated doses of rapid – but I did not want to risk that. I had been caught out once and needed to adapt my plan.

Which brings us to hypos. What exactly is a hypo? Is it a number? A fixed threshold? A sensation? In reality, it is a mix of all three. People with hypo unawareness must rely on numerical values, and CGMs have been a game-changer for them. Those of us with good awareness typically respond to how we feel.

I once ran a survey on my website mailing list and 45 people with type 1 diabetes responded. It was illuminating. The ketogenic diet significantly reduced the frequency of hypos. Seventy-eight per cent of those on keto had at least half the number of hypos compared to their non-keto peers, and half of that group reported at least a threefold reduction. That aligns well with a study published nearly 20 years ago by Swedish diabetes researcher Jorge Nielsen, who found a sixfold reduction in hypoglycaemia frequency. This is not a small number – for anyone managing type 1, that kind of reduction is transformative.

Comments from respondents on a ketogenic diet were consistent: hypos were not only less frequent, but they were also less dramatic. At least one person voiced a concern that this could lead to diminished awareness, but when I asked participants to rate their hypo awareness on a scale of 1 to 10, the results were telling:

- **Keto diet:** 8
- **Low-carb diet:** 7
- **High-carb diet:** 5

The high-carb group only had five participants, which is not a large sample, but the trend was clear: a keto diet improves sensitivity to hypo's.

As for hypo symptoms, they were varied. Everyone reported onset between 3 and 4 mmol/L (54–72 mg/dL). About half of the respondents mentioned shaking or tremors. Others described weakness, sweating, confusion, shimmering vision, and hunger. Around a third also experienced more nuanced symptoms: being argumentative, having nightmares, tingling lips or tongue, a strong urge to isolate, sleepiness, anxiety, and visual disturbances like seeing spots. A few even reported altered taste, pallor, nausea, headaches and tinnitus. It is a wide spectrum, and often multiple symptoms occur together – and let's be honest, anyone with type 1 knows how maddening it is to be asked, "Is your blood sugar low?" when you are simply indulging in an argument with a normal blood sugar.

The wide range of hypo symptoms can be difficult to spot by a third party, who might not be able to interpret them as a hypo anyway. It can be particularly dangerous for people with type 1 who are also dealing with mental health conditions or are under the influence of alcohol. While alcohol often contains carbs, it also blocks the action of glucagon, the injectable emergency hormone that raises blood glucose. So, if someone with type 1 has had a night of drinking and becomes aggressive or confused, it might not be the alcohol – it could be a hypo. But how would a police officer know the difference? Or a security guard? A glucagon injection will not work here: glucose must be given. This is why identification matters. If you are alone in that situation, make sure something about your appearance tells people you have type 1 – your CGM, a bracelet, necklace, etc. It might just save your life, because, who knows, you might be verbally abusing them at the time!

The lowest glucose level at which respondents remained conscious was about 2 mmol/L (36 mg/dL). There is even research to suggest people on keto can go lower without symptoms. In the Zerofive100 project, two participants without type 1 diabetes spent prolonged periods below 3 mmol/L (54 mg/dL) without any symptoms; one spent a full third of five days in that range.

Now imagine being involved in a car accident involving that individual. Your CGM data gets scrutinised, but they do not wear one. You could be deemed at fault, assumed to be "driving under the influence" – not of alcohol, but drugs: insulin. Your insurance company might refuse to help. That is a genuine problem people with type 1 need to be aware of. In my survey, 58% said they had needed to stop driving temporarily due to a hypo. Thankfully, nearly all respondents carried hypo treatments with them, and 90% said their CGM was essential for catching hypos in advance. And, of course, CGMs help us comply with current legal requirements that give us the privilege of driving.

The simple truth is this: hypoglycaemia only occurs when there is too much insulin in the body at a given time. A very low-carb or ketogenic diet reduces insulin needs – sometimes dramatically – and therefore reduces the risk of a hypo. The law of small numbers applies here: small inputs (carbs and insulin) result in smaller errors. And in type 1 diabetes, smaller errors mean fewer hypos.

The key message is to know your hypo level and work to avoid it. As far as I am concerned, the guiding principle remains: "As much insulin as necessary, but as little as possible." It is safer that way.

Chapter 9
Total Miles: 210

Day 3 – Matching Tye to Harwich & Hook of Holland, 67 miles

"Life is like riding a bicycle. To keep your balance, you must keep moving."
– Albert Einstein

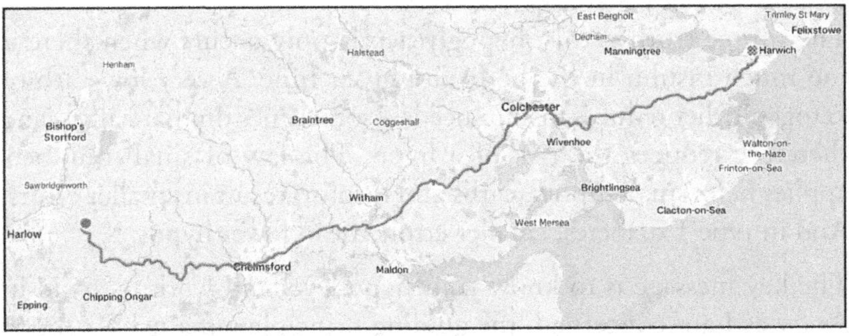

I drew back the curtains to find the rain still falling. There were puddles everywhere, rippling from the steady drops. I peered at the grey sky. Distinct higher-level and moving grey clouds were visible, rather than the depressing stratus clouds of a typically gloomy, overcast day. It looked promising; this was a weather front on the move. I reckoned that if I hung on, the rain would stop. I had a heater on all night, but some of my clothes were still damp, so I elected to put on some dry clothes and have breakfast to allow extra drying time.

Coffee, mushrooms, egg and bacon: my go-to breakfast. They are always on the menu in an English B&B. The proprietors must love people on a keto diet – a Full English becomes a Half English, with no reduction in price. Out went the sausages; while they can be a good source of macronutrients for a ketogenic diet, some are padded with wheat husk – presumably to reduce costs. There are several brands of keto-friendly sausages available. Some brands can have approximately 10 grams per sausage but that morning, I could not estimate the carbs in them. Out also went the tomatoes, hash browns, baked beans, black pudding, toast and, obviously, the marmalade.

I needed to decide on my insulin for today. A check of my glucose meter showed a slight decrease below three at night and a recovery to just under six at that moment. Yesterday, there were twelve units of Tresiba in total and four units of Novorapid, just for the evening meal. It was not a bad calculation, and despite a few hypos yesterday afternoon, I could not grumble. My CGM told me that my glucose had dipped in the night Last night's low reading was not a hypo that woke me, and I had no headache or anything that morning. I would have preferred it to stay around 3.5–4 mmol/L (63–72 mg/dL), but that is type 1 for you.

The breakfast macros for insulin counting were 19 g protein and 5 g carbohydrates. There might be an effect of the coffee as well. If I were sedentary, that would require one or two units of insulin. As I did yesterday, I elected to omit rapid and use Tresiba only. I went down a unit to five units that morning, and determined to assess the night-time dose upon arrival in Harwich.

Next, I struggled into my damp clothes. Dressing in damp, technical fibres and Lycra is a Pilates session and a good workout combined – lots of tugging, bending, and lying on the floor to coax the Lycra into position. I must have used up half my breakfast calories getting dressed. My shoes were still wet. When it is cold outside, as it was that morning, wet shoes can get very cold despite the pedalling, and I would have to pedal with numb feet for a while. I clipped on the pannier bags, summoned the sat nav, and attached my phone to the mount. A second Sainsbury's sandwich zip bag was necessary, as it is still raining; I did not want another episode of hogging a hand dryer. As I left the pub, the rain was easing. I retrieved my bike from the cellar and wished the landlord all the best – he was leaving pub ownership that week to start out in the building trade. Everyone is on their own adventure.

Amazingly, I was in open countryside, yet only 25 miles from St Paul's Cathedral in London. Now that I was in Essex, it would be a flat ride to Harwich and the coast. The change in weather as the low-pressure systems pass by, one after another, had brought another easterly wind, and it was a bit nippy coming off the North Sea but it was not too strong and the sun was breaking through the still heavily clouded sky. I set off under cloud cover, but the front was passing and would continue to clear as I headed east toward the port of Harwich.

The day would take me through the city of Chelmsford, northeast of London, and on to Colchester, finishing at the harbour – around 60 miles. I had already covered more than this distance, and was starting to get into my stride. There was plenty of flat agricultural land around, interspersed with small villages. Chelmsford came up quite quickly, and I followed the route around the outskirts. This section was the first where I had to ride on a couple of miles of trunk road full of heavy traffic, and it was narrow. There were soft grass verges, but they were about 30 cm high, and hitting them would send me back into traffic. All I could do was to get my head down and rush for the junction to a quieter road. This type of riding is not pleasant: large lorries holding back and revving their diesel engines as they changed gear to slow down. I tried to pull off the road onto driveways where I could let them pass. Then, of course, there were the cars that never saw me or, if they did, attempted to squeeze past, no matter what was coming the other way. I did not get angry; I am good at letting this stress go. In a few weeks, I will be in a car in a similar situation. There is room for all of us, if we cooperate – but then again, a few shouted expletives at inconsiderate drivers is never wasted.

Riding through a small housing estate, I spotted a long, unused cable tie. I pulled on the brakes and went back to retrieve it; I had not packed cable ties but I knew that at some point, this would come in handy. I put it in my handlebar bag and pressed on. Somewhere near Colchester, I hit National Cycle Route 1 – part of the North Sea Cycle Route. Yesterday, I crossed the canal I ran along last year, and now I had come across a route I passed by a decade ago. I really must expand my horizons!

I pressed on to Colchester. It was founded by the Romans and seemed a pleasant, historical city. I was already halfway to Harwich, and I was seeing the sun for the first time. I parked the bike up on the high street. It was lunchtime, and a man who was hammered with alcohol observed me from the pavement seating. He came over and had a chat. He wished me well and said he did not think he would get far nowadays, with the state he was in. I tended to agree. Then he went on his way, weaving through the street furniture and staggering across the road. He made it safely across into the pub on the other side. At some point, they would stop serving him; I suspect he was well known, and people were looking out for him. I hoped so.

Having topped up on some chain oil and a couple of phone charging cables – my wet one was unreliable – I sought out a sunny place in a pub terrace for some water and a coffee. I popped into a supermarket and bought some sandwich fillers with egg mayonnaise, chicken and bacon; they had around 10 g of carbs each and between 20 and 30 g of protein. If I had been sedentary for the rest of the day, I might have bolused some rapid insulin, but I planned to have one now and one in a few hours, so I elected not to.

My body was still adjusting to the trip, and I felt I still had some potential to become more insulin sensitive. After the shock of a single unit of insulin on the first day, I was still wary of Novorapid. For now, I would rely on the basal insulin and the increased insulin sensitivity to mop up the carbs. I felt it was unlikely that the protein would be converted to glucose. I suspected that, with muscle repair and new muscle being laid down by all this exercise, all of it would be used up. Only excess protein is converted to glucose. It can be a challenge to get it right; I am still working on it after a decade. It still seems a bit of an art to me.

After a leisurely half-hour soaking up the sun, I pushed off for the coast. Once out of Colchester, I spotted the EuroVelo 2 (EV2) Capitals cycling route. It is one of the 17 cycling routes organised by the European Cycling Union; they crisscross Europe, joining quiet roads and cycle paths to form a cycle route. EV2 runs from Galway to Moscow, but the marked part of the route is from Dublin to Berlin. The North Sea Cycle Route is EV12. For this trip, I toyed with the idea of EV5 London to Rome, but that was before I found the Rhine Route.

Looking at the map, I noticed I had been on the EV2 all day, and only then had I seen a sign marking it. I would be following it to Harwich. There was little of note in the countryside, and I pedalled out the miles. The last twenty were in sight; down to ten, and less than an hour to go. It must be psychological – it was the same yesterday – but I flew along the last 10 miles. I had three hours to spare as I approached the ferry terminal. The boat was already docked, but I was too early to embark.

I got back on the bike and rode a couple of miles away from the coast into Dovercourt, the nearest suburb to the terminal. I spotted a chippy. There did not seem to be any other options for eating in this part of town, so I stopped. It was busy and clearly local. People popped in, placed orders, then waited in their cars or lingered outside. It was a big menu, but for me, the choice was limited to fish or sausage. I could not trust the sausage – too processed-looking, and I had had enough processed food lately. The owner kindly agreed to fry an unbattered piece of cod.

I was now within an hour of check-in, so I packed up the fish and headed back. A brisk and biting easterly wind had picked up, and I needed to be indoors to stay warm. The reception building located outside the terminal was utterly faceless, unheated and grey, the atmosphere made worse by it being quiet. I had the place to myself, and sat down to enjoy a fish supper in paper and, to warm up, a coffee from the only vending machine in the building. It was bit late for caffeine, but I needed some internal heat. My glucose was 4 mmol/L (72 mg/dL), so I did not inject.

Gradually, a few more passengers arrived and that familiar buzz of anticipation built. As customs opened, I was waved to the front of the queue. Several cyclists had now turned up, and we swapped stories and routes. One was heading to Prague on a massive electric bike, another to Amsterdam for a short trip. A small group of young men were en route to Rome, probably on the EV5.

I rechecked my glucose; it was climbing – now around 8 mmol/L (144 mg/dL). That was due to the protein in the fish, I guessed. I needed to dose with insulin, so I wandered behind a building and discreetly injected six units of Tresiba and two of Novorapid into my thigh. It is still instinctive for me to hide my type 1 after all these years, it seems: be discreet and do not draw attention to yourself. I might get over it one day. I remembered too late that I had planned to drop to five units of Tresiba. Damn! The injections were painful – my legs were cold but not numb.

The embarkation was delayed – no sailing for a couple more hours. I was still in shorts and a cycling top, and I was getting cold. The sun was setting, and the east wind off the sea was biting. The temperature was down to 7 degrees Celsius. I slipped on my cycling jacket and paced around to stay warm. I had not packed trousers where I could easily access them and, honestly, I was not planning on needing them much for the trip.

Then word came: another delay – around 45 minutes. It was the ferry company doing expectation management, of course; an hour later, we were finally moved to the bottom of the ramp, and another 20 minutes passed while articulated lorries embarked. Then the cyclists were waved forward. I was cold and ready to move. The loading bay was a cacophony – engines, metal clanking, the echo of voices and fellow cyclists rushing for the cycle park. In the middle of the chaos, I paused, stepped back and let it all settle; there was no point adding to the frenzy. Once the riders dispersed, I grabbed my bags and navigated the narrow passageways to my cabin. Thankfully, it was not near the engine room. I have been there before, and it is no fun with all of the noise and vibration. I showered, washed my kit, and climbed into bed. The cabin had a heater, and I gratefully used it. I slowly warmed up.

Before turning in, I checked my glucose: 11 mmol/L (198 mg/dL), nearly two hours post-injection. That was unexpected. I could not do much about it at that stage. I needed to sleep and did not want to use more insulin and risk a hypo; but 11mmol/L (198 mg/dL) was a bit high. I had hoped to stay in a non-diabetic range for longer. Still, tomorrow was another day.

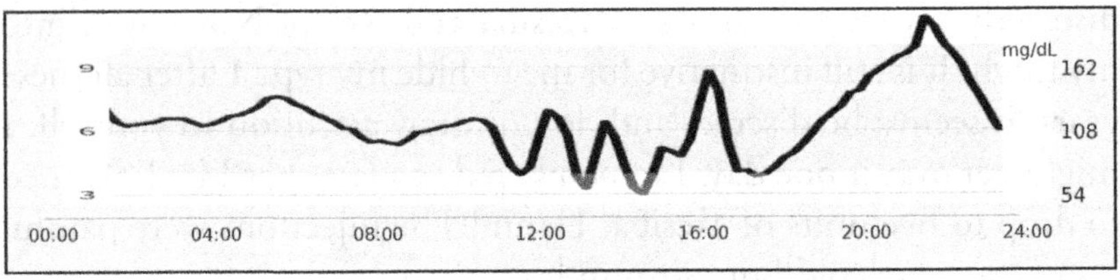

Chapter 10
How Are We Put Together?

Brian: "You are all individuals."
The followers (in unison): "Yes, we are all individuals."
– Monty Python's Life of Brian

There are around 400,000 people in the United Kingdom estimated to be living with type 1 diabetes – but there are also 400,000 ways to manage it, because every person is unique. Type 1 diabetes does not look or feel the same for everyone. What works for one person may not work for another.

To live well with type 1 diabetes, we need to understand how the body works. So, here is my overview of how it all fits together, which I think will be helpful when developing a practical strategy – while being in awe of our potential as humans.

Making Sense of Energy and Nutrition

We have all heard the usual phrases about food and energy. All together now:

"You need carbs for energy."

"Glucose is the body's main fuel."

"If you take insulin, you must eat carbs."

At first glance, these seem reasonable. But when you live with diabetes, things are rarely that simple. Advice can be confusing and even conflicting. There are countless messages online, in magazines and on social media. Some come from experts, but others are from people with products to sell or strong personal opinions based on their own experience.

After years of real-world experience, many people living with diabetes realise that these common statements are only partly true. The missing piece is context – knowing when, and how, these ideas apply.

For example, yes, the body can use glucose for energy; but glucose is not the only source of energy. To really understand what is going on, we have to look closer at how the body processes food.

How the Body Uses Food

Here is a quick recap: everything we eat contains a combination of macronutrients – protein, fat and carbohydrates. These nutrients are broken down in the digestive system into smaller building blocks:

- Proteins become amino acids.
- Fats become fatty acids and glycerol.
- Carbohydrates become simple sugars, mainly glucose.

Once digested, these components enter the bloodstream and travel to cells throughout the body. There, they are either used immediately for energy or stored for later use.

One of the most remarkable things about the human body is its flexibility. It can convert one type of nutrient into another:

- Carbohydrates can be turned into fat.
- Proteins can be turned into glucose or ketones.
- Fats can be used directly for energy, or converted into ketones.

This means that if the body runs low on carbohydrates, it can still make all the glucose it needs. The liver and kidneys can produce glucose from protein via a process called gluconeogenesis.

So technically, there is no minimum requirement for carbohydrates; the body can make its own. On the other hand, proteins and fats are essential because they contain certain amino acids and fatty acids that the body cannot make by itself. Without them, we cannot survive.

Carbohydrates can still be part of a healthy diet, of course – especially when they come from whole foods like fruits or vegetables that also provide vitamins, minerals and fibre. But it is important to understand that the body does not need carbs in the same way it needs protein and fat. This works in our favour when we try to live with type 1 diabetes. Carbohydrates are the primary fuel for raising glucose levels. Knowing this allows us to adopt strategies to use them in amounts more suited to the insulin deficiency state of type 1 diabetes and improve our overall metabolism.

The Role of Insulin and Metabolism

Insulin is one of the most important hormones in the human body. It acts like a key that unlocks the doors of our cells so that glucose can enter and be used for energy. Without insulin, glucose builds up in the bloodstream, leading to high blood sugar.

People with type 1 diabetes no longer produce insulin naturally, so they must replace it through injections or an insulin pump. Balancing insulin with food and activity is like performing a daily science experiment. When we eat carbohydrates, our blood sugar rises. Insulin helps move that sugar into the cells, where it can be burned for fuel or stored as glycogen or fat. Protein can also raise blood sugar slightly, though much more slowly. Fat has the least immediate effect on blood sugar – but it still provides plenty of energy.

Understanding how different foods affect blood sugar and insulin is key to managing type 1 diabetes. There is no single "right" approach for everyone. Some people prefer a low-carb lifestyle, while others manage well with balanced meals that include all three macronutrients. The important thing is to learn how your own body responds – and that takes observation, patience and time.

The Human Body: A Community of Cells

The human body contains approximately 30 trillion cells, all of which are alive and active. Even bone cells are constantly undergoing degradation and regeneration. We all start life as a single fertilised egg, which divides again and again to form all the tissues and organs of the body.

During this process, some cells become specialised – skin cells, muscle cells, nerve cells, and so on. Once a cell takes on its special role, it stays that way. For example, a liver cell cannot morph into a brain cell.

There are about 70 organs in the body, each performing its own task. The pancreas does two main jobs:

1. It produces digestive enzymes that break down food (this is the exocrine pancreas).
2. It produces hormones like insulin, glucagon and amylin (this is the endocrine pancreas).

These hormones are made in tiny clusters of cells called islets of Langerhans. In type 1 diabetes, the immune system attacks these cells, destroying their ability to secrete insulin; therefore, insulin must be administered as injections.

The Body as a Tube

In a way, the human body is like a long tube. Food enters through the mouth, travels down the oesophagus, through the stomach and intestines, and finally leaves the body as waste through the anus.

Until nutrients are absorbed through the intestinal wall, that food is technically outside the body. The inside of the digestive tract is "in contact" with the outside world, just like our skin is.

The walls of the intestine are covered in tiny folds called villi, and even smaller projections called microvilli. These create an enormous surface area – roughly half the size of a badminton court – allowing nutrients to be absorbed efficiently.

The lungs work in a similar way; if you could spread out all the tiny air sacs, they would cover an area about the size of a tennis court. This design allows oxygen to move into the blood and carbon dioxide to move out very efficiently.

Both the lungs and the intestines are lined with cells that interact with the external world. Both also host microbiomes – collections of bacteria and other microorganisms that play a big role in health.

DNA: The Code of Life

Every living thing on Earth shares the same basic genetic language – DNA. In humans, DNA is stored in the nucleus of almost every cell. It is made of four chemical "letters": A, T, C, and G. The order of these letters forms a code that tells the body how to make proteins.

Humans have 46 chromosomes, which are threadlike structures made of DNA and proteins that carry genetic information and organises it for cell function and inheritance. These are arranged in 23 pairs – half from the mother, half from the father. One of these pairs determines biological sex (XX for female, XY for male).

Only a small part of our DNA actually codes for genes. Most of it acts as regulatory material, turning genes on or off or controlling when and where proteins are made. Sometimes, during cell division, minor errors called mutations occur; most of these are harmless, but occasionally they can lead to diseases such as cancer.

Each specialised cell in the body uses only the genes it needs. A skin cell and a nerve cell contain the same DNA, but they use different genes to differentiate and perform the tasks unique to that tissue.

Mitochondria: The Powerhouses of the Cell

Inside almost every cell are tiny structures called mitochondria. They are often referred to as the powerhouses of the cell, because they convert nutrients into energy.

Mitochondria have their own DNA, known as mitochondrial DNA, which is inherited exclusively from the mother. This DNA helps the mitochondria make the enzymes and proteins they need to turn nutrients into energy. Mitochondria can use many different fuels – glucose, fatty acids and ketones – and they can multiply in number when the body needs more energy. For example, regular exercise can increase the number of mitochondria in muscle cells, making the body more efficient at producing energy. This ability to adapt, known as metabolic flexibility, helped our ancestors survive periods of food scarcity or unpredictability.

The Microbiome: Our Hidden Ecosystem

In recent years, scientists have discovered that humans are not just made of human cells. We are also home to around a hundred trillion bacteria, fungi and viruses – collectively called the microbiome.

These tiny organisms live primarily in the gut but also on the skin, in the mouth, and even in the lungs. Together, they weigh about as much as the human brain: 3 lb (1.3 kg). The bacteria in the gut are somehow recognised by the gut immune system as "friendly". We know about the potential for infection from bacteria in faeces, yet inside the bowel, the body can not only tolerate, but also form a symbiotic relationship with those bacteria.

The gut microbiome helps digest food, stimulates the immune system, provides the raw materials for nerve-transmitting and antioxidant molecules, and protects against harmful bacteria. Everyone's microbiome is slightly different, shaped by diet, lifestyle, environment and genetics. When the balance of bacteria in the gut is disrupted – a state known as dysbiosis – it can lead to inflammation and illness. Studies have found that people with type 1 diabetes often have lower levels of beneficial bacteria, such as *Lactobacillus* and *Bifidobacterium.*

The Gut-Brain and Gut-Lung Connections

The gut and the brain communicate constantly through a network of nerves (including the vagus nerve) and hormones, collectively known as the gut-brain axis. This is why stress can upset digestion, and why gut health can affect mood and concentration. The gut is sometimes called the "second brain" because it contains hundreds of millions of nerve cells. These nerves send signals not only to the digestive system but also to brain regions that regulate emotion.

This is an exciting new field, and researchers are exploring how the health of the microbiome might affect autoimmune diseases like type 1 diabetes.

Leaky Gut and Autoimmunity

One interesting theory about type 1 diabetes is the concept of a "leaky gut". Typically, the cells of the intestinal wall are tightly joined together by proteins called tight junctions. These keep bacteria and food particles inside the gut, where they belong.

In some people, certain foods – such as gluten proteins found in wheat – can damage these junctions. When that happens, tiny gaps open in the gut wall, allowing small food particles or bacteria to leak into the bloodstream. The immune system sees these particles as invaders and attacks them. Sometimes, this immune response can go awry and begin attacking the body's own tissues, such as insulin-producing cells in the pancreas.

Studies have found that people with type 1 diabetes often show signs of increased gut permeability. Researchers are now exploring whether reducing gut inflammation through diet could help. One research group in Hungary developed an anti-inflammatory diet composed mostly of clean, grass-fed meats and small amounts of pesticide-free vegetables. In one reported case, a child with type 1 diabetes experienced partial recovery of insulin production after following this diet. While it is just one case, it gives scientists clues about how gut health might influence autoimmune conditions.

Adapting to Modern Life

Human beings are incredibly adaptable. For most of our history, we lived as hunters and gatherers, constantly moving and adjusting to changing environments. Our bodies evolved to handle periods of feast and famine, and to get energy from a mix of fat and protein, with occasional carbohydrates.

Today, our world looks very different. We have constant access to food, much of it processed, and we spend most of our time sitting rather than moving. Modern lifestyles challenge our ancient biology.

For people with type 1 diabetes, these challenges are even greater. Managing blood sugar requires constant attention – tracking food, insulin, activity, sleep and stress. Each of these factors affects the others.

Learning how insulin interacts with metabolism can help us use this knowledge to our advantage. For example, physical activity makes the body more sensitive to insulin, while poor sleep and stress can make it less sensitive. Even the timing of meals and the body's natural day-night (circadian) rhythms can affect blood sugar control.

The human body is one of the most complex systems in the universe; we are made of trillions of human cells, surrounded by trillions of microorganisms, powered by the tiny mitochondria inside each cell.

We share about 50% of our genes with a banana and comprise 60% water, yet the combination of DNA, environment, and microbiome makes each of us completely unique. We are, quite literally, ecosystems walking on two legs.

Living with type 1 diabetes means becoming a careful observer of this system. It requires learning how food, stress, exercise, and sleep interact with insulin and blood sugar. It is a constant balancing act – part science, part art, and part intuition. And I am attempting to learn all of these things on this journey.

Chapter 11

Total Miles: 277

Day 4 – Hook of Holland to Wijk bij Duurstede, 67 miles

"The greatest illusion," said the mole, "is that life should be perfect."
– The Boy, the Mole, the Fox and the Horse

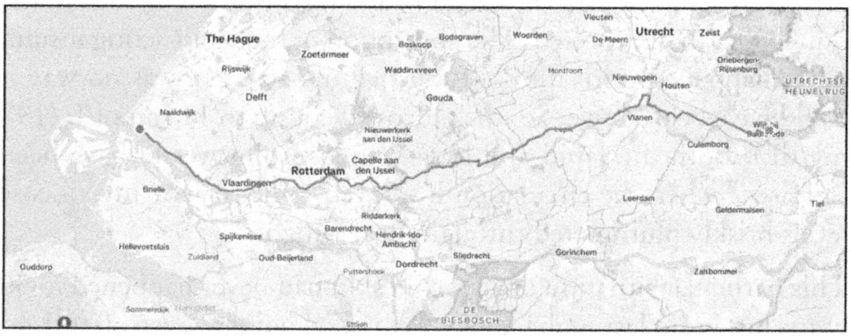

I had my alarm set but was beaten to it by Bobby McFerrin telling me, in a reggae-jazz-pop refrain, "Don't worry, be happy!" Fifteen minutes later, he prompted me again. I was out the door before the next call. I could not whistle along happily at that time of day.

I had slept well that night and, upon waking, went through my usual routine. Before all of the glucose management, I always check that I can move my limbs; my father had a haemorrhagic stroke when he was younger than I am now, and lived with significant disability for two more decades. My brother died instantly of the same kind of stroke when 54 years old, at a football match. Only my mum and I are left. I suppose that history sits quietly in the back of my mind, and having type 1 does not exactly calm the nerves. So, it was good to know I was okay that morning. I smile quietly to myself – all that medical knowledge, and I am still touching wood that both legs are working, at least for the moment.

I checked the CGM. Glucose had peaked at 11 mmol/L (198 mg/dL), drifted to 3.5 mmol/L (63 mg/dL) overnight, and risen again to 6 mmol/L (108 mg/dL) on waking with the dawn effect – the combination of growth hormone, cortisol and adrenaline (epinephrine) increasing in the early hours as part of our body's natural rhythm. I pondered what caused the glucose to rise last night. I am sure the insulin went in, and was fresh and not degraded; it was within the use-by date by a year.

Mulling it over at breakfast, the answer finally came to me: my legs were cold. The circulation was poor, and the insulin remained in the skin longer than expected. The absorption of the rapid acting insulin never happened until the skin warmed up, so there was no way it could have been active. So, the glucose went up to 11 mmol/L (198 mg/dL). Both the rapid and long-acting insulin would have been "released" when the circulation improved – that is why my glucose levels briskly plummeted throughout the night.

This particular situation of very cold skin had never happened in 30 years, but it did last night. Every day is a school day, even after three decades of diabetes. I have plenty of experience with erratic absorption of insulin – those days when you think you are doing everything right, day after day, and still get different results. There are many reasons for this, and I will explore many of them in this book, but the basics of insulin absorption are still significant. Those erratic traces can simply be due to absorption issues.

Research has found up to 25% variability in absorption when insulin is injected into the same person, and up to 50% variability between individuals. Types of insulin vary, even within the same profiles, such as rapid-acting insulins; of course, long-acting insulins are designed to be slow-acting and so are less of an issue. The volume of the injection does make a difference: larger volumes tend to be less predictable than smaller ones, which are usually absorbed more rapidly. Some claim that the site of injection is important, and many favour the abdomen because of its supposed reliability. I have never found this, but others might. Nor have I found that injecting into the thigh when running affects absorption. It does not really make sense, because we inject into the subcutaneous fat rather than directly into the muscle – so, while absorption might be faster due to the heat generated by muscle activity, this would be dispersed around the body in the bloodstream.

Subcutaneous fat itself is not a simple or uniform tissue; it varies in thickness, blood supply, temperature, local blood flow, and degree of scarring. Fat tissue can also differ markedly between individuals, and even between sites in the same person. Repeated injections can alter this tissue over time, creating areas of scarring that further disrupt absorption. Insulin injected into scarred fat may be absorbed more slowly or unpredictably, adding yet another layer of variability that is largely invisible to us in daily life.

Modern insulins are tweaked to try to improve uniformity of absorption rates, but variability still happens; and, of course, there are additional variables to explore, such as the internal effects of insulin, which are subject to many hormonal and metabolic events that affect its expression. Added to erratic insulin absorption is erratic food absorption, depending on the composition of the meal and the rate of gastric emptying – especially if one is stressed or has neuropathy of the gastric nerves, causing gastroparesis, or delayed and erratic emptying of the stomach. This will inevitably make insulin timing a challenge.

Of course, to someone living with type 1 diabetes, this is not a surprise, and we have to learn to adapt to this fairly common variability. One's unique expression of type 1 diabetes is something we all have to work out for ourselves. Do you have a more "erratic" metabolism than others?

Some people make it look easy and seem to have flat-line traces from day one; others find glucose is not so compliant, even with their best efforts. Never allow yourself to compare your diabetes with others. Each of us has to search for the best control we can achieve with the body we have – there is no single, uniform type 1 diabetes body. We might sometimes feel like lab rats – but unlike them, we are all metabolically unique. Lucky them, in that way!

The clothes situation was getting dire. Yesterday's socks were on their second day, caked in mud from the previous rain. They were pretty foul, really. I had packed only two cycling kits, a hoodie and one pair of trousers, as there was no room for anything else. I had expected a sun-fest heading south, so this rain was a real dampener. The shoes were still wet, edging toward biohazard territory.

I packed my bags and headed to the ferry's canteen, hoping no one would notice the state of my footwear. The smell of fried food in the air provided an excellent smokescreen. Beyond the condensation-streaked windows, the horizon glowed faint orange against grey clouds. I decided on some fresh air and popped out onto the deck to get a better view, joining the loners, the seasick, the excited holidaymakers, and the smokers.

We were heading east, and the dawn sky held promise – until I checked the weather on the phone app. A low-pressure system had settled over the North Sea, promising another cool mix of rain and sun. I checked a second app, more in hope than expectation. It said the same. I muttered something unkind about the Met Office – the UK's national weather service – we should set them targets.

Breakfast time – and calories of the right kind. Bacon, eggs, mushrooms: reliable staples, even at an outrageous, non-discounted ferry price. I haggled for extra bacon, grumbling about the lack of ketogenic foods and paying for less food at the same price. No toast, hash browns, fried bread or beans, yet I was still paying for them. Still, the coffee was cheap, refillable, and very drinkable. Clearly, the marketing team understood how to manipulate perception – that cheap coffee refills could make me feel better about blowing half of my holiday money on the breakfast.

And so, to insulin: Day Four, and I am settling in. Day Three had been a reasonably good one for control. Today would be a nearly identical day regarding physical activity. I needed to smash out about 60 flat miles. Bacon and eggs might or might not nudge things up. Type 1 can be unreliable, but I decided to skip rapid insulin, rely on exercise, stick with the six units of Tresiba, and see. It might prove a touch too much because, after all this exercise, I am more insulin sensitive. Eventually, it will stabilise. A half-unit pen or a pump would have helped, but adaptation is part of the type 1 life.

When the ferry docked, the usual scramble began. By the time I reached my bike, most people were already disembarking. I saw a couple of travellers from the night before – we wished each other well and went our separate ways. The pedal cleats on my shoes clanked across the metal deck, adding percussion to the roar of engines. As we disembarked amidst the smell of diesel fumes and hydraulic fluid, the fresh air hit me. There was a cool breeze and a glint of sunshine on the water of the harbour. I was officially on the continent. That sense of possibility that always greets me on foreign soil kicked in. It is hard to describe; it is not about where I *am* but where I can *go*. The familiarity of home now far behind, I clipped into my pedals and set off through the quiet roads of the Dutch port.

I set my Bikemap app and flipped open my Cycling the Rhine Route book, reading it backwards, since the authors started in the mountains of Switzerland. My route today: ride to Wijk bij Duurstede, just south of Utrecht in the Netherlands. A brief wrong turn took me onto a "Cycling Verboden" road, but a friendly shout from another rider waved me back onto the proper path. Once on-track, the Bikemap app approved. Everything here was designed for cyclists: proper lanes, courteous drivers, clear signs. I knew instantly this would be a good day.

Onwards then, towards the Rhine proper. Here in the Netherlands, it is a delta – where the river splits: the Nieuwe Maas north, the Oude Maas south, flowing to form the Lek in the north and Nederrijn in the south, and finally joining the Waal to form the Rhine, or Rijn, near Millingen an der Rijn.

The width of the Rhine at this point is as impressive as its statistics: 3,000 cubic metres of water flow through this delta every second in the winter. The Rhine is navigable all the way to Konstanz, where it widens into Bodensee. Metre-high black and white numbered boards mark the navigable section along the riverbank. The Rhine Kilometers markers were introduced in 1939, starting at 0 km in Konstanz and ending at 1,036 km at the Hook of Holland. I soon started ticking them off like milestones of my own.

After an hour, when the sun had begun to warm the land, I stopped at a quiet bench by a canal, took off my shoes and let my socks dry in the sunlight – a small but glorious moment. Physically, I was finding rhythm; mentally, I was calm. And I was metabolically steady: glucose in range, no hypos, and still in ketosis.

I merrily pedalled for an hour or so through typical flat Dutch farmland – green fields full of cattle, straight canals, brown-brick farmsteads with cream-framed shutters and lace curtains. Bridges and dams came and went. There was hardly anyone about, just the wind and distant cow bells. It was here, years ago on the North Sea Cycle Route, that I had discovered my "Dutch pace": 12 miles an hour. Everyone seemed to do it – parents, kids, dogs in baskets. Smooth, easy, efficient, and less chance of colliding as we were all going at the same speed. I adopted it then, and I kept it now.

Rotterdam was typically busy. There were too many choices for the sat nav; it dithered like a child in a sweet shop with not enough money. After it guided me round one too many loops, I rode with the river on my left and kept heading east, trusting the compass of the sun, which was now in the south and on my right. Eventually, the sprawl gave way to fields again.

My glucose behaved at first, then dipped – the dreaded down-arrow. I corrected twice with 20 g of glucose, 15 minutes apart, and paid the price with a rebound high. Still, it soon levelled. My insulin sensitivity factor is about 2.5 – one-unit drops glucose by 2.5 mmol/L (45 mg/dL) – so I now know how to calculate corrections, but prefer caution until I am fully in rhythm. I really should have held my nerve after the first rescue dose, but I was too impulsive and so overcorrected.

By the time I reached Schoonhoven, I was hungry. Shops were mostly closed for lunch but a local butcher sold me some cured sausage and egg-and-chicken salad; he swore there was no sugar, but the sweet tang of vinegar said otherwise. Still, waste not, want not!

Instinctively, I reached for the rapid insulin and injected two units without thinking. It is almost muscle memory now, but I cursed, as I had not at that point worked out the meal macros, and was doing macronutrient calculations in reverse order. It should be the calculation of macros followed by insulin; I was doing the opposite, unthinkingly.

I sat by the canal, weighing the meal: roughly 32 g of protein in the sausage, 17 g in the salad, 4 g of carbs. About 50 g of protein total. I usually bolus protein at half the carb dose – 10 g protein equals 0.5 units – so 2.5 units would have been right. As luck would have it, my insulin dose was okay. That is experience, I guess.

I knew a few hours of cycling would easily burn through the calories in the meal. Thirty years ago, before I was diagnosed with type 1, I could sit on that bench and simply enjoy the meal and the scenery; I had no thought for all of this. But because of type 1, calculations like this are part of my daily life. I am pleased to have discovered optimised insulin, which enables me more flexibility and tighter control. This trip is a working trip, so I have to record everything and it sounds obsessive, but if I were doing it for leisure, it would have been a breeze; it is still not difficult, and is far easier than fuelling on carbs all day. I would not like to do that.

By late afternoon, the sky had turned grey again, and a cool wind followed me to Wijk bij Duurstede. The B&B was perfect – an old town-centre, three-storey house with cream walls and a huge wooden door big enough to get a cart through. I had a top-floor room – half price thanks to a cancellation: warm towel rail (great for laundry), Nespresso coffee, and breakfast available. I was happy. After that filling lunch, I was not hungry for dinner, so I finished off some cheese and called it a night. My glucose trace stayed almost flat, drifting slightly low, but nothing concerning. Tomorrow's breakfast – and the glucose-raising effects of adrenaline and cortisol will lift it again.

I planned tomorrow to set off early, to use the natural glucose-lowering effect of exercise and reminded myself to be less trigger-happy with injections and glucose corrections. There was no need to be edgy. By now, I was getting settled – physically well, glucose steady, ketones calm, insulin tuned to the rhythm of the ride, the continent beneath my wheels, the day ahead...

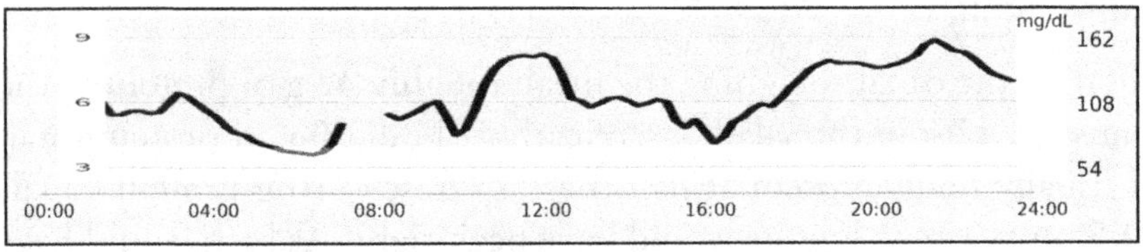

Chapter 12
Energy: The Life Force – How Do We Use It?

Our bodies are built from many specialised tissues and organ systems. To keep this whole structure alive – possibly for up to a century – we need a steady supply of energy. Food gives us that energy, but we can also use the energy we have already stored in our bodies, like when we are fasting or asleep. People often say the body "needs" glucose, fat, ketones or other fuels, but what does that really mean? To understand this properly, it helps to view it from the perspective of a single cell.

Fuel Reserves and What Blood Tests Actually Tell Us

Humans did not evolve to absorb food from the digestive system all the time. Instead, our ancestors experienced cycles of feast and famine, so the body developed practical energy reserves. We store glucose and fat, and we can access protein when absolutely required. These are our in-house energy supplies.

When we measure substances in the blood, we are really measuring what is *travelling through* the body, not what is happening *inside* the cells where energy is actually produced. Blood vessels are more like motorways or freeways: they move things from place to place, but no one "lives" there. So, whenever we check blood results, we should ask: what is this molecule doing here now? Where did it come from, and where is it going? For example, people with type 1 diabetes check their blood glucose often. If glucose is high, it is not being cleared quickly enough, so they act – using insulin or physical activity – to help move glucose out of the blood and into cells.

Some metabolites – molecules produced when we metabolise food – such as lactic acid, are easily measured. Fatty acids are rarely measured individually outside a research setting, but we commonly measure them indirectly as triglycerides. We also measure ketones via the blood, urine and breath, and we can estimate whether the body is mainly burning fat or glucose by analysing the gases we breathe out.

After We Eat: How Different Macronutrients Travel

After a meal, carbohydrates, proteins and fats enter the body through different pathways.

Carbohydrates and proteins enter the blood vessels of the intestinal wall. They are carried to the liver first, where sugars and amino acids are processed and regulated; only then are they released to the rest of the body.

Fat takes a different route. It first enters the lymphatic system, our second circulatory system. This means fat is delivered to tissues around the body before it reaches the liver. Because of this, the fat you eat can become part of your body tissues. We know this from comparing grain-fed and pasture-fed animals, which develop very different fat profiles. So, the type of fats we eat matter. Once digested, fats travel to the liver where they are processed and converted into other types of fats the body needs.

Capillaries, Interstitial Fluid, and Lymph

As blood vessels branch away from the heart, they become smaller until they form single-cell-thick capillaries. These tiny vessels have the ability to leak interstitial fluid – which is essentially blood plasma without the blood cells or most proteins. Every cell is surrounded by this fluid, which constantly bathes them in nutrients, electrolytes and minerals. Waste products return to the circulation for processing through small veins or the lymphatic system, which also supports the immune system and carries dietary fat. The lymph eventually drains into the left subclavian vein, just below the collarbone.

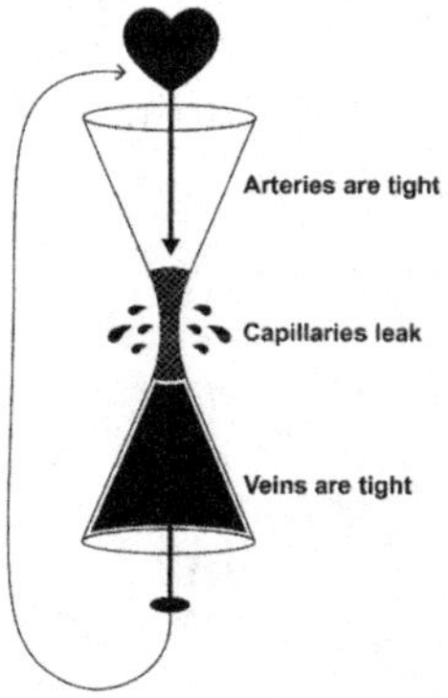

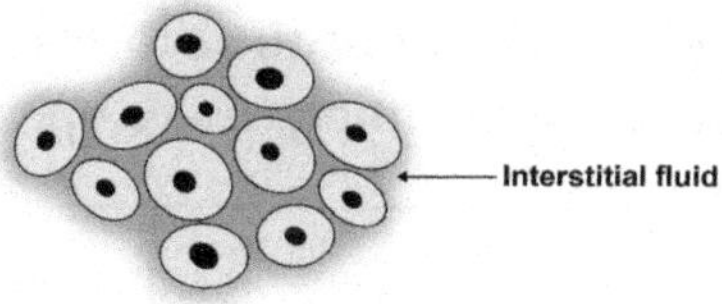

Interstitial fluid bathes cells in nutrients and signalling molecules — the cells choose their fuel from what is available

Nothing Gets Into a Cell Uninvited

Even though all tissues are bathed in nutrients, each cell decides what to take in. The digestive system delivers nutrients to the circulation, then to the cell surface via interstitial fluid, but the cell controls what actually enters. A good example is glucose. In a person without diabetes, interstitial fluid glucose stays between 4–6 mmol/L (72–108 mg/dL). Interstitial glucose is usually very close to capillary/plasma glucose, but is often a little lower and can lag by around 5 to 10 minutes if there is a rapid change. Continuous Glucose Meters sample interstitial fluid, and so the challenges of comparing this to the standard measure of capillary glucose become evident. Intracellular free glucose is usually much lower than either, because once glucose enters most cells, it is rapidly metabolised for energy.

The cell decides when to use glucose. Think of a cell as a house pantry. If your cupboards are already full, you do not bring more food into the house. If the cupboards are empty, you open the front door and bring in whatever is needed. Cells behave the same way. When energy is low, cells open "doors" in the membrane to let nutrients in; when energy is high, they close them. These "doors" are controlled entry points – receptors, channels, and transport systems. Some work like automatic doors, others like bolted doors, and others like escalators that require energy. Nothing gets inside without permission.

Your energy needs shift during the day. Sitting and reading require little energy. Running or lifting something heavy requires much more energy, but the process of energy entering cells is the same – the amount simply scales up.

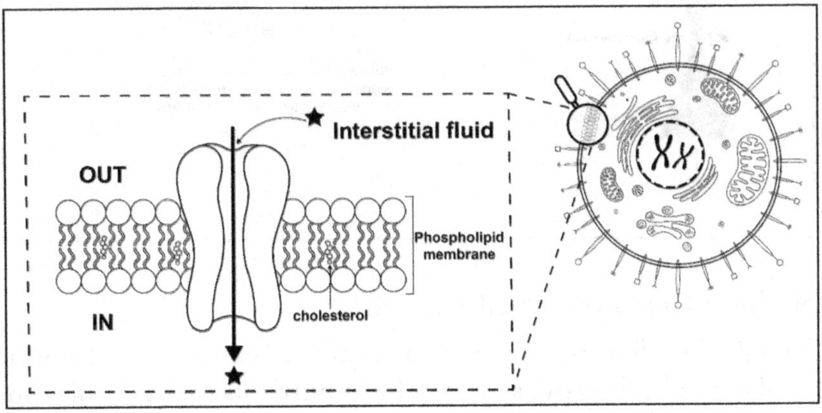

Some tissues specialise in storing energy. Fat cells and glycogen-storing cells open their receptors to take in fatty acids and glucose when levels are high. At first, fat is stored around the waist and hips. When those stores fill, fat begins to accumulate in the liver and other areas, such as the chin, jawline and chest, as well as around organs. This is called visceral fat. In large amounts, it is not healthy. When glucose stores are full, the liver converts extra glucose into fat. When energy supply is low, storage tissues release their contents in response to hormonal signals.

What a Cell Looks Like

Different cells have different jobs, but most share key structures:

- A cell membrane, made of a double layer of fatty molecules called phospholipids, with cholesterol helping to regulate fluidity. The phosphate side faces water; the lipid side avoids it.
- Proteins, proteolipids and glycoproteins that cross the membrane. These allow communication, form channels for nutrients and ions, and mark the cell as "self".
- A nucleus (except in red blood cells), which holds DNA.

- Networks of tubes near the nucleus where proteins are made, called the endoplasmic reticulum.
- Cytoplasm, the fluid inside the cell, where nutrients and proteins move about, and where glucose is also converted to energy.
- Mitochondria, the power generators of the cell.
- Lysosomes, the cell recycling centres.

Inside every cell, proteins carry out reactions that generate energy, build structures like muscle and nerve fibres, and send signals. Many signalling proteins sit in or just below the membrane, acting as communication devices that respond to both neighbouring cells and medications.

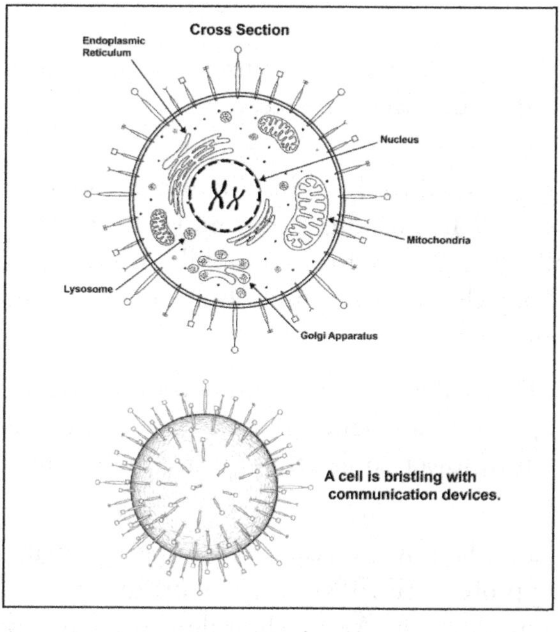

Glucose Transport: The GLUT Family

Glucose is a good example of how carefully nutrient entry into cells is controlled. Although glucose may be available in the blood, it cannot simply drift into cells; it must pass through special transport proteins called glucose transporters (GLUTs). There are at least 12 known GLUTs, each with a particular role. The most important ones for understanding type 1 diabetes and metabolism will be discussed here.

- GLUT1 is the main transporter, and is found in almost all cells. It works automatically, without insulin, providing a steady supply of glucose, which is especially important for tissues that rely heavily on it, like the brain and red blood cells. Under stress, cells can increase the number of GLUT1 to bring in more fuel. However, it becomes less efficient at very high glucose levels.
- GLUT2 is found mainly in the liver, pancreas, kidneys and intestine. Unlike other GLUTs, it allows glucose to move in and out of cells depending on blood levels. This makes it ideal for organs involved in glucose control, particularly the liver and pancreas.
- GLUT3 is the primary glucose transporter in neurons. It is highly efficient and ensures the brain receives enough glucose even when levels are low.
- GLUT4 responds directly to insulin and is abundant in muscle and fat tissue. When insulin is present, GLUT4 moves to the cell surface, allowing glucose to enter rapidly. This is one of the main ways the body clears excess glucose from the blood and stores it as glycogen or fat.

Other GLUTs also allow glucose to enter cells without insulin. Most work like open doors, letting glucose flow from areas of higher concentration to lower concentration, depending on the needs of each tissue.

Fatty acids have their own specialised transport proteins called fatty acid-binding proteins (FABPs), which allow them to enter cells in a similarly controlled way. Again, the rule is the same: nutrients are always available outside the cell, but entry is by invitation only.

Glucose Levels and Hormones

Glucose stays in a tight range: 4–6 mmol/L (72–108 mg/dL), rising to about 7.8 mmol/L (140 mg/dL) after meals, and higher in people with diabetes. Even if you do not eat carbohydrates, or if you fast for several days, your cells are still bathed in glucose; the body never allows glucose to reach zero.

Many hormones can raise glucose, including glucagon and adrenaline (epinephrine), but only insulin can lower it. It does this mainly in muscle, liver and fat tissue, which can take in large amounts of glucose.

Glucose is monitored by sensors around the pancreas. The islet cells – where insulin and glucagon are made – receive unusually high blood flow and have dense capillaries. They react quickly:

- Insulin rises when glucose goes above about 5.6 mmol/L (100 mg/dL). It lowers blood glucose by storing it in the muscle or the liver.
- Glucagon rises when glucose drops to around 3 mmol/L (54 mg/dL). It raises blood glucose by breaking down glycogen and producing new glucose in the liver.

Fuel Options for Cells

All cells can use glucose if necessary. Some tissues – such as parts of the brain, the retina, and red blood cells – depend on glucose exclusively and cannot switch to ketones. Other tissues can use ketones or fatty acids, and may prefer them when available; these include some brain regions, parts of the kidney, and some immune cells.

A flexible, multi-fuel environment allows each cell to choose what it needs. This is especially relevant to people with type 1 diabetes. Using well-balanced insulin dosing and avoiding extremely high-carb meals helps the interstitial fluid environment maintain access to all three major fuels: glucose, fatty acids and ketones. High carbohydrate eating floods the system with glucose, removing this flexibility and providing only glucose. This mono-fuelling can have long-term metabolic consequences.

Chapter 13
Total Miles: 349

Day 5 – Wijk bij Duurstede to Marienbaum, 72 miles

"Learn from yesterday, live for today, hope for tomorrow."
– Albert Einstein.

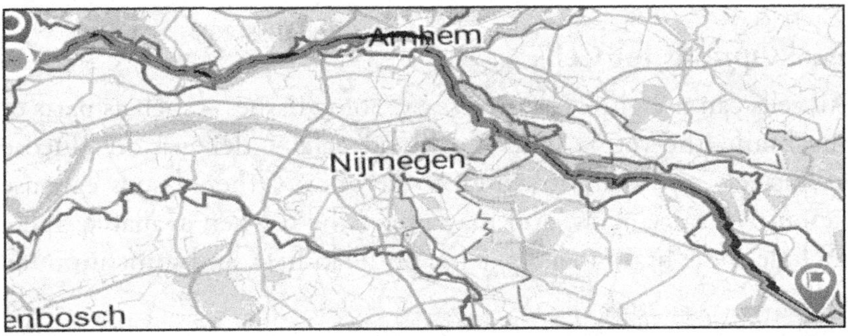

It was forecast to rain most of the day, but that did not materialise. In the end, it rained in the morning and again in the late afternoon, but for the most part, it was just cool and cloudy – something I could handle. With the weather, you can grumble for as long as you like, but it is not going to change.

Unable to control it, I adapted – but having type 1 diabetes is pretty much like that: every day, something turns up that requires attention. Mindfulness becomes the norm when you do not know what is going to happen from one hour to the next. The daily management of type 1 diabetes, and the curveballs of irritating glucose management challenges that are often unexpected, adds to the daily grind. But I am focused on the next three weeks, and that reduces my time to ponder my plight; I am getting on with the task at hand.

A routine is developing already, and it is becoming second nature to pack my luggage, calibrate the CGM with finger-prick testing, calibrate the ketone meter, clip on the heart-rate monitor, and fill the water bottles. As I was doing all of this, the hotel owner was bang on time with breakfast – scrambled eggs, yoghurt, and two bread rolls. The rolls were handed back but the rest of the food was pleasant. Of course, I had to weigh it and log it all onto the Cronometer app.

The pattern at the moment is to bookend the physical activity with a keto diet, plus or minus a light lunch. It seems right for this journey, and should work for my diabetes. I did worry about the yoghurt at breakfast, as too many hidden carbs can catch one out, but today's yoghurt turned out to be good.

I was setting off very soon after breakfast, and the decision proved a good one: six units of Tresiba basal insulin and no rapid insulin. The glucose had slowly nudged down overnight to a stable 4 mmol/L (72 mg/dL). Glucose peaked slightly, at 8 mmol/L (144 mg/dL), then steadily declined as the easy riding progressed and the basal long-acting insulin took effect. The route was flat; the predicted "hills" on the route's 3D mapping software were very shallow and did not require extra effort. This is the Netherlands – the "low lands" – the terrain is in the name.

Anticipating rain, I used Ziplock sandwich bags to waterproof my phone from the outset. The panniers were fully waterproof, but the handlebar bag was old and I had sprayed it to add some waterproofing. It worked for the most part, but was not perfect. I dressed in damp clothes and loaded the bike. I estimated three top layers today, and needed them all day. I set the sat nav and turned on Strava. I stuck with the Bikemap app, as there were few options around there for it to send me on a mystery tour. And so, for another day, the adventure began.

It was very rural Holland; there was a lot of agriculture, and everything was neat. I could quite believe that this manicured landscape, with grain silos and greenhouses dotting fields crisscrossed by canals, enabled the Netherlands to export half of the food it produced. It was not very "organic-looking"; I guess insects, small mammals and birds might not be the number one priority in the drive for what looked like volume at any cost. I do not know. But if you want food, then the Netherlands is your country.

After a few miles, it was time to hop on one of the many ferries that span the numerous natural rivers in this part of the Netherlands. It was not a problem; I was on the slow road, and taking a ferry was all part of the pace of life I settled into. Once disembarked, I fairly briskly pedalled towards Arnhem, in the east of the country. I was on the north river of the Rhine delta, which at this point had just two tributaries: the Nederrijn, which I was following to the north, and the Waal, the larger tributary about 10 miles south. At Arnhem, I would take a right onto the southbound road and head directly towards St Moritz.

Arnhem appeared on the horizon after only three hours. The weather had turned to light rain, and I headed straight for the centre, with its cobbled streets, tramways and cycle paths, and parked up opposite the most delightful café there could be. It was a stone-finished corner building with mini, semicircular red awnings over the windows, and inside, the subdued yellow lighting bathed the wooden floor, the veneered bar and the walls, while hanging on the ceiling and walls were old musical instruments. The Dutch are renowned for being the tallest people in the world, and the height of their urinals reflected this! It was a perfect place for a coffee and reflection; I would not have been surprised if Edith Piaf were singing at the bar, but she was French, and we were in the Netherlands...

The only other people in the bar were a couple having a lunchtime drink and the bar owner, who was quite young and told me she had owned the place for the past three months. She was enjoying running a bar. Her husband bought it for her; they were married just three months before. Having refreshed myself with a warm coffee, I wished the bar manager well in her new venture, and headed outside and into the light rain. It was steady but warm – but this was not the weather I had imagined for this late-spring trip.

The cycle chain had dried, and I was pleased to have bought extra oil at my stopover in Colchester a couple of days ago. I eased myself back onto the bike and headed back to the Nederrijn. When I used the brakes again for the first time, the pads squeezed away, boiling off the rainwater, and making a squeaking noise.

The sat nav stabilised and guided me towards the Arnhem Bridge, or "John Frost Bridge". John Frost was a commanding British Army officer; the bridge was named in his memory to honour his bravery in attempting to secure it at Arnhem against Nazi forces in the Second World War. It was a metal arch-span bridge that gained infamy for its role in a notorious World War II battle. That was 80 years and three months ago at the time, and there were still shrapnel scars on the older part of the stone foundation pillars on the town's side.

Operation Market Garden was the name given by the forces allied against the Nazis to the strategic offensive in the Netherlands, in an attempt to shorten the war. British General Montgomery hatched the plan: the intention was to establish a bridgehead over the River Rhine, from which a northern front could be opened, to support the western front and pincer the Nazi defences.

From the British perspective, it was a bloody but heroic failure. A small detachment, including John Frost, was supposed to hold the bridge while waiting for support coming swiftly from the main British and Polish army units; these were intended to be parachuted in or flown in on wooden gliders near the bridge, and to form up to support the advance troops. It never worked out like that. The troops landed too far away to provide timely support, and the fog hampered air support from fighter planes. It was a desperate fight, and after ten intense days of battle, the allied troops had to retreat.

Intelligence had assumed there would only be a light defence from the Nazis, but more troops than expected arrived, and reinforcements quickly followed. There were approximately 4,000 combined troop losses, and 6,000 British troops were captured. A further two operations, Pegasus One and Pegasus Two, were carried out to free the troops who had escaped capture and who were being supported by the Dutch underground. And, of course, less than a year later, Hitler surrendered.

Eighty years on from my last visit, I can cycle over the new bridge unimpeded. It is impossible, as I cross, not to imagine the atmosphere of what might have been going on in that conflict, and count my blessings that I never received the call-up to join the Second World War.

Once over the bridge, there was a floodplain, and a forest behind that; the challenge facing those soldiers in those ten long days of battle was immense on both sides. I took one last glance as I cycled past a rusting tank turret mounted on a concrete plinth as a piece of war art.

I had been cycling east, but now I was finally heading south. I needed only to follow the river and the sun all the way to Basel before turning east again. I would be there in a fortnight. It was a pleasant moment to be on the most direct route to St Moritz. Making swift progress on the minor roads, I spotted the confluence of the southern river Waal and my northern Nederrijn. I was now officially on the River Rhine. Soon after that, I passed the most ordinary, almost invisible, weather-beaten sign marking the border between the Netherlands and Germany. Blink, and I would have missed it – and to think that a couple of hours' cycling and 80 years ago, thousands of men were fighting a fierce, ten-day battle for this border.

I was enjoying this sat nav route. The Bikemap app had reconfigured itself, and I was on a direct route to my stopover in a village called Mariembaum, near a small town called Xanten. I had booked a B&B during the lunch break in Arnhem, and the distance was about right for a day. However, not long after that, the sat nav was back on the naughty step. In planning the route, it had factored in a ferry. Unfortunately, I had missed that detail; the sat nav had planned to get me across the Rhine to my stopover in Mariembaum only from the location I had ridden to – but no ferry was running until July. This was a bit of a blow. It was still May, and it was going to be a long wait until July. I cursed the app, but it was I who should have checked more thoroughly; I had assumed the crossing was a bridge.

I decided to head south along the road in hope – but also because there were not many opportunities presenting themselves just then. There was a bridge crossing approximately 10 miles, or an hour, away but it was well off the intended route I would need to head for. I had no option but to pedal on. The rain had stopped, and the roads were quiet. I had plenty of energy. All was going well. Then suddenly, out of nowhere, there was a dull thud, a scuffing noise, and the bike slowed.

I braked and looked around. The carrier, which held my belongings, had broken off the frame and was scraping along the road. One pannier had come off, and the rear light was in two pieces. I feared the worst – but luckily, apart from a couple of bolts missing, there was little damage. The bolts holding the rack onto the frame had come loose; it was poor preparation on my part. I walked down the road to recover the detached pannier. I had expected its plastic mounting clamp to be broken, but it had come away from the mounting point intact. It was a lucky day. The rear light had broken off; the welds had failed. I had to remove and store the light, but I had a spare. The damage was slight. I had been fortunate with this incident; all I needed to do was secure the upper pannier. I had no spare bolts, but did have the long cable tie I picked up in Essex. It saved the day!

The repair was strong, even though the bags were now located slightly forward, and my heels scuffed them as the pedals turned. But I was up and cycling again, and pleased for that. I would need to find a cycle shop tomorrow and do a proper repair, but for now, I could continue. If I prevaricated and had not picked up the tie, would the carrier have failed? Now, there's a thought…

But back to the mundane: I casually glanced at the CGM through the increasingly fogged-up Ziplock bag protecting the phone. I had a slight dip in glucose in the afternoon; this was the long-acting or basal insulin doing its work. One could argue that this reflected too much insulin, and that is fair, but I used basal as my main insulin, so I just needed to top up the carbs. I only needed 10 grams and the glucose trace nudged back into the normal range – something to work on, perhaps.

Getting the correct ratios of basal and bolus insulin was nearly there, but elusive today. I had no hypo symptoms. I was expecting to use small bolus doses when planning the trip, but had to adapt to the best solution for the circumstances, which, at the time, was to rely more heavily on basal insulin to do the work. However, when I reflect on this, I am juggling insulin for five foundations of health, and three, perhaps four, are more nuanced towards basal insulin. Maybe it was the most logical dosage, after all; I had not thought about it in that way until then.

I rolled into Mariembaum and was pleased to find that my accommodation was a whole apartment for the price of a single room. Such luxury on a budget trip cannot be wasted. I cycled to the only supermarket, indeed the only shop, open in the town, and indulged by purchasing an aged entrecôte of beef, some Greek yoghurt, and some bratwurst for my lunch the following day. I enjoyed my steak served on its own, cooked in butter, rare to medium. In 300 grams of steak, about a fifth is protein, or 60 grams – a lot of protein in one go. I had been exercising all day and would need some of that protein for muscle repair, and I am probably still making new muscle.

For me, protein is the trickiest of the macronutrients, as the amount of glucose derived from protein excess can vary depending on the circumstances. So, what to do with this large amount of protein in one go? Fortunately, I was eating well before my 8 pm deadline – that would help. I used three units of rapid insulin plus the usual basal six units of Tresiba. As it turned out, the insulin cover for the protein was an underestimate, and the glucose rose until midnight before slowly correcting towards dawn. It had been a good day overall.

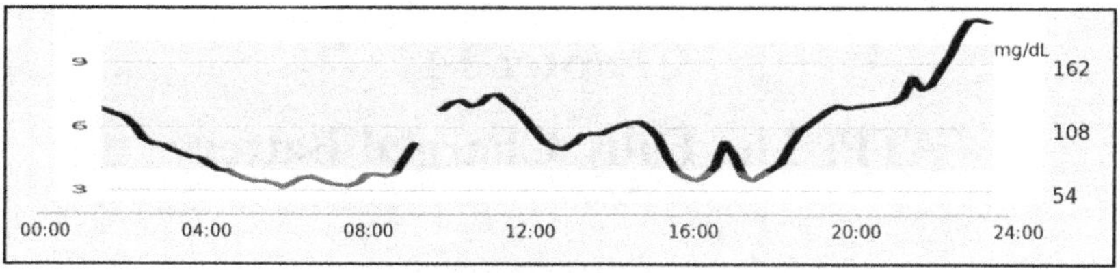

Chapter 14
ATP: The Fully Charged Battery

The cells of most tissues can use various fuels for energy, including glucose, amino acids, fatty acids, and ketone bodies. Most cells, however, have multiple fuel receptors available, so they have the potential to use multiple fuels. A few cell types have no choice at all. For example, red blood cells and certain brain regions can only use glucose. They take in glucose through special channels (GLUT transporters) which allow entry depending on insulin and the cell's energy needs. All cells bathe in the interstitial fluid surrounding them, a fluid rich in various fuels.

The fuel they take in depends on which receptors they open, and that in turn depends on their metabolic state – shaped by diet, activity, circadian rhythm and inflammation. At the interstitial level, the precise amount of fuel is tightly controlled; too much can damage the receptor function, too little may starve the cell of energy. For example, it is a function of insulin to ensure that the interstitial fluid has a glucose concentration ranging from 4–6 mmol/L (72–108 mg/dL).

Fuel provides a cell with the energy required to carry out the biochemical reactions that enable it to perform its functions. In the body, cells store energy from food in phosphate groups attached to adenosine molecules. Adenosine can carry one, two, or three phosphate groups. With one, it is called adenosine monophosphate (AMP), with two, it is adenosine diphosphate (ADP), and with three, it becomes adenosine triphosphate (ATP). ATP is the charged-up form that is full of energy potential.

Cells with plenty of ATP close their fuel supply receptors. Each time ATP loses a phosphate and becomes ADP, energy is released. That energy powers the cell. Most ATP comes from the mitochondria, the cell's tiny energy factories, which produce about 32 ATP per glucose molecule, while the cytoplasm generates 2 ATP through glycolysis. This process runs nonstop throughout life.

Energy in equals energy out, meaning the energy used to produce ATP is the same as the energy released when ATP is used. The fuel from our food is the input; the output is the energy released by breaking phosphate bonds. When ATP becomes ADP, fuel receptors reopen on the cell surface to take in more fuel to support this reaction. Although ATP gives the cell a fixed amount of energy, the fuel used to make it can come from sources with very different energy levels. Fat, for example, yields about twice as much energy as glucose, but ATP itself provides the precise, usable energy the cell needs for its delicate biochemical processes.

You can think of ATP like a mobile phone battery. When the battery level is low, you open the charging port by plugging it into a power supply to recharge. During charging, the battery powers the phone processes. When the battery is full, the supply from the charging port closes. The phone keeps working because the battery holds enough charge from the power supply. The battery's design provides a calibrated, constant power level that is safe for the hardware that operates the phone; it must avoid energy surges that might damage the hardware components. A human cell works the same way. It needs energy to make proteins, replicate, release hormones, and repair damage. Nothing happens without ATP. And once ATP is used, the cell needs to recharge it using fuel from the macronutrients we eat.

Some cells, such as those in the retina, can increase their energy requirements very quickly, up to ten times more in milliseconds. Luckily, ATP can also be recharged very fast. Every cell continually converts ATP into ADP and back again, consuming macronutrients in the process. In fact, we make and use about our entire body weight in ATP each day.

Too much insulin can cause problems because it can upset the balance of the other hormones that normally work with it. The cell will still function, but less smoothly. When this happens, some cells cannot work as well, and disease becomes more likely. Our cells are always ready. The energy system works. The fuel is available. Our job is to make sure the signals match the needs. Use "as much insulin as needed, but as little as possible".

Chapter 15
Metabolism in Action

Human metabolism is a flexible system that adapts constantly to diet, activity and energy needs. Several key pathways in the body work together to supply fuel:

- Glycolysis
- Lactate metabolism
- The Citric Acid (TCA/Krebs) Cycle and Oxidative Phosphorylation
- Gluconeogenesis
- Fat metabolism and ketone production

These pathways ultimately produce ATP, the cell's immediate energy currency, in two main places: the cytoplasm, which handles quick, simple reactions, and the mitochondria, which manage slower but far more efficient ATP production. In type 1 diabetes, these pathways still operate normally, but their coordination depends heavily on insulin.

Glycolysis: The First and Oldest Pathway

Glycolysis is the breakdown of glucose in the cytoplasm. It is one of the most ancient metabolic pathways, developed long before oxygen filled the atmosphere or cells captured mitochondria. Early life relied on glycolysis because it was simple, oxygen-independent, and fast.

Although glycolysis produces only 2 ATP per glucose molecule, it is extremely rapid. This speed compensates for the lower energy yield and is likely one of the reasons the pathway has been preserved for billions of years. It is robust.

Because it works without oxygen and requires no special structures, glycolysis remains the body's "first response" energy system.

- Red blood cells depend on it completely; they have no mitochondria.
- Muscles rely on it for sudden, high-intensity movements such as sprinting and lifting.

When oxygen is available, the end product of glycolysis, called pyruvate, moves into the mitochondria. When oxygen is limited, pyruvate becomes lactate, allowing glycolysis to continue without interruption.

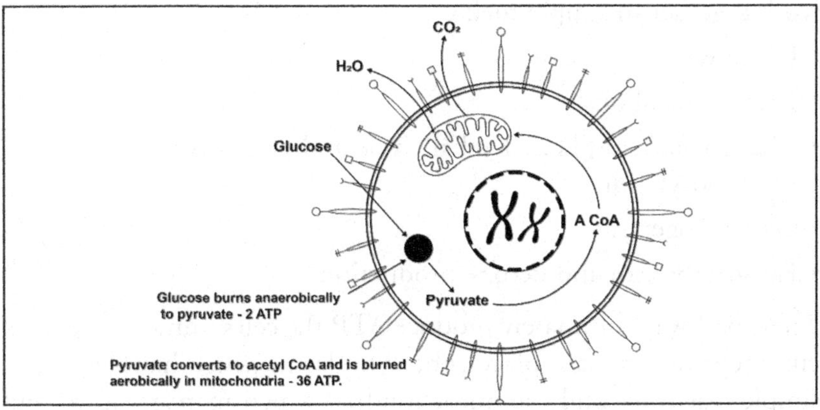

Lactate Metabolism

When oxygen levels fall, pyruvate is converted into lactate (often called lactic acid) in the cytoplasm. Lactate is not a waste product, even though we often think of it as such in sport. In elite short-distance sports, lactate can accumulate to unusually high levels that are rarely seen in everyday life. Lactate has several roles:

- It can be burned directly by the muscle and the heart.
- The liver can convert it back into glucose through the Cori Cycle.

Even with adequate oxygen, some tissues produce lactate as a flexible way of moving energy between cells.

The Citric Acid Cycle and Oxidative Phosphorylation

Most of the body's ATP is produced inside the mitochondria through linked biochemical processes that include the citric acid cycle (also known as the TCA Krebs cycle) and another pathway called oxidative phosphorylation. This system is slower than glycolysis but dramatically more productive in terms of ATP yield.

The Citric Acid Cycle Gateway

Acetyl-CoA is the molecule into which nearly all fuels – glucose, fatty acids, amino acids, and ketones – are converted. It is the gateway into the citric acid cycle.

The citric acid cycle itself produces only a small amount of ATP directly, but generates high-energy electron carriers, nicotinamide adenine dinucleotide (NADH) and flavin adenine dinucleotide ($FADH_2$), that drive oxidative phosphorylation.

NADH and $FADH_2$ feed electrons into the electron transport chain, powering the enzyme ATP synthase, which produces mitochondrial ATP by adding phosphates. Oxygen is required, hence the process is called "oxidative phosphorylation". Oxygen is essential at this step; without it, the system halts and the cell relies on glycolysis, producing lactate instead.

As a result, cells often use both anaerobic and aerobic pathways at the same time, even when oxygen is available: glycolysis for quick ATP production, and the citric acid cycle for slower, more efficient ATP production. During intense exercise, like sprinting, muscles rely mainly on anaerobic ATP production until increased heart rate and breathing restore sufficient oxygen for mitochondria to work – so, pyruvate is converted to lactate.

Under ideal conditions, glucose metabolism combines an initial anaerobic phase with aerobic mitochondrial processing, producing up to 38 ATP per glucose molecule.

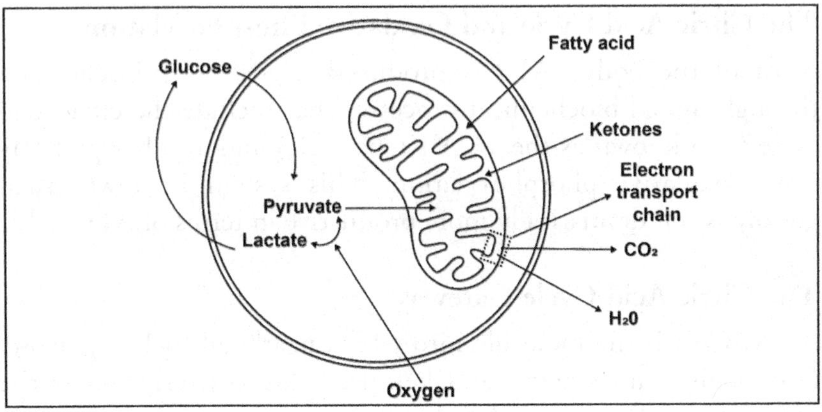

Gluconeogenesis

Gluconeogenesis is the production of glucose from non-carbohydrate sources such as lactate, glycerol and certain amino acids.

It becomes important during:

- Fasting
- Low-carbohydrate intake
- Prolonged activity
- Low-insulin states

This process draws on oxaloacetate, a key intermediate used to support glucose synthesis – one of the molecules within the citric acid cycle. When this molecule is diverted away from the cycle, metabolism shifts towards ketone production, described below. In states of glucose insufficiency, cells ramp up alternative energy production to meet their needs, while glucose is reserved for tissues that depend on it. It is an elegant system.

Fat Metabolism and Ketone Production

When the body needs long-lasting energy – overnight, between meals, during exercise, or during a ketogenic diet – it turns to fat.

Stored fat breaks down into:

- Glycerol, which can form glucose through gluconeogenesis, described above.
- Fatty acids, which undergo a biochemical breakdown called beta-oxidation in mitochondria.

Beta-oxidation produces acetyl-CoA by breaking down fatty acids two carbons at a time. For example, a common fat with 16 carbons undergoes eight cycles to generate acetyl-CoA, which then feeds into the citric acid cycle. Many tissues have receptors on their cell surfaces for fatty acids, just as others have receptors for glucose. These include fatty acid transport and binding proteins. Beta-oxidation makes fat a primary source of sustained ATP production. The acetyl-CoA produced can also be used in the liver to make ketone bodies.

The Liver: Switching to Ketones

During fasting or low-carbohydrate intake, oxaloacetate is diverted towards gluconeogenesis. As a result, the citric acid cycle slows and acetyl-CoA accumulates. Under these conditions, acetyl-CoA from fat burning is used to produce ketone bodies.

Ketone bodies:

- Are water-soluble
- Circulate easily
- Provide efficient mitochondrial fuel
- Reduce the need for glucose

The liver produces three ketones:

- Acetoacetate, used in mitochondria and measured in urine.
- Beta-hydroxybutyrate (BOHB), the most abundant ketone in circulation and the one measured in blood.
- Acetone, a by-product mostly exhaled and measured in breath, which gives the characteristic nail varnish smell in diabetic ketoacidosis (DKA).

The ketones:

- Are transported into cells by monocarboxylate transporter (MCT) proteins, which also transport lactate and pyruvate.
- Are converted from BOHB back into acetyl-CoA in mitochondria.
- Enter the citric acid cycle of target cells and feed into oxidative phosphorylation for ATP production.

Why the Liver Cannot Use the Ketones It Produces

Most tissues can utilise ketone bodies directly, but the liver lacks the enzyme SCOT, which is required to convert ketones back into acetyl-CoA for cellular use.

The absence of this enzyme results in export of excess ketones to tissues that require them, particularly the brain. The brain cannot use fatty acids because medium- to long-chain fatty acids cannot cross the blood-brain barrier in significant quantities.

On a higher-carb diet such as that consumed today, the brain relies on glucose. During low-carb intake, such as a ketogenic diet, glucose is reserved for glucose-dependent tissues, while ketones supply energy within the brain.

Ketone bodies:

- Cross into the brain easily
- Are burned efficiently by neurons
- Stabilise brain energy during low-glucose states

This system allows the brain to remain fully functional when carbohydrate intake is low. Ketosis should not be seen as an emergency state but as a normal, healthy physiological process, partly because ketones act as signalling molecules.

Ketones are not merely passive fuels; they also act as intercellular signals. BOHB, in particular, acts as both fuel and as a signalling molecule, with demonstrated anti-inflammatory effects.

BOHB helps:

- Reduce inflammation
- Regulate immune responses

These effects help explain why ketosis is often experienced as "clear", "steady", and "mentally stable". They also explain the growing interest in ketones beyond fasting and ketogenic diets – particularly in neuroprotection, ageing, and immune modulation.

Ketone Regulation and Transport

Ketone production is tightly regulated:

- Low insulin and high glucagon stimulate fat breakdown and ketogenesis.
- High insulin suppresses fat release and ketone synthesis.

Once in the bloodstream, ketones – mainly in the form of BOHB – are taken up by the heart, muscles and brain, where they are converted back into acetyl-CoA and oxidised via mitochondrial respiration.

In nutritional ketosis, ketone levels rise in a controlled, adaptive manner; and as long as insulin is present, they remain regulated. In people without type 1 diabetes, rising ketone levels trigger endogenous insulin production, which suppresses fat breakdown and limits further ketone production. This is a natural feedback loop.

Ketone levels in blood are typically in the range of 0.5–3.5 mmol/L. In type 1 diabetes, 75% of 150 people surveyed on the website type1keto.com reported levels between 0.5–1.5 mmol/L, although results can vary depending on insulin, diet and individual metabolism. The brain transitions to ketone use, sparing muscle protein and maintaining function. In contrast, DKA occurs when insulin is absent or critically low, leading to uncontrolled ketone production, acidosis, and potential coma.

Summary: Distinct Yet Interconnected Pathways

- Glucose is the only fuel that can be metabolised in the absence of oxygen. It is partially processed in the cytoplasm and converted into lactate or pyruvate to generate energy.
- Glucose (as pyruvate), amino acids, fats and ketone bodies are all metabolised in mitochondria.
- In mitochondria, the citric acid cycle and oxidative phosphorylation work together but are distinct: the citric acid cycle generates electron carriers, while oxidative phosphorylation converts those electrons into ATP.
- The end products of mitochondrial fuel oxidation are water and carbon dioxide, along with ATP as usable energy.
- Ketones are produced by the liver during fasting or carbohydrate restriction.
- Ketones act as both energy substrates and anti-inflammatory signalling molecules.

This interplay between oxidation, mitochondrial function, and ketone production demonstrates the elegance of human metabolism, which continually balances fuel use according to changing physiological demands.

Completing the Loop

Metabolism is a dynamic system that shifts between pathways in response to fuel availability and energy demand. Glycolysis provides rapid, flexible energy, while mitochondrial pathways deliver steady, long-lasting ATP. Gluconeogenesis and ketone production maintain energy stability when glucose is limited, with the liver playing a central regulatory role.

Acetyl-CoA and oxaloacetate sit at the centre of these transitions, helping determine whether the body burns glucose, fat or ketones. In type 1 diabetes, these pathways continue to function normally, but their coordination depends on appropriate insulin availability.

Understanding these processes brings clarity, reduces confusion, and helps support long-term metabolic health.

Chapter 16
Total Miles: 410

Day 6 – Marienbaum to Düsseldorf, 61 miles

"Rivers know this: There is no hurry. We shall get there some day."
– Winnie the Pooh

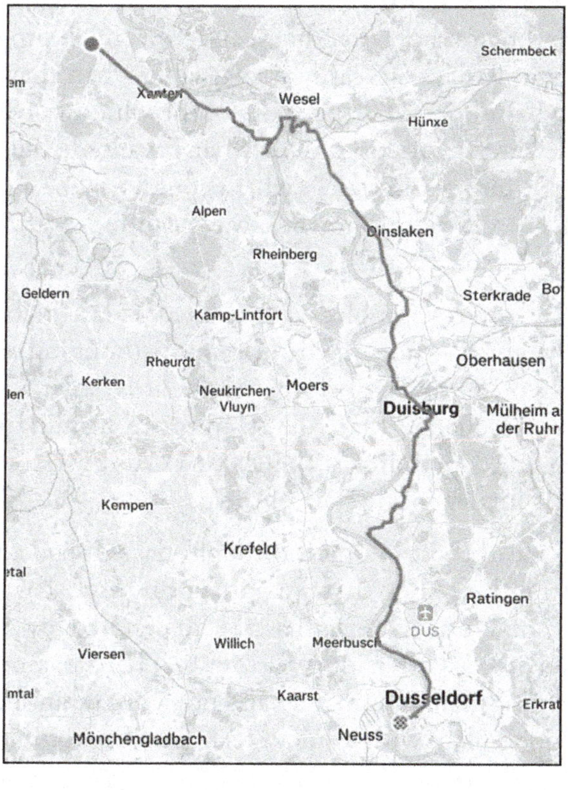

There are moments on some cycle rides when everything just comes together, and the last hour of today's ride turned out to be one of those moments. It was a welcome respite from the often cool, cloudy, and occasionally wet, days that have accompanied me on this trip. And this morning was no different: another three-layer clothing day. Unfortunately, I had forgotten to hang out last night's washing; it was still in the shower tray, thoroughly wet. I had been expecting a soaking, based on the forecast, but things looked slightly more hopeful now.

I wrung out the clothes, turned on the heating, had breakfast, packed up, and then pulled on the still-damp but partially dry gear. My shoes were now close to becoming unusable, and had to be handled with care. I had given up on the idea of dry shoes altogether.

Today's target was Germany's western city of Düsseldorf, but I had not booked anywhere to stay. I always see how things go and then book, depending on how tired I am, and how much progress I have made. Sixty-mile days are easily manageable when they are spread out over daylight hours. I glanced out of the window: overcast skies, drizzle and wind in the trees. Not what I wanted. But the breeze meant the weather was moving, which could only be a good thing. The clouds were heading north; I was heading south. There was room for optimism, at last.

Breakfast was three scrambled eggs cooked in last night's beef fat, and half a yoghurt – not much for a multi-thousand-calorie ride, but I usually prefer fasting before exercise; it is easier. On this trip, I am having to change that rule to improve insulin and glucose management. Adaptability is the key. My AeroPress coffee ritual added a little luxury to the start of the day.

Today was one of those "think it through" days. It had all been a bit frantic getting here, but that was just a mindset. I was not fully settled yet; my food choices had been dictated by last-minute supermarket sweeps after long, wet days. There was not much in Marienbaum: a small supermarket and not a restaurant in sight. Last night had gone okay with a juicy steak, but I overcompensated at breakfast, to get the calories in. Two boiled eggs rather than three scrambled eggs would have been sufficient, but it was at least something fresh, rather than a selection of cured meats. I was skipping fish and fresh meat too often; for the past couple of days, I had been drifting back into student-traveller mode.

I had two coffees, mindful that the combination of protein and caffeine can be tricky for glucose control. I had settled into six units of Tresiba twice a day, which was working for now. I got on with my routine: set up the satnav, clipped on the heart rate monitor, logged breakfast, calibrated the CGM and ketone meters, filled the water bottles, and struggled into my damp gear.

It was a cool morning, and I was cold from the start – but at least the bike was dry. My host had kindly let me store it in their shed, neatly lined up alongside the family's own bikes. I love seeing active families, kids gaining independence through cycling. Having a bike as a child meant freedom for me; we would cycle to the river, to fields, to nowhere in particular. At primary school, every Monday, we were told to write about our weekends – probably a subtle way for teachers to check on home life. I often wrote about my bike. I still have one of those early essays, written in the tall, thin pencil script of an eight-year-old:

"On Tuesday night, Geoffrey and I played on our bikes. Mine was the fastest. It was a sports bike, and it was red and gold. The tyres were half black and half white. Last Saturday, I cleaned it with oil. I oiled the chain and the wheels and tightened all of the screws so it would go faster. It was called Sports. Geoffrey's bike was blue, with black tyres, and called a James Sprite. It had smaller wheels and different brakes. We played until it got dark, then had to fetch Peter from David's house. On the way back, Geoffrey went in. Peter and I put our bikes away and went to watch television. The next night, we played on our bikes and then went to my dad's smallholding. We played with my toy rifle, threw stones in the river, and climbed a pile of straw, where we watched the pigs eating. Then we played in an empty pig pen before heading home for tea."

That appears to be an active life to me – plenty of references to bikes. And, oh my goodness, how competitive I was!

After reminiscing, it was time to load up. I needed to make an early stop in Xanten, a few miles away, to get bolts for a bike repair; that is partly why I had taken an extra unit of insulin – I knew I would have a slow start today, and without activity, my glucose would likely rise. I breezed into Xanten in half an hour, only to find all the cycle shops were closed for another hour – it was Saturday, after all. Even at 9 am, the market stalls in the town square were still setting up. I was not going to hang around in the grey and cold, so I decided to find somewhere in Duisburg instead. I estimated it was 20 miles away, but the route turned out to be twice that. I had not checked accurately, and the psychological impact of realising I had another unexpected 25 miles to go was demoralising.

The steady passage of clouds overhead meant a headwind, but the roads were flat. The lush countryside slipped by on minor roads with few vehicles. The Rhine was fast flowing, and water had already breached the flood plains and woodland areas. Clearly, the swollen river reflected the unseasonal heavy rainfall the region had endured recently. There was still a cycle path in this part, but it was uneven, and the ride was not the smoothest. Tree roots had lifted the tarmac, and my tyres occasionally slid on them, making it difficult not to fall off. At junctions, there were kerbs with one-inch lips – tiny, but jarring when my bike's heavy back end crashed. I hoped the cable tie holding things together would last a bit longer. It was becoming a worry. I was increasingly aware of how thin the cycle frame was; it was certainly not built for this relentless punishment.

I was now a third of the way to St. Moritz, feeling optimistic, and with a newfound respect for my bike. But on the approach to Duisburg, there were many junctions and transitions from one side of the road to the other, slowing progress and sapping the enjoyment. Bikemap was not helping either; it directed me to another ferry that did not exist, adding an unnecessary loop. I found myself shouting at my phone. When I startled birds from the trees,

I realised how cross I was. Time for a bit of calm. Switching to Google Maps was the only solution, if only to spite Bikemap.

I continued on to Duisburg, a major steel town with the largest port on the Rhine, dominated by gigantic steelworks, ducts, chimneys, and railways feeding coal into power stations. Many plants were being decommissioned, but it was still a true testament to past industrial confidence and engineering. The tall chimneys disappearing into the misty sky made for an impressive sight.

Priority number one was bike repairs. The panniers were catching my heel, and the rhythmic scrape had become annoying. The cycle shop was a giant warehouse of perhaps a thousand cycles, mostly e-bikes priced at approximately €5,000 each. The mechanic replaced the bolts, gave me spares, added four extra spare cable ties, and refused payment.

E-bikes seem to be the thing right now. My own rough estimation of the ratio of e-bikes to non-e-bikes on this trip, based on nothing but my own lazy observation, was that around a third were e-bikes. They are convenient for those who want to extend their range and get from A to B more quickly than pedal power alone allows. I met a cyclist in Harwich who intended to cover 200 km per day on his top-of-the-range, very heavy-looking, dual-battery bike. It did look bombproof, and he told me he had deregulated the motor. He was hoping to reach the Czech Republic in six days. I am covering that same distance in double the time.

One massive advantage of an e-bike is on hills. With e-bikes limited to 15 mph, I can easily keep up on the flat with my human power. Of course, I have the secret weapon: a keto fuel additive, which seems to give me boundless energy! But on the way out of Duisburg, on a wide cycle track, I overtook a bloke about my age, dressed casually and riding an e-bike in the same casual, unrushed manner. He was not in a hurry. He was well behind me when a steady but sustained incline required me to shift into the easiest possible gear and stand on the pedals to put in the effort. He bowled by without so much as a sweat and left me for dust.

Some people feel that an e-bike is somehow cheating. I would not have wanted one on this trip, as I have an agenda that rules out motor assistance. However, people have a wide range of ailments and needs. If it means they can extend their cycling life, that reduced-effort pedalling helps them explore new areas or simply get to work and keep in shape at the same time, then why not? If, horror of horrors, my good health fails me, I might well repeat this trip on an e-bike.

Lunch consisted of the remaining cheese, four chipolata bratwurst and two hard-boiled eggs, eaten on a bench in a large, paved concourse outside the station and next to the cycle shop. I felt hungry and wanted to split up my protein a bit. Too much in the evening risked high blood glucose; my new strategy was breakfast, then get three-quarters of the ride done, take some protein, and have an end-of-ride main meal.

I was surprised to find I had already covered 40 miles today, and that was a boost, but I felt tired and slightly achy, a bit like a cold was coming on. I had 20 miles to go and was digging in to get to the end of the day. I set up Google Maps, booked a stay, and made my way to Düsseldorf.

I did not feel in tip-top condition as the day progressed. I had not slept all that well for a few days, being excited to get going, micromanaging insulin and overcorrecting, keen to get the numbers right. And doing last-minute accommodation and meal planning, and generally getting dragged down by the weather. All mindset issues.

With glucose hovering around 8 mmol/L (144 mg/dL) and feeling less than 100%, I concluded it was due to the poor sleep. An infection would have sent the glucose higher. Mostly, I find that infection causes insulin resistance, so insulin injections become far less effective. When I had COVID-19, even though it was very mild, the first indications were an uptick in glucose, followed by a low-teen glucose for three days despite a triple dose of insulin. When the COVID infection receded, the glucose level came down. The trick, then, was to be aware of the possibility of too much insulin suddenly becoming responsive and causing a hypo. In that case, glucose tablets would be needed in large quantities. People without type 1 diabetes do not realise they, too, are insulin resistant at times – but they can make their own insulin. We could teach non–type 1s a lot about insulin.

After 10 miles or so, the wind had dropped and the sun was out. For the last hour of riding, it stayed out. It was the first proper sunny evening, and the wind was warm. I had been cold and bedraggled, tired and achy today, so the sun and warmth perked me up a bit. Added to this was the lovely, direct, quiet, and well-signposted ride to my accommodation for the night. There was still a headwind ride to dig into, but the sun made it very pleasant. I was able to take off my waterproof jacket and absorb the warmth. It made such a difference to the ride, and I felt that the weather I had imagined when I planned this trip had finally arrived. Now I could be warm all night and have warm, dry clothes to start the day. It is the small things that make the difference. It is amazing how mindset impacts activity.

I had sourced a shop just before arriving at the hotel, and used some of my purchases as a snack before my intended evening meal. It consisted of a small goat's cheese, 100 g of – unbeknownst to me – uncooked bratwurst (which I had to eat raw), one remaining egg, and a pot of Greek yoghurt. I also snuck in a small glass of prosecco, to kick back and contemplate the day. I calculated two units for this meal and opted for the now-usual six units of Tresiba at night. I had considered five units for a few days, but six had become the optimal number. Everything remained well controlled with respect to glucose levels.

After the snack, I did not feel hungry, which was fortunate, because I ended up falling asleep for a couple of hours. Upon waking, it was already too late to eat; I typically aim to have my last meal by 8 pm or earlier.

My insulin requirements had dropped from a total daily dose in the mid-twenties to a consistent fifteen units a day – about eight units below my normal daily dose. Life adapts to prevailing circumstances, and so does the need for insulin. I reflected that this recent reduction in insulin had nothing to do with food but everything to do with physical activity, being outdoors and relaxing from the daily grind. Paying attention to the five foundations of health has reduced my total daily insulin requirement by at least six units.

The standard advice is to focus primarily on food, and insulin volumes are set by the amount of food. It is all about managing glucose levels. These days, I have completely flipped that approach. Understanding the core issue of type 1 diabetes – the lack of insulin – requires a deep dive into the subject. High glucose is simply a symptom of type 1 diabetes, while the cause is insulin deficiency. It is not as difficult as it sounds; I have not had to change much – just fine-tuning habits like sleep preparation and the timing of food and exercise. It is not an imposition. I see the improved results, and that is the motivating factor. I feel so much healthier now, and this trip is a way of celebrating my good fortune in discovering the ketogenic diet, purely by accident. I look forward to exploring the foundations of health in greater depth as I continue on this journey.

A decade ago, on the North Sea Cycle Route, I used to ache. Back then, high glucose and higher insulin doses, I now know, were a recipe for inflammation, and with additional exercise, that combination made my joints ache. On that sugar-fuelled trip, I ached most mornings. Nowadays, every morning I wake up refreshed and free of muscular or joint aches.

Düsseldorf was looking good. It was Saturday night. It is an attractive university town and was vibrant that night. Its nightlife seems to revolve around party boats. Boats full of around 150 party-dressed people, getting drunk and singing out loud to mostly German pop songs and oompah band music, were quite a spectacle.

Having popped out for the evening to look around, I took in a fantastic orange sunset over the river. It was the first visible sunset of the trip, but well worth the wait. But there was no peace; three party boats were chugging along the wide river in full, thudding loudspeaker mode, and festooned with disco lights. The upper decks were heaving with revellers, glasses in hand, as they plied the waters just south of the city. At every bridge, a boat did a pirouette, much to the pleasure of the cheering crowd; it seemed to lean a bit, but never toppled over. All had a good time, no doubt. It was indeed a sight not to forget. A smaller boat, lurking under a bridge about a mile out of town, was lit up in lurid blue and red, on the far bank. It was hardly moving and was putting out a lot of smoke, and a throbbing beat. I can only assume they were hotboxing weed in that one, and occasionally had to open the door for air. In any other town, you would have rung the fire brigade.

I wandered back to my hotel after sunset, feeling warm and relaxed, and went to sleep – and sleep I really did!

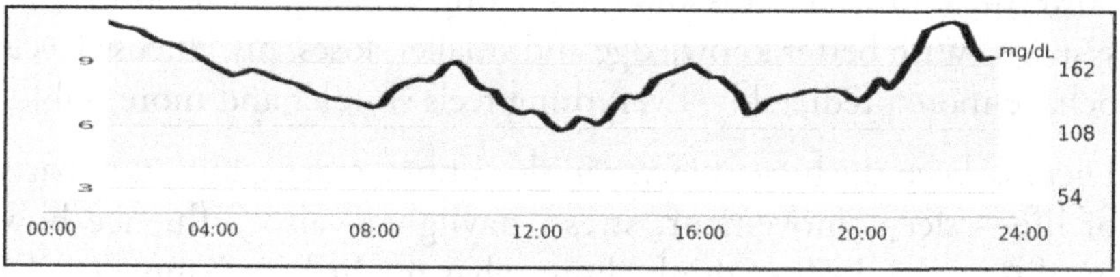

Chapter 17
Insulin: Hormone Replacement Therapy

When I reflect on my first 20 years with type 1 diabetes, I can see how much I did not understand. My glucose control was only modest, and I relied on far more insulin than I really needed. At the time, taking more insulin seemed logical. Now, I realise how powerful a hormone it is and how strongly it shapes the body's fuel systems. With better knowledge and smaller doses, my glucose levels behave more predictably. Everything feels simpler and more stable.

Diet has been the biggest factor in this improvement, but other parts of life – sleep, movement, stress, daylight – also influence how insulin works. I often think about what might have happened if I had learned these principles earlier. I cannot change the past, but I can make better choices for the years ahead. A long, healthy lifespan is preferable to a long decline. Understanding insulin gives me a better chance of achieving that.

Metabolism may seem complex, but once you see how insulin acts as the main switch, the pathways become much easier to understand. Two questions guide everything:

- How does insulin shape our metabolic pathways?
- And how do our daily choices shape insulin?

Before Insulin

Before insulin's discovery, type 1 diabetes was a fatal disease. Children became thinner each day, even under strict starvation diets designed only to delay the inevitable rise of glucose. The hope was that removing carbohydrates and suppressing glucagon (which raises glucose) might slow the progression of the condition. Adults were sometimes given meat and whiskey, since alcohol lowers glucagon and briefly stops glucose from rising. But nothing could replace insulin, and life expectancy was short. Without insulin it was a hopeless situation.

Scientists had already suspected that the pancreas produced something essential. In 1889, using animals was a normal part of medical research. Joseph von Mering and Oskar Minkowski removed a dog's pancreas and watched it develop type 1 diabetes almost immediately. That experiment confirmed the pancreas's role. Researchers believed the islets of Langerhans produced a chemical that controlled blood sugar. They called this substance "insulin", from the Latin *insula*, meaning "island".

The Discovery That Changed Everything

For decades, researchers tried to extract insulin, but digestive enzymes always destroyed it. Frederick Banting solved this by tying off the pancreatic ducts, so the digestive part of the gland shrank while the islets remained. It was a simple idea, but it overcame the main barrier that had stopped others researching the problem.

Banting worked in a small lab with ten dogs, alongside Charles Best, a medical student. The early experiments were rough: dogs died, extracts varied from day to day, and equipment often failed. Some days they felt close to success; other days they felt they were starting over. Everything changed when biochemist James Collip joined the team. Collip had the chemical expertise to purify the extract into a form safe enough for humans – without him, insulin might never have progressed beyond the lab.

They eventually showed that their insulin could reduce blood glucose. A research dog called Marjorie, who had insulin-dependent diabetes induced by surgical removal of her pancreas, received the first dose of insulin on July 30, 1921. She lived for 70 days more. Unfortunately, severe injection-site infections caused by impurities in the insulin meant she had to be put to sleep. Even so, it was a significant breakthrough.

Just a few months later, in January 1922, the team treated a boy, 14-year-old Leonard Thompson. The first dose was too impure and caused an adverse reaction. The second, purified by Collip, worked. Leonard's blood glucose fell, his colour returned, and he began to regain strength. Doctors described this as "a resurrection". The family called it a miracle. News spread quickly, and pharmaceutical company Eli Lilly helped scale production, allowing insulin to reach thousands more people. Early insulins still had problems – short duration, abscesses, unpredictable potency – but compared to certain death, they were miraculous.

To standardise insulin potency and make injections more accurate, a "unit" of insulin was proposed. It was defined in a crude way: the amount needed to lower a 2 kg fasting rabbit's blood sugar to the point of convulsions within three hours. It seems shocking now, but it was the only reliable method at the time. Nowadays, of course, we spare the bunnies and use other measures to standardise insulin potency. A British scientist called Dorothy Crowfoot Hodgkin published the first accurate three-dimensional structure of insulin using a new technique of X-ray crystallography. One unit is now defined as 34.7 nanograms of pure crystalline insulin.

Banting and Macleod received the Nobel Prize in 1923. Banting shared his prize money with Best, and Macleod shared his with Collip. Best was retrospectively awarded the Nobel Prize as recognition of his efforts. Banting sold the insulin patent for one dollar, saying, "Insulin belongs to the world, not to me." Ironically, the insulin that Banting believed should remain accessible has become a multi-billion-dollar industry.

Today, a small number of large pharmaceutical companies control most of the world's insulin supply – from manufacturing to patent protection. Prices remain high despite insulin being essential for life. The irony is hard to ignore: a lifesaving discovery meant for everyone is now unaffordable for some who depend on it.

Progress and Tools

Researchers later discovered that adding zinc or protamine (a protein) could extend the duration of injected insulin. Protamine was originally isolated from fish sperm and was later used clinically to reverse anticoagulants such as heparin. When added to insulin, it enabled the first long-acting insulins to be produced. Premixed insulins followed, containing a mixture of short- and long-acting insulins.

Glucose testing also evolved. Glucose was initially measured using chemicals on urine, giving only a rough estimate of blood glucose. This method was inherently delayed, often by an hour or two, as glucose first had to pass from the bloodstream to the kidneys before appearing in urine. Can you imagine having to add sodium citrate and sodium carbonate to a urine sample, then slowly add blue copper sulphate and wait to see whether it turned into red cuprous oxide precipitate in response to glucose? How lucky we are today to have constant glucose readings through our fire-and-forget continuous glucose meters.

Richard Bernstein, a medical equipment engineer with type 1 diabetes, played a major role in our modern understanding of it. He obtained one of the first home glucose meters, and recorded and compared every glucose reading with what he ate. This showed a clear link between carbohydrates and high blood glucose. Doctors in the pre-insulin era had noticed this, but Bernstein quantified it and applied it to modern insulin therapy. He was one of the earliest proponents of the very low-carbohydrate diet in the insulin era, but was largely ignored by the medical profession. As a result, he retrained as a doctor and wrote the iconic book Dr Bernstein's Diabetes Solution, which has been the go-to resource for type 1s seeking an alternative to standard care for the past 40 years.

Insulin pens were introduced in the 1980s, improving ease and accuracy of dosing. Later, more rapid-acting insulin analogues became available. Combining this with long-acting basal insulin led to the basal-bolus approach that remains the foundation of treatment today. Pumps and closed-loop systems build on the same principle: stable background insulin with flexible mealtime dosing.

How Insulin Is Made and Stored

Insulin is a peptide (protein) hormone, made from 51 amino acids arranged in two chains. In someone without type 1 diabetes, when blood glucose rises above about 5.6 mmol/L (100 mg/dL), pancreatic beta cells increase insulin production. Insulin is initially synthesised in the beta cells as proinsulin, which contains the A-chain, B-chain, and a peptide called Connecting peptide (C-peptide), which joins the A and B chains together. Before release, C-peptide is removed. Inside beta cells, six insulin molecules are electrostatically held around a zinc atom to form a structure called a hexamer (hex = 6).

These hexamers are stored in granules along with C-peptide and another hormone called amylin (see next chapter for details). Each granule contains hundreds of thousands of insulin molecules. When glucose stimulates insulin secretion, hexamers enter the bloodstream and fall apart into single, active molecules due to the higher acidity of blood compared to the granules. C-peptide may help reduce oxidative stress and discourage arterial plaque formation.

Some evidence suggests insulin may also be produced in the brain, though this remains under study. It is known, however, that insulin crosses the blood-brain barrier and plays a role in brain metabolism. Beta cells can multiply when needed, such as during pregnancy or in response to insulin resistance. Some reports suggest that beta cells can recover, at least in the early stages of type 1 diabetes, but ultimately they may fail as the immune system attacks them.

How Insulin Works in the Body

Insulin is often described as the hormone that lowers blood sugar – and this is important to keep both blood glucose and the interstitial glucose surrounding cells at levels optimal for cell function. However, its role is much broader. Insulin acts as a master switch that decides whether the body stores energy or releases it. Every major fuel pathway responds to insulin. Insulin is essentially an anabolic – or growth-promoting – hormone.

Insulin: Those Without Type 1 Diabetes vs T1s

Healthy people release insulin in two phases. The first phase response is immediate upon sensing raised glucose, lasting about 10 minutes, and involves releasing the stored insulin hexamers from the granules. The second phase response is slower, lasting several hours, and involves insulin being synthesised by beta cells on demand. Regarding macronutrients, glucose triggers the strongest response; fat and protein also stimulate insulin, but more slowly and over a longer period. A standard 75-gram glucose load used in clinical investigation can raise insulin tenfold within minutes. Protein and fat raise insulin twofold but take longer to achieve the effect.

Insulin injected into the skin has an onset of action from around 15 minutes and lasts up to 33 hours, depending on the type of insulin used. Even the fastest-acting insulins remain in the circulation for up to 5 hours, irrespective of glucose levels. Compare this to the 10 minutes or so of insulin duration in those without type 1 diabetes. It is this quality of short-acting artificial insulin that presents the challenge; it simply is too slow to react and hangs around for far too long. But right now, it is the best we have, and it is lifesaving. We should celebrate it and learn to work with it as best we can.

Glucose Pathways

Insulin moves GLUT4 transporters to the cell surface in muscle, heart and fat, increasing glucose uptake by more than thirty-fold to help normalise blood glucose. Once inside the cell, glucose is bound together as glycogen under the action of insulin, which, of course, prevents glycogen breakdown. Glycogen is preserved for sudden, intense activity but can be recruited for everyday use should the need for glucose arise.

In the liver, insulin shuts down glucose production by blocking enzymes that raise blood sugar. It also suppresses hormones that increase glucose, including glucagon and adrenaline.

Fat and Ketones

Insulin helps decide whether the body stores fat or burns it. It does this through its effect on two important enzymes. The first is lipoprotein lipase (LPL). This enzyme sits on the walls of small blood vessels and breaks down fat carried in the bloodstream. In fat tissue, insulin helps LPL move this fat into fat cells, where it can be stored. And the second is hormone-sensitive lipase (HSL). This enzyme works inside fat cells. Its job is to break down stored fat so it can be released and used for energy. Low levels of insulin enable HSL to function.

So, when insulin levels are high, fat is stored through its action of LPL. This means insulin pushes the body towards fat storage. It helps move fat into fat cells and slows the breakdown of fat that is already there. When insulin levels are low, the balance changes. HSL becomes more active, so stored fat is broken down and released into the bloodstream as fatty acids. These can then be burned for energy. The liver also turns some of these fatty acids into ketones, which can be used as fuel by the brain and many other tissues.

This is why insulin is often called a fat-storing hormone. It does not just lower glucose – it also tells the body to store fuel and makes it harder to use stored fat.

Protein and Muscle

Insulin supports protein synthesis by facilitating the entry of amino acids into cells. It reduces muscle breakdown. Without insulin, muscle wasting increases.

Electrolytes

Insulin moves potassium into cells. It also increases sodium retention in the kidneys, which can raise blood pressure by increasing water retention. With a well-managed insulin strategy, blood pressure is usually better controlled. Magnesium and phosphate, which are important for bone health, are similarly affected.

Circulation and Inflammation

At normal levels, insulin helps blood vessels relax by increasing nitric oxide. It also reduces oxidative stress. These benefits decline when insulin is chronically high. Insulin also increases a growth factor called VEGF, which can worsen diabetic eye disease by promoting the formation of new blood vessels (see Chapter 21).

The Brain

Insulin influences appetite, memory, mood and cognitive clarity. Its transport into the brain is reduced in states of long-term high insulin, such as diabetes. Lower insulin levels increase ketone production, which can improve mental clarity, reduce migraines and stabilise mood. Ketogenic diets are increasingly being used for mental health and have shown promise in bipolar disorder, depression and migraine.

How Insulin Is Cleared

Natural insulin lasts only minutes; the liver removes most of it, the kidneys clear the rest. Injected insulin is cleared mainly by the kidneys. After insulin binds its receptor, it enters the cell and is degraded by the insulin-degrading enzyme (IDE).

Genetic Variants

Rare insulin variants such as Chicago, Los Angeles and Wakayama bind poorly to insulin receptors. These are naturally occurring insulins with genetically altered amino acid sequences that change their shape and reduce their ability to be recognised by insulin receptors. These conditions can resemble type 2 diabetes, but the issue lies with the glucose transport response, not with a lack of insulin.

Moving Forward with Understanding

Insulin affects every major system in the body. It shapes glucose, fat, protein, electrolytes, blood flow, and brain function. When we understand how insulin works, type 1 diabetes becomes far more predictable. Instead of fighting chaos, we begin to work with the body's design.

Using insulin with intention brings clarity and stability. It does not remove the condition, but it provides a steadier path forward.

Chapter 18
Total Miles: 475

Day 7 – Dusseldorf to Unkel, 65 miles

"The doctor of the future will give no medicine, but will instruct his patients in care of the human frame, in diet, and in the cause and prevention of disease."
– Thomas Edison

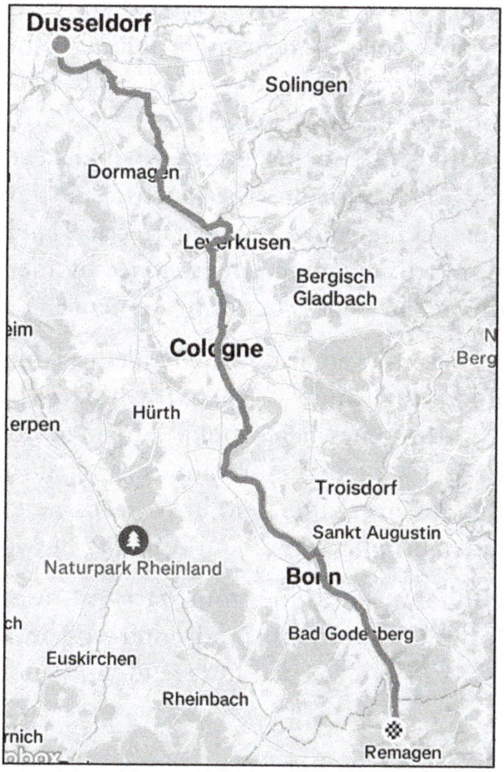

What a difference a good night's sleep makes. I woke late, at 07:30am, to sunshine and a sense of being refreshed. I brewed a coffee on the small terrace outside my room and sat looking out towards the top of a Rhine bridge and a handful of houses nestled among the trees. Brewing coffee on my camping stove has become part of the ritual; steam rising from the pot is always inviting. The joy of my setup is its versatility: coffee anytime, anywhere – often with magnificent views.

Breakfast was the usual continental spread of cured meats and cheeses, but with the welcome addition of fresh salmon. Some real, fresh food felt like a treat. Continental breakfasts tend to be carbohydrate-heavy – muesli, cereals, bread, fruit, fruit juice – but I can usually assemble a keto-friendly plate, even if it leans towards the processed. Beside the salmon sat a scrambled-egg smiley face, with cucumber slices for eyes and cherry tomatoes for pupils. It was amusing and oddly uplifting. A touch of imagination in food presentation can bring joy at any age.

I settled on my now well-tested six units of long-acting Tresiba, and pondered the rapid-acting insulin. Two units felt right for the protein, the coffee and a tiny dawn effect. I was starting to trust the rapid insulin again, since my insulin sensitivity had stabilised. I was still attempting to smooth out the glucose. However, that extra insulin in the morning needed a hypo correction later – I overdid it a bit. I cursed myself: too much interference by me, and too little attention to my insulin sensitivity improvement.

A glance at the map showed just over 60 miles to Unkel, a town that sits on the bank of the Rhine – a place I had never heard of. It was a Sunday, so I hoped somewhere would be open for food. I expected to pass through Cologne before lunch and skirt Bonn mid-afternoon. Both are great cities, and it was a shame to pass through so fleetingly, but this journey is about reaching St Moritz on time.

Today's route follows the Rhine from start to finish. I am leaving the Lower Rhine (Niederrhein) and entering the Middle Rhine (Mittel Rhein), a region steeped in legend, and adored by writers such as Goethe and Lord Byron. Artists like Turner were captivated by its landscapes, as were winemakers. This is the "Romantic Rhine", where the steepening riverbanks give way to a 70 km stretch of valleys carved by powerful water and lined with more than sixty castles. The area has UNESCO World Heritage status. Vineyard after vineyard covers the slopes; Riesling dominates here, with red varieties becoming more common further south. For the remainder of my ride through Germany, I would rarely be far from a vineyard.

One reliable feature of this leg of the trip is that, until Basel, I would be heading almost due south. The sun was my compass: left in the morning, in front during the day, and drifting right as evening approaches. The Earth spins on, indifferent to our concerns; we merely interpret that rotation as the sun's movement from east to west.

Over the past seven days, my insulin-optimised strategy has worked well, and as I move into Day Eight, I feel well-balanced. It is a profound shift in approach. The key is to integrate insulin management seamlessly into life rather than constantly planning around it. Before I optimised insulin, everything revolved around preparation, pre-planning, planning and post-planning: glucose checks, carb calculations, constant adjustments. Now, I glance at my CGM only occasionally, and adjust diet or insulin as needed. Today I powered on, at times forgetting the physical effort of turning the pedals. My fitness has finally caught up with the challenge.

As I cycled, I reflected again on how the body's regulatory systems are analogous to the weather – both are dynamic, ever-changing balances of multiple forces. Atmospheric conditions shape the weather. In the same way, a complex interplay of hormones shapes blood glucose. At that exact moment, on a cycle path south of Cologne, I was experiencing weather that was a balance of millions of tiny atmospheric variables aligning, and at that exact same time, millions of biochemical reactions were adjusting my metabolism. A fraction of a second later, one variable would shift, then another, until the equilibrium shifted again, producing a new balance – and on and on.

Living with type 1 diabetes means constantly adapting insulin in sympathy with the metabolism, much as we adapt to shifting weather on a long ride by adjusting our clothing to suit. My glucose is influenced by countless factors, not just carbohydrates. The lifestyle habits of metabolically healthy people offer clues: stay active, exercise regularly, maintain a normal weight and low blood pressure, incorporate fasting, avoid overeating and ultra-processed foods, spend time in pleasant environments, and cultivate supportive social circles.

For me, the strategy is clear: keep insulin "as much as necessary but as little as possible" – it simplifies everything. Lower insulin levels mean more time in range and less cognitive burden. Our bodies are ecosystems responding to the environments we create. If we provide the right conditions, we give ourselves the best chance of thriving. That is why I try to keep insulin low; it is entirely achievable once you understand it. Low insulin is the natural state in a healthy human; why not try to mimic it?

I switched on the satnav to guide me to Cologne. Once I had escaped the suburbs of Düsseldorf, the riding became smooth and easy. Leaving the suburban maze, I reached my happy place: open countryside. It felt freeing. The route was straightforward, and I let my mind wander. I avoided headphones; I preferred to be alone with my thoughts while cycling, and podcasts were too distracting. Music might have been nice, especially in the built-up areas, but I wanted to be fully aware of the traffic. So, I travelled inside my own head – possibly the most hazardous place of the entire trip.

It was a beautiful day. A scattering of white cumulus clouds puffed across the sky. We were likely in a gap between fronts – the brief calm that follows a warm front before a cold one catches up. I suspected another system was building. I pictured the swirling cloud masses on satellite images; I was somewhere beneath them. Warm breezes blew from all directions. I had hoped for a stable high-pressure system all week, but it had never arrived. With clouds thickening lower in the western sky, another front seemed imminent. Fronts usually mean rain. I pressed on while the sun still shone.

I was making good progress, feeling fit, and enjoying the ride. The hills were beginning to rise gently but the morning remained mostly flat, with long stretches of agricultural land and woodland. The Rhine was flowing faster now, and I had heard that some areas were flooding – it was no surprise, given the weather I had endured downstream. It all added to the sense of adventure. I never truly knew what weather I would meet next and by lunchtime, I only ever had a vague idea where I would end up sleeping each night. I hoped for some camping if the conditions improved, but the trip was busier than expected – and I needed time each evening to write my diary and record the details.

I reached the outskirts of Cologne only after cycling past a massive Ford factory – two miles long from end to end – which was silent on a Sunday morning. A car plant had stood here since 1931, producing some of Ford's best-known cars: the Capri, the Fiesta, and the first petrol Puma. Now, the site has been converted to electric vehicle production. I pedalled on toward the city. Cologne is lovely, especially on a Sunday when the sun is out.

I stopped on the waterfront by the city-centre bridge, a huge double-arched structure humming with the life of the tiny-looking people crossing it, emphasising its size. I had a view of the cathedral from where I was – one of Europe's finest twin-spired structures. A beer festival lined the waterside, with around fifty stalls offering craft beers. Germany, sunshine, exercise and cold beer… the temptation was strong. But I had a mission to stick to: St Moritz on an insulin-optimised diet.

I rummaged in my pannier for my coffee kit. I love coffee far too much, really, but I limit it to mornings only – two or three cups max. More than that, and my glucose climbs. Caffeine is a stimulant; it triggers hormones like adrenaline, which in turn raise glucose. I can increase by around 2 mmol/L (36 mg/dL) with black coffee alone. I sat between two closed ticket booths, leaning on the railing by the riverbank, watching the world drift by, and reflecting on how fortunate I was to have discovered caffeine's subtle effect on my blood sugar. In the old days of pure carb counting, that subtlety would have been masked by the noise of carbs and large insulin doses. When I turned off the metabolic chainsaw, I could finally concentrate on the small details that make all the difference.

Two impossibly long river cruisers pulled into the jetty, ready to disgorge tourists who would soon be weaving through the beer and frankfurter stands. I packed up, growing cold in the bridge's shadow, and set off once more. Onwards, through lush pastures and fields along the Rhine, towards the tidy ancient city of Bonn, with a quick stopover to refuel. Skirting Bonn, I realised no shops were open. Thankfully, I had had a big breakfast, so I could opt for a delayed meal – but I was aware of the need to get some calories in.

I checked my Cronometer food app. I have been logging everything each day, recording weights where possible, and using packaging information for the rest. After a week, I have been consuming just under 3,000 calories per day. I had estimated that six hours of cycling, combined with the rest of the day being relatively sedentary (aside from a bit of walking), meant I would need closer to 4,000 calories to maintain energy balance. Of course, I know not all calories are equal in metabolic terms, but when it comes to the sheer physics of moving 100 kg of cycle, kit and rider against friction, wind resistance and gravity, calories are calories. Physics does not care where they come from. Biology, however, does, and that is why I am paying attention to the type of calories I consume.

In the end, this becomes a mathematical calculation: 4,000 calories out, 3,000 in over a planned 18 days; that is an 18,000-calorie deficit. It does not matter that fat has more calories than carbs, I still need to find that number of calories from somewhere.

This is where the ketogenic diet truly shines: I can make up the difference by eating more to maintain my body weight or, if I prefer, I can draw from my own fat stores. With around 120,000 calories in stored body fat, equivalent to 17% of my 78 kg weight, I could lose 2 kg. That 2 kg of fat equals 18,000 calories, and I could still function perfectly well. I would not notice it in terms of tiredness – after all, that is what fat is stored for: to be used for a "rainy day".

Ironically, today was the first day it had not rained, but you get the point.

From the previous chapter, we will remember that insulin activates an enzyme called lipoprotein lipase (LPL), whose action is essentially to move fat into storage. It also inhibits the counter-enzyme hormone-sensitive lipase (HSL), which prevents fat breakdown.

For me, fasted sport is better. I do not think we were designed to eat when exercising. Humans can be lazy by nature. I'd wager that our ancestors would only get off their butts if there were an advantage to it; a human with a fresh animal carcass in the yard would be unlikely to go for a run for pleasure. They would need to be hungry first. They would need an incentive. And with no freezers around, there would be little point in catching more animals than were needed, unless they salted or smoked their food. They would be conserving energy for the next hunting trip. I think fasting exercise makes sense, and is certainly easier for glucose control. Birds of prey are the same. Falconers who do demonstrations at county fairs have to keep the birds below a crucial weight; otherwise, those birds would not see the point in delighting us by catching a dead mouse flying around on a wire.

I stopped at a petrol station, the only option on a Sunday here, and pieced together a light snack of keto-friendly junk: gouda in plastic, mortadella, a few bratwurst, and the plain yoghurt I had tucked into my bag at breakfast. It is entirely possible to build a ketogenic meal from junk food when needed. I even folded the foil lid into a spoon, quietly proud of my improvised toolmaking – though the handle buckled as I scraped the last of the yoghurt from the pot.

The food was more processed than I would normally choose, but I felt like a top-up, to avoid a potential hypo later. I had taken a total of eight units that morning, and paid the price of overdosing on insulin with a rescue snack. The initial hypo had subsequently caused a peak of 8 mmol/L (199 mg/dL), but it was now on a downward trajectory, heading towards 4mmol/L (72 mg/dL); I needed to pick this up. Tresiba has a slow, steady background effect. For me, it gently lowers glucose throughout the day, which works beautifully on long rides but can be tricky to fine-tune. A pump might make life easier, especially with the option of tiny incremental doses, but my current pen only delivers whole units. A half-unit pen would have been useful. It is all experimental, but then I am here to do just that. I have a strategy that sort of works, but today I was interested in having a play.

Typically, I see one noticeable rise – more of a plateau than a peak – each day, usually a few hours after eating. It is probably the protein from my meals being converted into glucose. The rest of the time, my levels stay steady or drift slightly downward thanks to Tresiba's background action. For now, this system was working well. I stay within conventional targets (4–10 mmol/L / 72–180 mg/dL) for most of the day, though I would like to spend more time in the physiological range of 4–6 mmol/L (72–108 mg/dL).

I wondered whether a different approach would work even better – perhaps reducing Tresiba or using it only at night, then relying on rapid-acting insulin during the day. The downside would be constant dose adjustments to match food intake and varying physical activity levels. It is a viable option, though.

The real key is understanding insulin intimately: how it behaves under these particular, slightly unusual conditions, and working with it, rather than around it. No system is perfect. Pumps are intuitively more accurate, but even they have quirks. Most pump algorithms are designed around high-carb eating patterns rather than fat-based metabolism. I have met people who abandoned pumps during endurance training and returned to pens for simplicity. Each device has its advocates.

For now, I was making gains. I had reduced my total daily dose to around fifteen units – ten below my usual – and it was fairly stable now that my fitness had adapted to the challenge. If I were an engine, I would be called fuel efficient: more miles per litre. In my case, that meant more glucose stability per unit of insulin. Perhaps this lifestyle really was the optimal one. My "office" on the banks of the Rhine certainly beat a twelve-hour clinic shift under harsh lighting, staring at rectangles of glowing glass screens, where my only exercise is walking a patient to the door or briefly standing to examine them.

I had booked a B&B in Unkel, which was a small village with a charming medieval centre. My room was in an old, timber-framed house at a very reasonable price; even better, the property had a cosy restaurant housed in a densely planted orangery. I rewarded myself with a rare steak and salad. The salad arrived pre-dressed, heavy with balsamic, as is the fashion here, and tasted sugary, so I left half. It is always better to ask for dressing on the side, but I had forgotten. I took four units of insulin for the meal. It was early enough in the evening that any misjudgements could be corrected before sleep.

I had packed enough glucose for a packet a day, but approaching Day Eight, I had only used two packets. I was already about a third of the way to St Moritz, and making solid progress. If everything held together, I would take a short break in Lindau, a pretty tourist town on the southeast shore of Lake Constance. I had built in three spare days for rest, recovery and anything unexpected – such as injury, illness or mechanical issues. So far, I am bang on schedule.

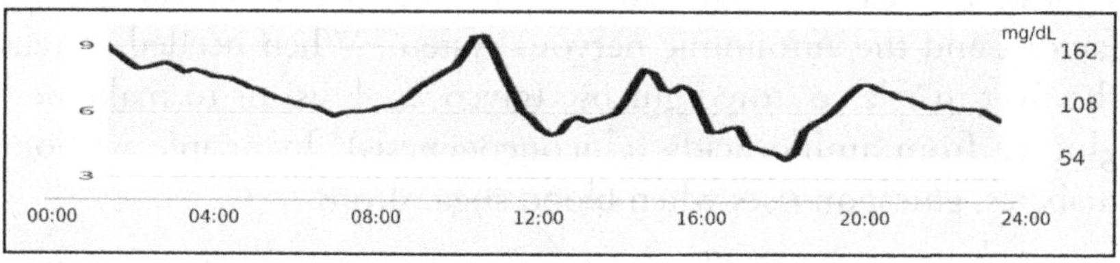

Chapter 19
Hormones That Interact with Insulin

Insulin interacts with many other hormones in the body, and together they help control energy, blood sugar, and how we respond to food, stress and activity. For people with type 1 diabetes, understanding these hormone systems helps explain why blood glucose can rise or fall for reasons unrelated to carbohydrate intake.

Glucagon

Glucagon is insulin's main opposing hormone. Its name comes from "glucose agonist", reflecting its ability to raise blood glucose. Glucagon is made in the pancreas by alpha cells of the islets of Langerhans, and works mostly on the liver. It is secreted especially in response to low blood glucose, prolonged fasting and exercise. Glucagon release is regulated by hormonal pathways, nutritional factors, and the autonomic nervous system. When needed, it tells the liver to release stored glucose (glycogenolysis) or to make new glucose from amino acids (gluconeogenesis). In people without diabetes, glucagon rises when blood sugar drops.

In type 1 diabetes, the glucagon response to low blood glucose can stop working, sometimes within months of diagnosis. The alpha cells still exist, but they do not release glucagon during a hypo unless some beta-cell function remains (for example, in latent autoimmune diabetes in adults [LADA] or not long after diagnosis, during the "honeymoon" stage, when beta cells still produce some insulin). Glucagon still responds to exercise, stress and protein, so it is mainly the hypo response in the pancreas that is missing. Adrenaline remains an effective backup hormone for raising blood glucose.

Glucagon itself is made in the gut as well as the pancreas. Glucagon-like peptides are also made in the gut. Even animals without a pancreas show glucagon-like activity, suggesting the intestine also plays a role. Emergency glucagon still works because it is injected directly.

Glucagon is broken down quickly – after about five minutes – mainly by the liver and kidneys. The enzyme DPP-4 also contributes and breaks down glucagon-like peptide-1 (GLP-1) (see below).

Adrenaline & Noradrenaline

Adrenaline (epinephrine) and noradrenaline (norepinephrine) are stress hormones made in the adrenal glands. They are part of the catecholamine family, along with dopamine, their biochemical precursor. These hormones raise blood sugar by:

- Blocking insulin release, decreasing glucose uptake into glucose storage cells by altering the sensitivity of GLUT4 receptors
- Raising glucagon

  Releasing stored glucose from the liver
- Increasing fat breakdown

This is why stress, fear, or even excitement can send a person with type 1 diabetes unexpectedly high.

Dopamine

Dopamine is usually seen as the "reward-seeking" chemical, but it also helps regulate insulin. Insulin-releasing pancreatic beta cells contain dopamine receptors, and when activated, they reduce insulin release in the same way as adrenaline. Because dopamine is converted to noradrenaline and then to adrenaline, it sits at the top of the catecholamine family. Changes in dopamine (due to stress, illness or medication) can therefore influence energy and glucose levels.

Cortisol

Cortisol is the body's long-acting stress hormone. It naturally rises in the early morning (part of the dawn effect) and can raise glucose by:

- Lowering insulin release
- Raising glucagon
- Increasing glucose production by the liver
- Reducing glucose uptake into muscle

Short bursts help the body survive stress. Long-term elevation, however, can lead to insulin resistance. Cortisol also suppresses inflammation, which is why steroid medicines given for inflammatory conditions such as asthma and rheumatoid arthritis often raise glucose dramatically. Steroids are useful medicines for inflammatory illnesses, but they have glucose raising effects which is problematic especially when treating someone with diabetes.

Growth Hormone (GH)

GH rises during sleep and puberty. It increases glucose production and reduces glucose uptake by muscles, making blood sugar management harder. It also contributes to the dawn effect, which is the natural early-morning rise in blood sugar.

Leptin & Ghrelin

Leptin and ghrelin are the body's main hunger and satiety hormones.

- Leptin, made by fat cells, signals the brain that energy stores are sufficient. Higher leptin usually reduces appetite. People with type 1 diabetes can have disrupted leptin responses when glucose levels swing or when insulin doses vary. Leptin regulates appetite, weight, fertility, and even bone health – but its main job is energy balance.
- Ghrelin is the "hunger hormone", rising before meals and falling after eating.

Both hormones are tightly linked to sleep. Poor sleep lowers leptin and raises ghrelin, increasing hunger and making blood glucose harder to manage.

Osteocalcin (Bone Hormone)

Osteocalcin is a hormone made by bone-forming cells (osteoblasts). Its main job is to support bone structure, but it also helps regulate metabolism by boosting insulin sensitivity and supporting healthy energy use.

Insulin normally activates osteocalcin in bone, but in type 1 diabetes – where insulin inside bone tissue is low – osteocalcin can become less active. This is one reason why people with type 1 diabetes have a higher risk of bone fractures. In short, the insulin-osteocalcin partnership is important not only for strong bones but also for good metabolic health. Bone broth is a good source of osteocalcin.

Somatostatin

Somatostatin acts as a brake on many hormone systems. It slows the release of insulin, glucagon and GH, keeping the body from over-responding. It is produced in the pancreas, gut and brain.

Sex Hormones

Sex hormones are transported in the bloodstream attached to sex hormone binding globulin (SHBG), a protein. There is evidence that insulin lowers SHBG levels, which, in turn affects the activity of the sex hormones it carries.

Oestrogen

Oestrogen improves insulin sensitivity. When levels drop – before a period or during menopause – insulin resistance rises, and blood sugar can rise. Puberty, pregnancy, hormonal contraception, and hormone replacement therapy (HRT) all alter oestrogen levels and may require significant insulin adjustments.

Progesterone

Progesterone tends to increase insulin resistance, especially in the week before menstruation or during pregnancy. Many women with type 1 notice higher glucose during this phase.

Testosterone

Testosterone improves insulin sensitivity when in the normal range. Low testosterone (common in men with type 1 diabetes) increases insulin resistance. Excess testosterone (as in polycyctic ovary syndrome, or PCOS) also worsens glucose control.

Melatonin

Melatonin controls sleep and interacts with insulin receptors. Night-time melatonin rises can slightly reduce insulin sensitivity.

Thyroxine (T4)

Thyroid hormones control metabolic speed.

- Too much T4 = higher glucose, more insulin needed.
- Too little T4 = lower glucose, slower metabolism, risk of hypos.

People with type 1 diabetes are more likely to develop autoimmune thyroid disease, so regular testing is recommended.

Gut Peptides

There are many gut peptides involved in digestion and metabolism. Peptides are proteins with a small number of amino acids. Insulin has 51 amino acids; hormonal gut peptides are typically around 20 amino acids long. A few of the better-known ones are GLP-1 and GIP. GLP-1 and GIP are gut hormones released after eating.

- GLP-1: boosts insulin (if you can make it), lowers glucagon, slows digestion, and reduces appetite.
- GIP: stimulates insulin in those without type 1 diabetes, but in type 1 its insulin-boosting effect is lost; it can still raise glucagon slightly.

Medicines that mimic GLP-1 or GLP-1/GIP (like semaglutide, tirzepatide) are now major weight-loss drugs, but the body produces these hormones naturally. It will not be a surprise by now to know that insulin blocks their release.

- CCK (Cholecystokinin - chole, bile; cysto, bladder; kinin, activity): this gut hormone is released in response to fat and protein. Its effect is to increase satiety, stimulate the release of digestive enzymes, and cause the gallbladder to contract. Injected CCK can trigger anxiety, suggesting that its effects extend beyond digestion. It is not yet clear whether naturally produced CCK has the same effect, but it is possible.
- PYY (Peptide YY): reduces appetite and is more sensitive to protein. It has the same type of action as the GLP-1 peptides.

Chapter 20
Total Miles: 534

Day 8 – Unkel to Bacharach, 59 miles

"The greatest glory in living lies not in never falling, but in rising every time we fall."
– Nelson Mandela

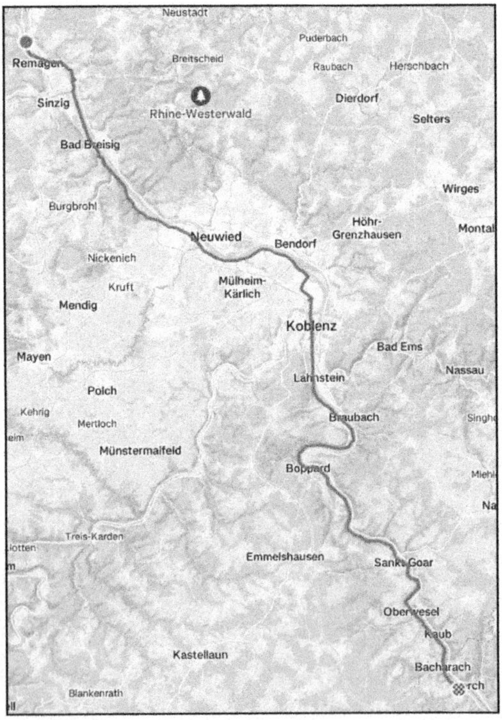

It was a bright and sunny day – a great start to the second week of riding. Another warm day was in prospect, and even though the forecast for the foreseeable future was mixed, today was a good day. And, being a mindful type, the present day was the only one I needed to worry about, so I was very happy. Breakfast was typical fare: eggs, cheese and cured meats in small amounts. I added a plain yoghurt, wondering if it was a good idea. The label stated 4 grams of carbs and 20 grams of protein, so perhaps I would use one unit of rapid insulin with six Tresiba. I was suspicious of Greek yoghurt, hence including the rapid. Some yoghurt brands do not appear to be very low in carbs on the label, but the effect on glucose is inconsistent across brands. I was not hungry, but had to make a gesture toward calorie intake without dumping it all into one meal; I had tried once-a-day meals before, and it could work but the protein could be a problem. I have found that, for me, the best daily routine was no breakfast, a late lunch, and an early evening meal at seven. That is a typical day. Other people will find their own sweet spot – excuse the pun! However, this trip has required a tweak to the usual routine, and breakfast fits it well.

After a couple of hours, the protein kicked in and my glucose rose from 3.5 to 8 mmol/L (63 to 144 mgl/dL). I took another single unit of rapid insulin; it proved effective, and for the rest of the day, the glucose hovered around 6 mmol/L (108 mgl/dL).

It was getting hilly all around me, and the Mittelrhein was in its full glory; the route was becoming very pretty. Also noticeable was a very slight uphill gradient – not enough to require hard work but enough to know that coasting was not an option. I would ascend less than 1,000 feet all day, so it was a very shallow gradient compared with what lay ahead, but it was still flat, really; I needed to drop only a gear or two to maintain cadence and stay comfortable. The gradient was visible in the river, too: it was running rapidly, the water swirling and rising up around buoys and bridge supports. There was a lot of water moving that day. I had first-hand experience of this in several places where the water was flowing onto the cycleway – not enough to impede progress, but another few feet and it would have been flooded.

I was stymied after a couple of miles when the intended ferry crossing was closed. It operated from 07:00am to 07:45am, then at lunchtime, then in the evening – but it was not much help to me at that time. I continued along the east side of the river, hoping to find a bridge at some stage. I was headed for Koblenz for this part of the ride, and was confident there would be a bridge there, as it is a big and historic town – however, about another five miles further on, another working ferry crossing appeared unexpectedly. It was not on the map, but was a significant crossing. Luckily, there was only a ten-minute wait. It was worth it for the entertainment.

The current was strong, and on its way towards my side of the crossing, the ferry kept its nose upstream and almost went sideways and slightly upstream, with its engine at near full throttle to avoid drifting back, before dropping the throttle to ease back to dock at the jetty. It was a demonstration of real skill. Our crossing was as eventful as the one we had witnessed.

After all that excitement, it was an easy, pleasant ride into Koblenz along well-maintained paths, with little navigation required. The centre of the city was old and beautiful, with elegant squares and their fair share of coffee shops and restaurants. I had covered 30 miles without a break, so it was a good time to fuel with water and coffee. As I rested, I thought about how easily the delicate balance of glucose-affecting hormones can be disturbed. Stress alone is enough to throw everything off. Every stress hormone, from adrenaline to cortisol, leaves measurable fingerprints in the bloodstream. Their metabolic effects are well known, and we can measure their levels in the blood with great precision. Yet insulin is treated differently; we still tend to dose it bluntly, often in amounts that overwhelm the body's ability to integrate it with the rest of the hormonal mix.

Dozens of hormones interact with insulin, nudging glucose up or down, raising or lowering appetite, tension, heart rate or energy use. When insulin is pushed too high, the ratios shift, and the whole orchestra loses its harmony. It makes sense to try to keep the metabolic dose near optimal. When cooking a dish with many ingredients, you notice immediately after tasting if you made a mistake in reading the recipe and added a teaspoon instead of a tablespoon. We have all done it. The same applies here, and balance matters. Synthetic insulin comes with its challenges, but understanding its interactions gives us a fighting chance. I have no intention of returning to the old "eat what I like and inject regardless" approach. "As much as necessary, as little as possible" remains my guiding principle.

The ride through the Mittelrhein was very pleasant: nice cycle paths, hills, vineyards, castles, passing a mediaeval crane on the riverbank, and some sun – a perfect day. I glimpsed a white, square board with black letters: 539. It was a Rhine kilometre marker, indicating the number of Rhine kilometres from the start of the navigable Rhine in Konstanz to the North Sea at Hook van Holland, at kilometre 1,036. I was now in the five hundreds, so halfway along the Rhine. Vineyards in this area named their wines after kilometre markers, such as a Riesling 555. People also use these markers as meeting points, and for fishing. I did not stop to take in much culture; I was on a mission, but a re-visit would be pleasant. A fortress of a castle on the opposite bank was served by a cable car. There was a university and some old-town charm.

I had lunch on a bench in a park by the river – a few leftover squares of sweaty cheese and warm salami from the garage stop yesterday, plus a couple of boiled eggs from a shop in Koblenz. I eked them out over a few hours in the afternoon and avoided any glucose spike. It worked well. Sometimes it felt as if I were living like a student. Nothing wrong with that; I had a happy student time, and eking out food is no bad thing. I like this aspect of the trip: being frugal and opportunistic. Remember that cable tie? It still gave me a certain pleasure.

Within minutes of setting off for Bacharach, dark clouds gathered and the heavens opened. This was a proper summer storm. The clouds had pushed up over the gorge, the Rhine supplying moisture, and the heat mixing everything up. It was impossible to ride; the raindrops were so heavy they splashed back up inches above the ground. I stood under a broad-leaved tree with my hood up; I decided to sit it out for half an hour. It was cold rain, but only a local storm. I realised too late that I had left my phone on the bike with no cover, and once again the charging port filled with water. I was stuck. I had a backup phone, but it was not set up with all the apps I needed.

After the rain stopped, I positioned the port in the dry air, and the warm wind from the ride dried it within an hour. The relief was short-lived; soon after, the port failed to charge. I had to go to the backup phone and start the laborious process of loading apps. The CGM refused to load, as did the ketone meter, but I had some functionality – the mapping was ready to lead me to Bacharach.

I decided to go for it. I had just booked the accommodation, and there were not many alternatives around. Tomorrow I would be in larger towns, with a chance of phone repair. I pedalled on uneventfully to Bacharach. Nothing to do with Burt – he was from Kansas! The guidebook told me it was the prettiest town on the Rhine.

The overnight stay was out of town on the south side, for a good start the next morning. It was a strange place but comfortable. Decorated in a Southeast Asian style on several levels, it seemed incongruous with its 1960s plain, rendered exterior. The bar and dining area were very German, with curvy pine and heavy benches. A circle of light bulbs was mounted on an old wooden wheel and suspended from the ceiling by chains. The owners seemed to be an odd couple, on first appearance. The man was a shadow presence, appearing only when needed, with a pasty complexion, a rough beard, sliders on his feet, and wearing baggy trackie bottoms and a very old, heavy metal-style T-shirt. The person running front of house was, I think, his partner: Asian, and completely the opposite appearance. That would explain the eastern Asia décor. She did the food and billing.

I was the only diner in the restaurant that evening, and had a perfectly rare, succulent, tasty steak. It came with salad and a few other small dishes, some looking quite sweet. I really appreciate well-cooked beef. The freshness of real food seems to infuse me with health. The sweaty cheese earlier seemed a dead food by comparison, but it did contain calories and the correct macros of protein and fat, with no carbs – it is possible to stay ketogenic with convenience food. I sometimes substituted real food with convenience food. Sometimes a compromise between the two is required.

I used four units of rapid and seven of Tresiba, as I suspected a higher carb amount in the side dishes, and the steak had plenty of protein. I had initially planned on five units of Tresiba, based on the previous night's slow glucose decline, but I ended up taking slightly more, out of instinct – that's type 1 for you. The glucose trace was smooth all night, so I had got that dose spot-on.

Tomorrow I would try to be more proactive with shopping and source fresh fish or something similar. I noticed while checking my food app that I was getting low on my fat intake. I was also a bit protein-heavy, and that might have made glucose management unnecessarily challenging. I think that low-fat recommendations mean that packaged food has less fat. Buying some butter, olive oil or coconut oil might help increase the fat intake; I was well supplied with protein, around two grams per kilogram, which felt right – but I noticed my calorie deficit and saw potential to add fat. On the other hand, I pondered, should I just let body fat run down slightly? Adding fat for the sake of calories when protein was right seemed like being a slave to macro ratios. I would think about it, but for the moment, I would err on the side of letting the body fat drain down. I do not know if body fat has a "use by" date like the fat we buy in the shops, but it sounds like it should. It is one to ponder on.

The more I thought, the more I was comfortable sacrificing some body fat; I had enough, after all, to continue my journey all the way to Africa if called upon. I had calculated earlier that I would only lose a couple of kilograms. I would see how it went. It was not a crucial decision either way – but dividing the daily protein intake into three meals was definitely the right decision, and was rewarded with stable glucose levels; at least for today.

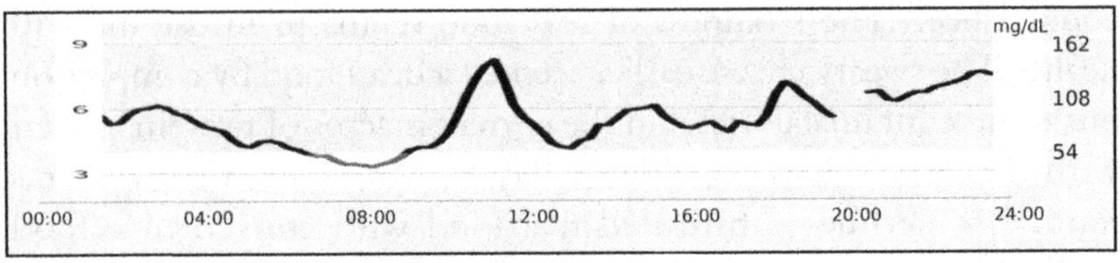
mg/dL
9
6
3
162
108
54
00:00
04:00
08:00
12:00
16:00
20:00
24:00

Chapter 21
Insulin: As Much as Needed, as Little as Possible

The hormones and pathways we have looked at so far give us a good picture of how type 1 diabetes works, and that is enough to help manage it well. But science keeps moving. One new discovery or an odd result in a lab can change the way we think. For example, the microbiome was discovered in the 1800s, but only recently have we learned how much it affects almost every disease. The process of breaking down glucose, called glycolysis, was only mapped in 1918 because people wanted to understand how yeast works in brewing. The Krebs Cycle, another key process, was not discovered until 1937. Science keeps changing – but what we know right now about metabolism and insulin is more than sufficient to guide everyday life with type 1 diabetes.

One area I find especially important is how injected insulin compares with how the body normally uses insulin. In people without type 1 diabetes, the pancreas releases insulin straight into a blood vessel called the portal vein, which goes directly to the liver. Because of this, the liver gets more insulin than the rest of the body. That balance matters. However, when we inject insulin into the skin, it travels through the body in a different way. The liver gets less of it, and the muscles and fat tissue get more of it. This means the normal "insulin gradient" is lost; the liver does not receive the same signal it normally receives. If we could safely send insulin to the liver first, it could fix some of this problem. But right now, that is not practical for everyday use.

The liver plays a big role in blood sugar control. After a meal, it stores sugar as glycogen. If there is extra energy, it can turn some of it into fat. When you have not eaten for a while, the liver makes and releases glucose to keep blood sugar from dropping too low.

Because injected insulin reaches the liver less effectively, people with type 1 diabetes can have a harder time shutting down the liver's glucose release. They may also store less glycogen. As a result, they often need more insulin overall to keep glucose in range.

This can matter both in the short term and the long term. In the short term, blood sugar can sometimes rise during stress or high-intensity exercise, partly because the liver releases more glucose. Stress hormones like adrenaline (epinephrine) can push glucose up, too. Over the long term, needing more insulin can contribute to weight gain, insulin resistance, and other metabolic problems.

One study stayed in my mind because of what it found during sleep. Researchers took blood samples all night from people with type 1 diabetes and compared them with people without it. As expected, the type 1 group had higher glucose and higher insulin levels through the night.

Long-term studies also tell an interesting story. The "Golden Cohort" includes people who have lived with type 1 diabetes for more than 50 years. Many of them did not have perfect blood sugar levels, yet they still lived long, healthy lives. A key pattern stood out: most were of normal weight and used relatively low insulin doses. Another study, the Jubilee Study, showed similar findings. People who had lived with type 1 for more than 40 years were also using modest insulin doses and had good overall health. These studies show that long-term survival is possible even without perfect numbers, as long as weight and insulin use stay closer to normal.

Another study looked at healthy women following a ketogenic diet. When their ketosis was stopped with a high-carb diet, their insulin levels rose sharply, and inflammation markers increased. When they returned to ketosis, insulin and inflammation dropped again. This suggests that lowering insulin, when safe to do so, may help the body run more smoothly.

High insulin levels, known as hyperinsulinaemia, are also linked to cancer risk. Insulin is a growth hormone and can make cells divide more quickly. High insulin can also raise IGF-1, which is a strong growth signal, and both can push cells towards uncontrolled growth. Cancer cells fuel on glucose, and high insulin helps feed them. It makes sense that managing insulin carefully could lower some of these risks. In type 1 diabetes, new vessel growth in the retina is partly driven by elevated insulin levels, because insulin promotes the action of a blood vessel growth promotor VEGF. Poor-quality new blood vessels cause proliferative retinopathy, which requires laser treatment to control (this eye condition will be discussed more fully in a later chapter).

For me, all of this supports one clear idea: keeping insulin as close to normal physiology as possible is key to living well with type 1 diabetes. The usual advice – eat whatever you want, count the carbs, then inject – may work in the short term, but what is the long-term cost of constantly flooding the body with insulin? Even with modern tech like hybrid closed-loop systems, a perfect HbA1c means little if it requires large amounts of insulin.

My journey is about understanding the foundations of health – food, movement, stress, sleep and environment – and how each one influences the amount of insulin I need. I want to understand what aspects of daily life, as well as food, drive my insulin needs so I can make better choices. And that is where the freedom is. Not in restriction, but in awareness; not in control for its own sake, but in empowerment to live better, fuller and healthier with type 1 diabetes.

Chapter 22
Total miles: 598

Day 9 – Bacharach to Worms, 64 miles

Chacun à son goût (each to their own taste)
– attributed to William Cowper

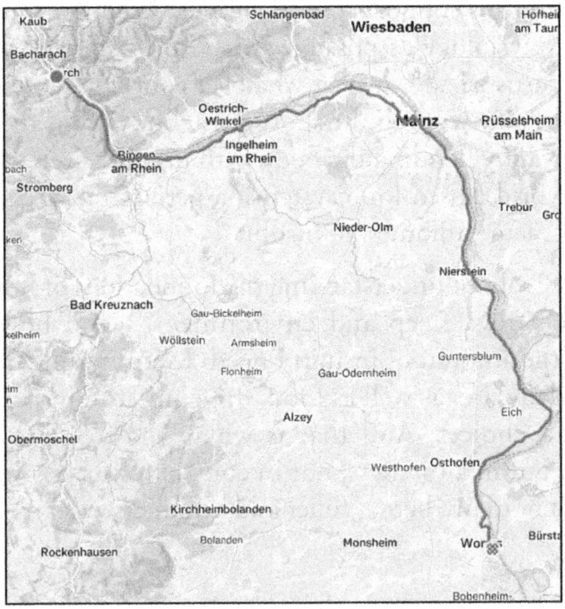

Have you ever taken your car to the garage to have the mechanic diagnose a rattle and when you get there, the car refuses to play the game and behaves perfectly? The mechanic sits in the driver's seat, revving the engine with *that* look on their face – a mixture of triumph and the suggestion that you are a complete moron. Well, just after 9 am, I arrived at the town of Bingen and looked up the only phone repair shop that was open at the time. It was full of an eclectic mix of household decorative items such as vases and floral teapots, towels, and several of those gold, smiley cats that are always waving. I told the shopkeeper my charging port was not working. He plugged it into his fancy charging station and, hey presto, it started charging. To double-check, he did it twice more while smiling in "that" way, and I thought, "he thinks I am a moron!" He plugged in my cable, and it worked. Then he plugged that cable into my charging brick, and it provided flawless charging port performance. Well, what could I say? Deep down, I was grateful I could save an hour and get back on the road. I bought a charging cable from him as a spare and set off on my way, feeling like a right fool.

The breakfast provided that morning only had flavoured yoghurt, and I dismissed this almost without thought, skipping yoghurt for breakfast from that moment for the rest of the trip. Instead, I had one egg and a selection of fish, meat, and cheese, served on a three-tier cake stand. I injected six units of Tresiba and a single unit of rapid insulin. There were, of course, bread and cereal options, which I did not give a second thought.

I hardly notice carbs these days; after a while of living a keto lifestyle, I find that my food radar is set only to those foods of interest to me. For someone whose staple breakfast for the first 20 years was porridge, this is not a problem. I don't "see" these as foods relevant to me these days, so I overlook them.

In the early days of transitioning to keto and on those days when I feel sorry for myself and crave something "carby", I now have the ability to resist. The reward of a carb 'hit' is short-lived compared to the hours of dealing with erratic glucose levels, so the trade-off for me makes sense. With a quick scan of a buffet, I immediately zone in on eggs, fish, cheese and meat, and zone out the breads, cereals, fruit and juices, porridge and yoghurt. I never really "see" them. To the unconverted, it seems like a lot to sacrifice. I would agree that it can be in the early days – perhaps the first few months to a year – however, over time, one develops the knack of navigating the food space. A croissant with jam or a pain au chocolat with coffee would generally be considered a treat. The sweet taste can be difficult to lose once acquired and, in my experience, it is something I would rather not get into. It is, of course, possible to still indulge and tinker with the rapid insulin and the pump settings, and get a reasonable result but I focus on foods I know will work well with my routine and minimise my insulin use. In the long term, low insulin use might extend my healthy years – and that is worth resisting some temporary craving. We have enough information to know the downside of higher-than-necessary insulin use. The immediate reward of low insulin is stable glucose levels, so this is also a motivator.

I remember long ago when, at a hotel buffet breakfast, I had a standard keto breakfast – bacon, eggs, mushrooms, etc. I locked eyes with someone having muesli, croissants and orange juice. What passed between us was priceless. We both were convinced that our breakfast was the healthiest. And this encapsulates the problem with dietary advice: the woman had no clue I had type 1 diabetes, and if she did, she might have been more horrified – and if she had type 1, I would have been equally horrified!

I am one of the lucky ones in that I am able to resist carbs without too much problem. Others I know are more addicted to sweet foods and suffer more than I do. It is likely that sweet foods do encourage us to eat more. From an ancestral point of view, in temperate climates, carbs are only available in the summer and autumn months. When we taste sweet foods such as fruits and berries, our brain is stimulated to tell us to eat more; the more we eat in these months, the more carbs we convert to fat, which will sustain us through the winter when little food is available. In the summer months, we store fat, which contains the fat-soluble vitamins A, D, E, and K. In the winter months, fat-burning during lean times would release those vitamins for use. But now that food companies have refined the science of palatability and shelf life, we have ready availability of carbs all year round, and in refined quantities that subvert our ancestral instincts. We are "eating for the winter that never comes".

If we continually eat carbohydrates throughout the year, we are continually in fat-storage metabolism, and the fat-soluble vitamins are locked away. So it is no real surprise that, with most of the world trying to avoid heart attacks while eating a high-carb, low-fat diet, we are deficient in the fat-soluble vitamin D, which is stored in fat. We are unable to access it, even though it is locked up in our bodies. So then we take supplements. Vitamin D is derived from the conversion of cholesterol-type substances through the action of sunlight, which creates the chemical reaction needed to convert inert vitamin D into the active form. When we burned fat in the winter, as our ancestors did, we released this sunlight-derived vitamin throughout the winter. It is a romantic thought that emphasises that we indeed are creatures of the universe. Sure, we can focus our medicines on affecting single molecules and changing the numbers, but panning out to view ourselves through a wider lens, I think, is also helpful. The basic foundations of health will always be the cornerstone of our well-being.

Nevertheless, the range of food choices for a keto diet is still wide, and recipes can produce excellent mimics of carb-rich foods, which some people prefer during their transition to a keto diet. I stick to the basic eight food types: green vegetables, fish, eggs, dairy, berries in small amounts, 85% minimum dark chocolate, meat, and tree-derived nuts (which are lower in carbohydrates). It is perfectly possible to have a meat-free keto diet where eggs, nuts and dairy take up the load.

It is not difficult to be a carb-basher and talk about overdosing, unseasonal eating of carbs, etc. I think the main problem with carbohydrates is the sheer amount we eat when we are not genetically set up to do so – or in the case of type 1 diabetes, hormonally set up. For those with a potential addiction to ultra-sweet foods, it is not unreasonable to use sugar substitutes to help with a transition.

Others choose a hybrid diet to add in some sweet food and work it out that way. Yet others have carb days, and others go low-carb rather than keto. There is no right way. As long as we have the information, we can make the choices that suit us. There is no science supporting a 50% carb diet; it came off the back of low-fat recommendations, as we know. A lot of people eat carbs without apparent ill health – but I do not think people with type 1 diabetes have that luxury, in the main. The things the long-lived type 1s share are all the general markers of health: blood pressure, weight, favourable lipid profiles, etc., but also low insulin volumes. I think that this is a very significant measurement, and that, for me, is the route to vitality and, hopefully, longevity. But feeling vital will suffice for me, and a ketogenic diet helps reduce insulin levels to a healthier range, where insulin is better able to interact harmoniously with the metabolic processes it affects. And the ketones rev up my brain in a good way.

If we ate seasonally, we would be limited to a constant supply of meat, fish and dairy. Eggs are, in the main, seasonal, and up in the Arctic and down in the Antarctic, the choice for most of the year is meat only, including, of course, fat. The people who live there appear to have a good health record. Ernest Shackleton, on his fated voyage to the South Pole, left his crew marooned on an island while he and another sailor rowed to South Georgia; it was an epic adventure, and his crew survived on seal meat and blubber, fish, and the occasional albatross for several months. But then, whilst I live in temperate zones, did my ancestors do the same? Were they originally from the equatorial regions of the world? These big questions are a lot to take in over breakfast, and I do not have an answer to them.

What I do know is that many people living in the UK and many developed Western nations consume a significant amount of what I consider unhealthy food and appear to live long. I know people who have lived for 60 years with type 1 with no complications, and they have a totally different, higher-carb diet than me; they wonder what the fuss is all about. I can't take that chance. Overall, type 1 diabetes reduces lifespan by several years, and I have found a method that helps me take out the chance factor. I can only work out what seems to be the most reasonable, sustainable diet for my own situation of type 1 diabetes. There will always be a compromise between the purity of living and what is available, acceptable or practical; it depends on how far you want to take it. Reducing this argument to absurdity, of course, requires hunting down and slaughtering your meat, and growing your own vegetables. "Chacun à son goût", as they say – each to their own taste. And I agree.

To me, the basic keto foods in their most natural form seem reasonable. They are nutrient-dense, and it seems that our bodies sense nutrients in addition to calories – these hit the brain's reward centres. I choose ketogenic foods to minimise my insulin requirements; others will make a different choice and still live well. It depends on the unique expression of our type 1 diabetes. Natural, minimally processed, nutrient-dense, ketogenic food is my aim.

Even so, some keto foods do not suit. Almonds, for example, can make my joints ache, especially if I take them in volume, such as in a pastry. It might be the oxalic acid or even the cyanide that forms during the digestion of the chemicals in that particular nut. We have to find our own way. The basic keto foods will give us all of the nutrition we need – I am confident of that. For this trip, some compromises are necessary. I rarely eat cured meats at home – I do have some – but there is a lot of this on offer in Germany. I have not dedicated enough time to enjoying real food during the trip and am eating "on the hoof". Will three weeks of cured meats affect my long-term health? I do not think so – but it is what I would call unhealthy keto. There is zero carbohydrate in cured meat, so this contributes to a ketogenic diet. I would rather be in ketosis than not, so the compromise is acceptable to me for this trip.

With an early start and excellent roads, I made swift progress to Mainz. It must have been bombed heavily during the Second World War, as nearly all of its historic buildings had been destroyed, replaced by largely modernist Bauhaus-style, Modern Movement structures and a road system that seemed impenetrable to me, as a first-time visitor. I decided to have some fat and protein for lunch, and, having promised myself quality food, found myself in an organic supermarket chain called Biomarkt. It was a proper supermarket, specialising in organic and artisan food, and was, of course, relatively expensive. I bought fresh salmon, cheese and some sparkling water, and ate them at the café. I used a couple of units of insulin for that.

I needed to make some plans for the rest of the route. I was on Day Nine and halfway through the journey. That night, I was going to meet my friend Martin, whom I had met at Keto-Live conferences in the past. Martin was retired but had worked in the chemical industry in the area during his career. On hearing about my journey, he volunteered to host me for an evening, and I was looking forward to catching up with him – but first, I needed to cover the distance between Mainz and Mannheim.

It was a lovely day with light winds, and the cycle track was empty as it wound through gently rolling hills covered with straight rows of vines. In this area, there are a few bullet-shaped recumbent bikes; it is perfect for them, and the rider is hidden behind a tiny cockpit, peeping just above a smooth, streamlined shell. These are rapid forms of transport indeed – they flew past, sounding a little hollow and rattly as they sped over the bumps. Highly specialist, I would not like to tackle a hill on one, but they added interest to an otherwise unmemorable stretch of the route.

Just as I was relaxing into the ride on smooth tarmac, the track became gravel and then grass. It was soft, and the bike's thin wheels dug in and mushed about, making it difficult to steer. And shortly after, I found myself on a path with a concrete base formed of interlocking hexagons as a binding structure for the soil inside them, each about 20 cm in size. This would have been okay, but the soil had shrunk or been washed out. It was a rough ride, and the wheels were juddering into the holes. I was concerned about the rims at this point. When I was on my trip around the North Sea, I had a wheel rim crack – and the wheels on that bike were made for heavy lifting; these lightweight road bike wheels were not designed for this terrain. Then it happened – a crash into a deep hexagon, followed by an unstable back end and a flat tyre. The tube had become pinched by movement in the rim and punctured in two places.

I was in the middle of nowhere, relatively speaking – although one is never really isolated in this part of Europe. It was no big deal, as I had a spare tube and the wheel rim was undamaged except for a slightly jagged edge where it had scraped the concrete; this was easily smoothed out with a knife blade.

All of the luggage had to come off the bike. I knew all of the tools were at the bottom of one pannier, but which one? Well, not the first one, obviously! I found the pump, though. I had not thought I would need a tube repair. Ten years ago, I rode the whole North Sea Cycle Route without any punctures on wonderful Schwalbe Marathon Plus tyres; with those particular tyres, punctures are not an issue. These Continental tyres had a good puncture rating but, of course, this was not the penetration of the tyre casing that the puncture rating referred to; it was a pinch-tear of the tube, so it did not really count. I removed the tyre and tube, and replaced it with the only spare I was carrying. I intended to repair the damaged one at the end of the day. Because I was packing as light as possible, I had only brought one spare tube.

Within half a mile of setting off again, I had another flat! So now I had to repair the tube before I could proceed. I needed some water to pump up the tube and find the hole by looking for where bubbles were forced out. The Rhine was literally ten metres away, with millions of gallons of water, but it was inaccessible, being down a steep bank full of thorny bushes – and after all that rain, puddles were scarce, as the sunny weather was drying things up.

I spotted a puddle a little way up ahead and carried the wheel to it. Then the problem began: I could not inflate the tube fast enough to get any pressure into it to blow air out of the tube and form bubbles that would show me where the tear was. This typically means that there is a big cut somewhere. Yet, try as I might, I was unable to find it. A detailed visual inspection followed, and I ran my hand along the inner wall of the tyre to find any thorns, but nothing gave me a clue. What to do? My options were to ride with a flat tyre or walk the bike out. It was at least two miles to the next hamlet, and I was unlikely to find a bike shop there – but I would find a road and then, hopefully, a passing car for a lift.

Casting around for inspiration, I finally saw a solution: by lucky chance, my clear water bottle was full. I folded the tube into sections and dipped them into the water, then used the pump to blow air in; I could then see the bubbles and locate the holes. I spotted them – the two tell-tale holes of a pinch puncture. I checked the rest of the tube thoroughly, and patched the holes. I then took advantage of my lucky streak of lateral thinking and repaired the second tube as well, just in case. The final tube change was done, and off I went, reasoning that the nice thing about all this was the number of people who stopped to check I was okay.

I phoned Martin, who was already on his way. I could not make the distance in a reasonable time, so we agreed to meet in a town a forty-minute ride away, so that he would not be inconvenienced. I smashed out a good time with strong power and speed. It was sunny, the roads were smooth and dry, the sat nav had few decisions to make, and I was in the town of Worms at the rendezvous point, near a bridge with a red stone tower, in seemingly no time at all.

Martin was there to greet me. Soon, we were passing the vast BASF chemial plant where he had worked. With a cat's cradle of stainless-steel pipes, gantries, chimneys, and myriad shiny metal staircases, BASF is the largest chemical factory in the world, and has a history of great inventions. Martin worked in paper technology, using chemicals to enhance paper quality for specific requirements. He subsequently moved into polymer chemistry and won an award for the invention of a monomer that could be scaled up to produce many types of plastic. He was rightfully proud of that, and I learned a lot from him about everyday items where chemistry is applied; for instance, the reverse end of a Nespresso aluminium coffee capsule has a small area of polyester that melts at the coffee maker's operating temperature and pressure, allowing the coffee to be extracted. It is amazing how complex some deceptively simple-looking everyday objects are.

That evening, Martin barbecued a wonderful entrecôte steak and served it with herb butter and a glass of red wine. The steak was big, and I used two units of insulin to cover the protein. The wine would not be a problem, but alcohol can inhibit other glucose-raising mechanisms, so I did not want to over-inject insulin and cause an unnecessary hypo. It proved to be a good decision.

I was now in a routine of twelve units of long-acting insulin per day, in two doses. It seemed to suit the requirements of this trip: six units of Tresiba twice a day and around four units of rapid. At some point, I thought I would reduce Tresiba but in reality, I elected for an extra unit out of a sixth sense, really; it worked well for this lifestyle.

Physical activity, on this adventure, is becoming significant in optimising insulin, and is second only to diet as a way of managing type 1. It is not equal, in my opinion – but it is significant. I reckon that for me, physical activity is worth several units of insulin saved.

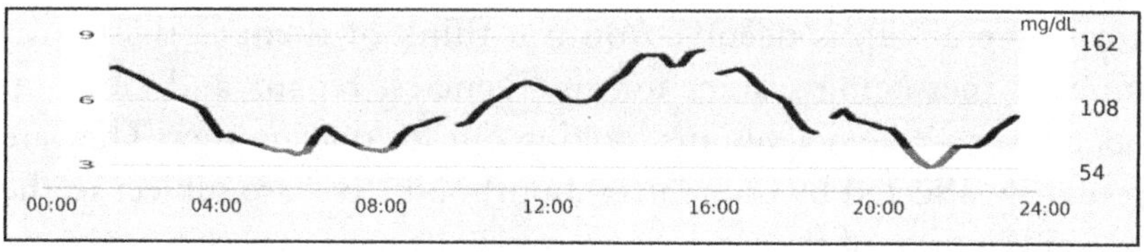

Chapter 23
Inflammation: Helpful *and* Harmful – The Search for Equilibrium

You have probably heard the word "inflammation" mentioned often in discussions about health, particularly in relation to metabolism, diabetes or heart disease. But what does inflammation actually mean, especially when it comes to type 1 diabetes? To fully understand it, we need to examine the key messengers of the immune system: cytokines.

Cytokines are small proteins released by cells – particularly immune cells. Their role is to help cells communicate, sending signals to ramp up or tone down an immune response, or to direct immune cells to areas where help is needed. You can think of them as the body's internal messaging system for emergencies, repairs and clean-up operations – like neighbours looking out for one another. They are primarily affected by their "neighbourhood", but are subject to the prevailing rules of the land.

Importantly, cytokines are not inherently "good" or "bad"; their effects depend entirely on context. When balanced, they help the body stay healthy and respond appropriately to challenges. However, when this balance is disrupted or the challenge persists, it can contribute to disease.

When the immune system is activated – say, by an infection or an injury – specific cytokines such as interleukin-1 beta (IL-1β), interleukin-6 (IL-6), tumour necrosis factor-alpha (TNF-α), and interferon-gamma (IFN-γ) are among the first to respond. These pro-inflammatory cytokines recruit immune cells to the site, stimulate further signalling, and sustain the immune response. This is an essential part of defence and healing. But if this response does not switch off, or is triggered unnecessarily, it can cause long-term harm. Chronic inflammation is the result and plays a central role in conditions such as arthritis, heart disease and diabetes. Even poor dental health can promote a chronic inflammatory state, because diseased gums shed bacteria into the circulation, thereby activating the inflammatory cascade.

Thankfully, there is a natural counterbalance: anti-inflammatory cytokines, including IL-10 and transforming growth factor-beta (TGF-β), act as brakes on the immune system. They help quieten the immune response, promote tissue healing, and return the body to a steady, balanced state.

Cytokines are not only involved in classic immune defence; they also regulate nutrient metabolism, making them essential in metabolic diseases. In obesity, for example, adipose tissue becomes inflamed as immune cells infiltrate and release cytokines. This creates a low-grade, persistent form of inflammation called metaflammation – a kind of hidden fire linked to insulin resistance, type 2 diabetes, and cardiovascular disease.

How Does This Relate to Type 1 Diabetes?

The current consensus on the cause of type 1 diabetes is that it is an autoimmune disease in which the immune system mistakenly attacks the pancreas's insulin-producing cells. Cytokines play a central role in this process. IL-1β and TNF-α, for example, help recruit aggressive immune cells to the pancreatic islets, making the beta cells more vulnerable to destruction. So, the immune system is not just physically attacking the pancreas; it is also creating a toxic environment that speeds up the damage. Additionally, beta cells have a notably weak capacity to resist oxidative stress and related injury.

The inflammatory activity does not stop once the pancreas is compromised. People with type 1 diabetes often show signs of ongoing immune system activity, even when they are not ill. Their cytokine profiles may remain imbalanced, influenced by factors such as blood sugar fluctuations, oxidative stress, insulin dosing, and more. For example, sharp increases in blood glucose can trigger temporary rises in IL-6 and TNF-α – small inflammatory surges that, over time, can contribute to complications such as nerve damage and heart disease.

TNF-α is known to damage insulin-producing beta cells in type 1 diabetes and is also elevated in the fat tissue of people with insulin resistance. It interferes with insulin signalling, making it harder for insulin to work even when blood sugar levels seem normal. This has implications for people with type 1 diabetes on insulin therapy (i.e. all of us): background inflammation may affect how well insulin works, regardless of glucose levels.

Here is where it gets even more interesting: cytokines do not always behave in the same way. Take IL-6, for instance. It is commonly labelled a "pro-inflammatory" cytokine. However, during exercise, muscles release IL-6, which has almost the opposite effect – it reduces inflammation and improves insulin sensitivity. It helps the body use glucose more efficiently and promotes fat burning. So, the same molecule can be harmful in one context and helpful in another. It is all about the situation.

High Glucose, High Insulin, AGEs and Fibrosis

In both type 1 and type 2 diabetes, it is not simply glucose that damages the body over many years. Insulin has a role here, too. Normalising glucose helps, but only if insulin is normalised as well. "Eat what you fancy and shoot up what it takes" is not a good strategy.

Let's dive deeper. When glucose is high, it attaches to proteins in the body and forms sticky molecules called AGEs – advanced glycation end products. Red blood cells bind to glucose, which we can measure as HbA1c, but because red blood cells are short-lived, they provide only a limited view of long-term tissue damage. Glucose does not attach only to red cells; it affects tissues that are longer lived such as muscles, tendons, collagen and cartilage, which become stiffer and less flexible. These changes also trigger more inflammatory cytokines, adding stress to nerves, kidneys, blood vessels and the eyes.

High insulin can be just as harmful. Insulin is not only a glucose-lowering hormone but also a growth signal. When insulin levels stay high every day, it can activate cytokines that lead to fibrosis. Fibrosis is the slow build-up of stiff, scar-like tissue in cartilage, connective tissues, and major organs such as the kidneys, liver, heart, eyes, and even fat tissue. This makes tissues harder, less elastic, and less able to do their job.

Put simply, high glucose leads to AGEs, which trigger inflammation and cause damage. High insulin levels also activate cytokines, which promote fibrosis and stiffen tissues. Think about this in the eye: high glucose levels begin the process of damage to the structures that provide energy to the retina. The blood vessels leak slightly, creating background retinopathy. Meanwhile, AGEs combined with the high levels of insulin seen in a high-carb diet lead to the continuation of inflammation and cause fibrosis, with the potential for retinal detachment. In the poor-quality tissue that results, insulin promotes new blood vessel growth and proliferative retinopathy. It is therefore important to address not only glucose but also insulin.

Metaflammation – the low-level, persistent type of inflammation – does not produce classic symptoms of illness, like fever. It quietly disrupts metabolism, damages blood vessels, impairs mitochondria (the cell's energy generators), and gets in the way of tissue repair. It is driven by factors like overeating, physical inactivity, poor sleep, and constant low-grade stress.

Interestingly, insulin itself – not just glucose – can influence the immune system. Immune cells have insulin receptors. In acute illness, insulin can reduce inflammation. But when insulin levels stay high for extended periods, especially in a high-carb environment, it can push the immune system towards a more inflammatory state.

Among all the markers doctors use to assess inflammation, C-reactive protein (CRP) is useful and easily accessible. The liver produces CRP in response to cytokines, particularly IL-6, and to a lesser extent IL-1β and TNF-α. CRP binds to the surface of damaged cells and to pathogens such as bacteria. This binding acts as a pattern recognition mechanism, flagging targets for immune clearance. In medicine, it is used as a general signpost of inflammation. CRP levels can soar during acute infections or trauma. People with type 1 diabetes often show raised CRP levels, especially when blood glucose control is poor or complications are present. But the encouraging news is that people who are active, eat well, and manage their diabetes effectively can have CRP levels no different from individuals with no type 1 diabetes. This suggests that inflammation is an avoidable part of type 1 diabetes; it is shaped by how we live.

Chapter 24

Total Miles: 688

Day 10 – Worms to Eggenstein-Leopoldshafen, 90 miles

"Getting lost along your path is a part of finding the path you are meant to be on." – Robin Sharma

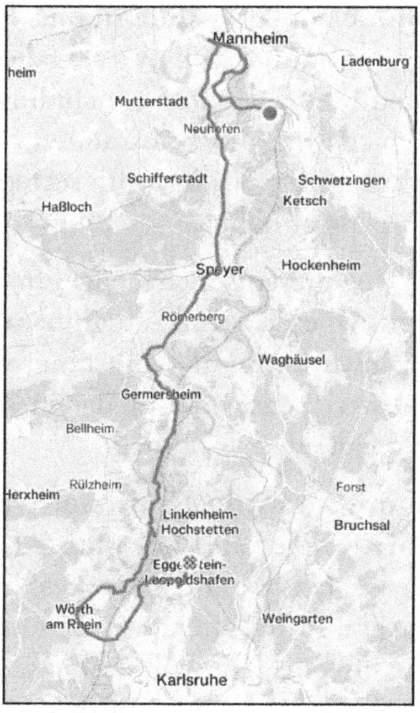

The day began well. Martin made an early breakfast. He has adopted a keto diet, too, so he knows exactly what I want: a three-egg omelette with chives. That is a good start to the day. I opted to take the usual six units of Tresiba for this meal, and no rapid. There were around 20 grams of protein, and I would let this be consumed for muscle growth and repair, especially as I was going to be doing a fair bit of riding from the start. Martin had planned a lightning tour of the local area by bike. On a sedentary day, it would have attracted a unit of insulin – but then again, on a sedentary day, I would personally miss breakfast and extend my fast to late morning.

The act of waking is complex, and cortisol plays a part. Cortisol is a strange one in type 1. It is a steroid hormone that follows a circadian rhythm; its level will naturally rise in the early hours, peak just after waking, and then decline in the mid-morning and throughout the day, reaching its lowest point at midnight. Cortisol is partly responsible for the glucose-raising dawn effect, along with adrenaline (epinephrine) and growth hormone. Insulin secretion in someone without type 1 tends to follow a circadian pattern also, but this will be disrupted by many things, including meals. However, because insulin interacts with other hormones, insulin sensitivity is generally higher in the mid-morning, with secretion peaking in the afternoon and decreasing at night.

For us with type 1, this presents a challenge. Insulin will not be as effective unit-for-unit when cortisol is high because cortisol causes insulin resistance. However, by mid-morning, we will be back to normal insulin sensitivity, as cortisol declines; this is why the adjustment for the dawn effect is needed.

As we know, insulin in individuals without type 1 diabetes lasts around a quarter of an hour, and our injected insulin has barely started by then. Cortisol lasts around one to two hours. So, it is likely that if we have a breakfast just after waking, some of our morning insulin will not be as effective, but will start acting more potently at the time cortisol levels are declining. In this situation, we will be vulnerable to hypos, and this is a common experience for many. It is not necessarily a miscalculation of carbohydrates, but the timing of the insulin and the meal. After a bad start in the morning, the rollercoaster often continues, as the sugar for rescuing a hypo rises so much that a correction dose is needed. I should know. Every morning, I used to start the day with porridge oats, and the glucose was challenging to get right reliably. Now I know why that is.

A morning fast, or a light keto breakfast taken a couple of hours after rising, makes life easier. The advantage of a ketogenic diet at breakfast is that insulin is not required in large quantities; therefore, the rapid morning insulin injection needs only a small amount to counter the dawn effect. If we do eat carbs, we can improve our chances by having a slightly later breakfast. On this trip, I am choosing to rely on long-acting insulin to cover the dawn effect and then use physical activity to manage my glucose levels. By the time I get started on my ride, about an hour or so after waking, my circadian cortisol is on the way down; on a normal, more sedentary day, I would use rapid-acting insulin to correct the dawn effect.

After breakfast, I had another puncture-repair session. I could see that air was coming out of one of the initial repair sites, lifting a bit where the glue had failed. I reinforced the repair with three patches, which would surely do the job. Martin was keen to show me his local area by bike, and we set off towards Ludwigshafen, leaving my gear behind. It was great fun on the bike, luggage-free. It was doing what it was designed for – it felt light and lively, and was clearly enjoying itself, as was I. The ride was rapid and relatively effortless, without any baggage to haul; I could feel the wheels accelerating on the tarmac.

We rode for 17 miles, and Martin provided a running commentary on the local area, interspersed with nuggets of detail, including that a few years ago, during a drought, the Rhine at this point was so low that the ferry we were waiting for could not run. It was now at the opposite extreme and in some places was spilling over onto the cycleway. He also gave some mind-blowing numbers for the local power station, which I forgot to write down – but they were big, believe me. As was the local power station itself.

It was time to say goodbye, and we set off by car back to where I was picked up yesterday, near the bridge tower in Worms. I waved Martin off with grateful thanks for his hospitality. He had also supplied me with some cured sausages, which had effectively zero carbs, so I was set up for the day. It was now half past two in the afternoon, and progress had been slow. I had to stop to top up on spare inner tubes, which required a detour. I was slowly chomping through the sausages and experiencing a rise in blood glucose from the conversion of protein; I needed an occasional unit of rapid, but overall, the trace was good, with a maximum of 9 mmol/L (162 mg/dL).

I expected a delay in reaching my destination today because of Martin's kindness in taking time out to ride with me, but the previous hour of riding was a definite demoraliser, having to search for inner tubes and then wait for the shop to open. I wanted to get to the town of Speyer at least, by which time most of my daily target distance would be achieved, but got there at 4 pm, which was early – too early for a stopover.

Speyer is twinned with Spalding in Lincolnshire, the nearest town to the village in which I grew up. I attended secondary school in Spalding, and local families exchanged social visits with people from the twin town of Speyer. Twinning British and German towns started after the Second World War, to encourage cultural exchange. My family never took part in these exchanges, so I was curious to see what I had missed – and I was not disappointed. There was a large, wide cobbled town square, framed by tidy medieval buildings in various pastel shades, and a grand town hall with an imposing tower. I did not hang around for long. I felt rushed that day, and it would have been sensible to stay there and rest, having covered my planned daily distance; however, if I were to do so, I would fall behind the targets I had set based on the guidebook. My daily target for each stopover was based on its recommendations. I decided I needed to get another couple of hours in. I stopped to regroup in a café, to have a think and hatch a plan.

Karlsruhe was the target in the guidebook – it was only a guidebook, for goodness' sake, but I had set the daily target for each stopover based on the book's recommendations. The city was another two-and-a-half hours away. That would be three hours in practice, based on my experience on this journey – and rain was forecast in the evening, so that would mean an eight o'clock finish. I felt that was too far. I settled on a hotel with a restaurant in a town 45 minutes north, Leopoldshafen. It was roughly on my route; I just had to follow the river on one side and cross over to the town on the other side at my destination. So off I went.

It was now raining, but only lightly – enough to be felt on the face and make it wet. The sky was grey, and the headwind was brisk, occasionally gusty, and it was incessant. Out on the open road and by the vast expanse of the river, with no trees for cover, there was nothing to stop the wind, so it was a case of digging in, shifting gears to accommodate the resistance, getting my head down, and getting the job done. The thing about the headwind was not just the extra effort required to pedal, but also the constant sound of it whistling in my ears; it was a distraction and a stress.

Onward in the cold wind and spitting rain, the miles slowly counted down through the featureless agricultural landscape. It was an effort but I had put in a good shift and had just twenty-two minutes to go. I started focusing on the minutes, so keen was I to finish the day's ride. I was on a quiet road shaded from the wind by poplar trees and coasted around a bend towards the river crossing when: stop! This crossing was by ferry, not by road – and at 6:38 pm, the ferry was no longer in operation. It had completed its last journey at 6:30 pm, and the pilot was packing up, carrying a lunch bag on his shoulder and lowering the barrier. I double-checked the map; this "bridge" was a ferry! I should have zoomed in and taken more care when planning the place to stop. It was a mental disaster, at the very least. I was in the countryside on the wrong side of the Rhine and was now committed to a trip to Karlsruhe.

There was no other option; I would have to ride downriver, then dogleg back up to the same point to reach the hotel, which was within touching distance from where I was now. Booking a hotel in Karlsruhe was my first choice earlier in the day, in order to follow the guidebook, and I would have now to add the extra hour to my journey anyway as a result of this detour – but I did not want to do it; the hotel I had already booked was not cheap, and I was in the mood to be frugal. So, I set off in the rain and tried to follow the river. There was no direct route, so I took a detour into the open countryside. The satnav was having none of it; it spent 40 minutes trying to reroute me back to the ferry, but finally gave up on that idea and sent me towards the northern outskirts of Karlsruhe.

I was using Google Maps at this point, and it had been good enough for the past few days, but I was cross that I had not double-checked the river crossing. This was the second ferry crossing I had been inconvenienced by. My new time was estimated to be 8 pm – but the satnav had not finished with me yet; it had another surprise in store. The route it had calculated took me through a grassy, overgrown track for half a mile. I duly complied, and the thin wheels dug in. It was a tough and slippery ride; I prayed not to have another puncture right now. Then I found myself down a not-so-obvious road to an informal overnight lorry park, and was guided along an undulating footpath with tree roots that led to a fence that had clearly been deliberately broken to extend the path. I was unsure whether Google had intended this route, as I seemed to be going nowhere, and was starting to curse it loudly when I spotted a couple of people – lorry drivers – coming through that broken fence carrying shopping bags.

We exchanged cursory, non-committal nods. What a stroke of luck. There must be a shop nearby. I took the chance. Through the overgrown, barely identifiable path, I carried and dragged the bike over tree roots, three disused railway lines, and finally onto tarmac. A brief ride out of the woods, and I spotted a fuel station and then a supermarket. Tomorrow was a local holiday, and I had been warned that everything would be closed. But I did not want to waste any more time shopping; I still had at least 40 minutes to go, so I pressed on in the hope of finding something the next day.

Finally, I reached the bridge. I was wet, sweaty, tired, and still had a way to go – plus, I had some irritating stings from the nettles I had brushed past. Twilight was setting in. I was done in. But I had no option but to turn and ride along the opposite riverbank and head to my destination. I dug in and pedalled along a gravel track through an endless wood, watching the raindrops form perfect circles on the river to my right.

The final straw was arriving at a village and realising I had entered the wrong zip code; I had another five miles to go. It was dark as I finally checked into the hotel, which looked as tired as I felt – but it was warm and dry, with an excellent shower. It fulfilled all the functions I needed right now, and I was not complaining. I headed straight for the restaurant as it was closing in half an hour, and I was the sole diner on a wet Wednesday night. Another couple briefly joined and picked up a takeaway pizza. I ordered a mixed grill and salad.

I allowed four units of rapid for the mixed grill, as some of the salad dressing seemed sweet. I had forgotten to ask for a separate pot of olive oil. The four units did the trick. It is surprising how a mixed grill can start the warming process – all that internal heat gets the warmth to where it is needed. Half an hour later, it was aided by a hot shower and the familiar routine of writing, washing clothes and charging up every device I could.

I was glad that day was over. I calculated that I had done 90 miles, and I had felt every one of them that day. I was light on food, and apart from the mixed grill, I had only nibbled my way through two small packs of cured sausages. So much for my clean-eating plan! When I finally settled, I reflected that this had been a good challenge; in fact, the last two days had been the most challenging so far. I had been exercising for around eight hours today, if not more, and was fairly continually on the pedals. Yesterday, I did six hours or so, punctuated by punctures, so the activity was a stop-start affair. For an adventure of any kind, the unpredictable will happen, and we must be ready to react. Adventures are therefore more difficult to plan for. A park run, a marathon, a long cycle race, swimming gala, or a team football, hockey, rugby or basketball game, are fixed and relatively predictable, and insulin management can be planned more easily.

The last two days highlighted the limitations of physical activity guidelines for type 1 diabetes when you can't plan ahead. While we do need to plan, in most unplanned events in life, we need to learn to adapt to survive. I think that prioritising insulin rather than glucose is a good strategy because it helps us understand what insulin requirements actually are; we are not spending time hoping that our insulin on board will be too much or not enough. And when we know and *love* our insulin – if that is possible – our glucose will fall into line.

I could not begin to imagine how today would have panned out if I had been fuelling on carbs. I would have eaten a lot, that is for sure, intermittently injecting insulin, and likely getting far greater swings of glucose than I did on an optimised insulin strategy. And I would probably have run out of food.

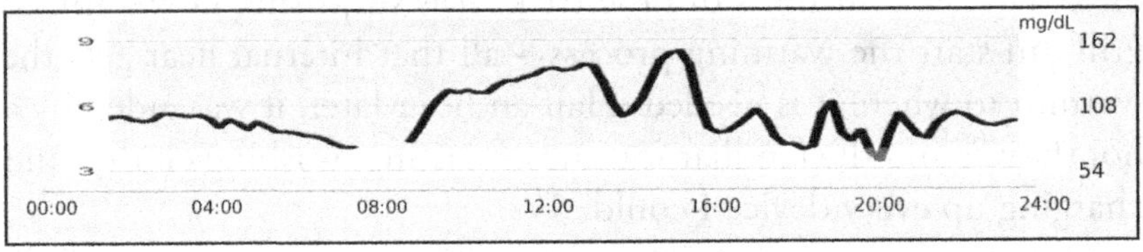

Chapter 25
Foundations of Health: Physical Activity

"Physical fitness is not only one of the most important keys to a healthy body, it is the basis of dynamic and creative intellectual activity."
– John F. Kennedy

I have made excellent progress on my adventure so far, and remain on schedule; I should be able to take a short break before the final push to St. Moritz. There will likely be challenges between here and there – there always are – but whatever crops up, my type 1 will be well controlled. I have spent much of this journey exploring how diet affects insulin volumes. Now it is time to explore the other foundations of health that influence insulin.

You can choose as many foundations of health as you like, but I think five are particularly relevant for type 1 diabetes: nutrition, physical activity, mindset, our lived environment, and circadian rhythms, which includes sleep.

Physical Activity and Type 1 Diabetes

The advantages of physical activity are no different from those for the population without type 1 diabetes, and are well known: improved muscle mass, reduced tiredness, better stamina, improved cardiovascular health, enhanced sense of wellbeing, and reduced joint pain – the list goes on. The challenge in type 1 diabetes is to ensure normal blood glucose without straying into hypoglycaemia. It is the concern about hypos that drives guideline recommendations.

I looked at a consensus statement – a report that looks into medical topics to discuss evolving research – from 21 international experts, who all concluded that reducing insulin was desirable the night before and on the day of the activity to cope with the improvement in insulin sensitivity with exercise. They also advised that the person should consume more carbohydrates during and after the activity, as insulin sensitivity would persist through the night. It is a complex balancing act that can negatively impact doing the actual sport itself. Indeed, every box in the algorithm addresses insulin reduction, glucose ingestion, or both. If we have too much insulin on board – either from overestimating doses or from increased insulin sensitivity after activity – our only option is to add glucose to avoid a hypo.

In the days when I fuelled with carbohydrates, I followed the sport-specific algorithms created for people with type 1. I believed they represented the best evidence; after all, they were developed by experts. But they were built around the assumption that sugar burning is the only viable fuel for physical activity. What a surprise, then, to realise they had not even considered multi-fuelling strategies.

The algorithms are designed for high-carb diets, and they are complicated. Every time I looked at one, I saw more boxes than you would need for a house move. These sugar-based algorithms all warned about the risk of hypos after exercise, and advise checking glucose overnight and eating glucose before bed. Imagine disturbing your digestive tract when it is meant to be resting – something I had to do every night for twenty-one nights on this journey. It would not just be disruptive; I would have been exhausted and metabolically depleted. You have to keep one eye on your glucose meter and a stash of glucose on your person.

Barriers to Exercise for People with Type 1 Diabetes

There is evidence to show that 60% of people with type 1 diabetes do not schedule exercise into their routines at all, and the main reasons given for this are fear of hypoglycaemia, work schedules, loss of control over diabetes, and low fitness levels. Despite the undoubted benefits of physical activity in type 1 diabetes, the medical profession seems to be failing to convey to T1s the advantages of exercise.

Even with guidance, an algorithm is designed for a single episode of sport. If your event is cancelled or rescheduled, or if, like me, you are doing a long-duration activity, you will need to look for one of the many small-print information boxes that accompany algorithms.

Because of the variety of sports available, algorithms can only be general. And, of course, not all physical activity counts as a sport. Dancing, gardening, and most muscle-stimulating activities can improve insulin sensitivity and are excellent options for someone with type 1 diabetes. Even pottering or regular movement can affect glucose levels – but these are not deemed worthy of an algorithm. Sport, by contrast, is a formalised, competitive, and physically demanding form of activity. Exercise can, of course, lead to blood glucose going up or down depending on the intensity, but it will mostly go down after about half an hour. I am really not surprised by the fear of hypos.

The research paper also explored the reasons people do not exercise, and I was not shocked to see the following: "Factors associated with barriers to physical activity included basic knowledge about insulin pharmacokinetics."

For me, this hits the nail on the head; it is the missing link in the chain. When I teach optimised insulin, the issue comes up repeatedly. Most people can manage the basics of carbohydrate counting, insulin estimation, and correction doses, but few are aware of how insulin works beyond this. I do not think that people can ever be confident unless they know about insulin. This is not a problem of clinical staff shortages or lack of resources; it is more about attitude.

Rethinking Fuel: Beyond Carbohydrates

Mono-fuelling on glucose alone is not ideal – denying tissues access to ketones, which many readily use, is bound to cause problems eventually. I set out on this journey to test optimised insulin and, therefore, multi-fuelling in the real world, and I am pleased to say that the practice matches the theory. I feel fit, lively, and free of injury. Each morning of my ride, I have started out fresh – no aches, no stiffness, no hesitation. I pedal off with ease and strength. It is working. And it is becoming clear to me: the algorithms need an update. Indeed, if you flip the paradigm on its head and change the fuelling method, it is likely you will not need algorithms at all.

At every half-marathon I have run, glucose is on offer throughout the course. Energy bars, gels, sugar-laced drinks – promoted by sponsors and handed out by volunteers who believe in sugar fuelling. Meanwhile, every article or documentary about sports performance seems to show top athletes refuelling with sugar mid-event. That is the visual language of sport now: athletes sipping glucose between sets or games, tennis players nibbling bananas after just two games. It all looks very technical, very scientific. But I would wager that a top-ranked player on a water-only hydration and keto fuelling strategy could match the performance of an equal-ranked player.

Sugar fuelling does work as a fuel for sport, undeniably, and I do not want to give the impression that glucose is not an excellent fuel. The sports diabetes specialists often come from athletic backgrounds themselves, so their enthusiasm makes sense. No other fuel has been found to surpass it for pure sports performance. It is true that it is readily available, and the body has highly efficient pathways that enable glucose to be used in both aerobic and anaerobic exercise; there are at least 12 glucose transport receptors – which must indicate their importance in metabolism. The science of sugar burning is mature and well established.

Limitations of Glucose Fuelling

However, glucose fuelling poses challenges for people with type 1 diabetes, because it ignores the root problem of our condition: insulin deficiency. It also assumes insulin delivery is as precise as in someone without diabetes – which it is not. Injected synthetic insulin, even the fastest types, is a blunt instrument compared with the elegant precision of the pancreas. And that matters. For someone without type 1, insulin is entrained to glucose levels. It rises and falls in perfect symphony. But for us, it lingers – even rapid-acting insulin lasts three hours, compared to the 15 minutes for insulin in those without type 1 diabetes. So, our margin of error is much greater... and the consequences are more immediate.

When you inject insulin, you inject it into the wrong part of the body, as mentioned in a previous chapter. In people without diabetes, the liver sees insulin first, and in higher concentrations. For type 1s, it is the opposite: our muscles see more insulin than our livers do. During exercise, as blood flow to the skin increases to cool the body, insulin absorption changes. This adds another variable, another layer of complexity – as I found out while waiting for the ferry, when my legs got cold.

Ketogenic Fuelling

So, if the problem is too much insulin, wouldn't the logical solution be... less insulin? On a ketogenic, fat-burning metabolism, insulin volumes are low. Fat is accessible, ketones flow, and the tissues that prefer them, like the brain, get what they need. You can't store fat and burn it at the same time, and high insulin, driven by high-carb fuelling, completely blocks fat burning. Glucose fuelling makes things harder for us. This is why optimised insulin matters – because we live in that wide margin of error of matching injected insulin to glucose levels. But when insulin is matched to the right fuel, at the right time, the system works. That is what a ketogenic diet allows. Minimal carbs mean minimal insulin. Therefore, the risk of insulin overload is low; you have less risk of chasing low glucose with sugar; you are not waking up to chew glucose tabs at 3 am.

For balance, people who consume glucose to manage their physical activity come to no harm. Glucose is an excellent and versatile energy molecule. From a calorie density standpoint, it is up there with ketones and protein – and all of these are half the energy density of fat. But we have been sold the idea that it is the only fuel worth having, and that is simply not true. I have fasted for days. I have exercised for hours on ketones and fatty acids. I have never run out of energy or hit a performance wall. And no, I am not a world-class athlete; I am just someone who wants to feel good and keep moving. I aim for consistency and would rather adopt practices that will preserve health than to "go for gold".

Muscle, Metabolism, and Longevity

The more muscle you have, the more resilient you are, health-wise. As we age and become more sedentary, many muscles are simply not being used. It is like having an arm in plaster – the unused muscles wither away, only to rebuild again once the plaster is off and function returns. Someone carrying a hod of roof tiles up a ladder a hundred times a day will build more muscle than someone performing spreadsheet calculations all day. Use builds capacity. Even the muscles used to smile – more than those needed to scowl – will atrophy if not used.

The ability to build muscle diminishes with age; some suggest muscle bulk peaks as early as age 35. Yet the human body carries large muscle groups, especially in the pelvis and legs, that hint at functions far beyond sitting. According to the Healthline.com website, muscle mass accounts for 32–44% of body weight in males and 27–33% in females in adulthood. These muscles serve functions beyond locomotion; they act as metabolic engines, which are highly relevant to type 1 diabetes.

Muscles grow with use, and their mitochondria multiply and enlarge to meet energy demands. More muscle means more glucose receptors – GLUT4s – allowing muscles to take more glucose out of the blood and into the glycogen stores. It is another route of glucose disposal, complementary to the liver's efforts. Even into old age, muscle can be rebuilt, as anyone who has had a cast removed knows. But, crucially, only with use – you can't drink protein shakes and expect a six-pack. Muscle growth requires work.

Health can't be banked, either. Fat can be stored, but it was only ever meant to be a backup energy reserve, not a permanent, enlarging mass. Muscle must be maintained in real time. The goal is to keep as many of our 700 or so muscles as possible toned and functional; if not, we pay the price in poor posture, weak joints and compromised mobility – and possibly a permanent scowl. Muscle tone and joint flexibility shape posture. Unexercised joints lead to reduced range of movement, and when core muscles atrophy, even standing up may require arm strength to push out of a chair, as they lose their ability to support body weight. The message is clear: use muscle or lose it.

The fix is not complicated. It means incorporating regular movement into daily life. Brisk walking, cycling, swimming, running – any aerobic activity will help. Resistance training builds core strength, just as joint movement maintains flexibility. Even simple balance training, like standing on one leg, is valuable. Try doing it with your eyes closed for a real challenge. Dancing is excellent for both coordination and joy; there is probably a better happy hormone profile in energetic dancing than pounding the streets in a time trial. Gardening – real gardening, not strolling with a glass of wine whilst deadheading the odd rose – also counts. These activities use skeletal muscle and improve insulin sensitivity.

Should we build new muscle or maintain what we have? It depends! What is your current fitness level? Do you have room for improvement? The answer is usually "yes". Physical activity of any sort is helpful, and many people with type 1 diabetes need encouragement, not fear. If you build muscles and fail to maintain them, they will shrink back to their optimal size for the use to which they are put. Athletes look like athletes because of the muscles they build to train for a specific sport; but, of course, your genes will define your skeletal shape – you might be a weightlifter or a 1,500-metre runner.

Optimised Insulin and Fat-Adapted Training

Many people with type 1 diabetes understand carb counting, correction doses, and mealtime boluses but very few truly grasp how insulin works. This is where optimised insulin changes things; it gives people the knowledge to manage insulin on their own terms, with confidence. It changes the question from "How do I avoid a hypo?" to "How do I fuel smartly?"

I learned the hard way. During a year of monthly half-marathons, I thought I had to fuel ahead of the run, even on a ketogenic diet, to replace the calories I was about to burn – that was the old carb-fuelling idea breaking through. I tried English breakfasts, then Bulletproof coffee. I felt bloated and sluggish.

Eventually, the lightbulb came on. I stopped eating before runs. I realised I was already fat-adapted. The stomach is not an energy store; it is a delivery system. For fat-adapted people, the fuel is already in the tank – the fat store. I did not need replacement fuel immediately; I had tens of thousands of calories already on board. That was a turning point.

Since then, I have relied on fasted training. Occasionally, I reduce basal insulin the night before if I am putting in a mammoth shift. My blood sugar stays stable. I do not get glucose spikes. I am not watching my CGM every kilometre, I am just moving. I have done it long enough now to trust the method. Sometimes I need a little glucose or a little insulin – but rarely. The fear is gone.

There have been experiments on super-athletic men that have shown that small glucose supplements extend time to exhaustion by around 20%, which is useful information. But I do not think I will ever need to use that information myself; I am usually exhausted from the start!

Fat-Burning and Understanding Your Body's Needs

Physical activity means anything that moves your muscles and raises your heart rate. It does not have to be a sport – even walking the dog or moving boxes counts. The type of activity does not matter as much as consistency. And the basics matter most: when you move, and how hard.

Here is a simple reference for estimated calorie burn per hour:

Activity	57 kg (125 lb)	84 kg (185 lb)
Cycling	500 kcal	700 kcal
Aerobic dance	400 kcal	600 kcal
Casual swimming	400 kcal	600 kcal
Jogging	400 kcal	600 kcal
Hiking	350 kcal	500 kcal

The fuel stores in the body are generous: about 2,000 calories of glycogen and 100,000 calories of fat. Unless you are elite-level, you do not need to top up anything for a short- or medium-duration workout; in fact, fuelling before exercise may be counterproductive. For long, three-hour efforts, sugar burners will need to eat. Fat burners will not, because fat is their primary fuel, but they might need small glucose supplements if their glucose levels dip.

Glucose-fuelled cyclists and runners must refuel constantly, otherwise, they "bonk" – or hit the wall. In the end, it is about understanding your body's needs. There is no single answer. But with optimised insulin and fat-adaptation, physical activity becomes less daunting and more joyful.

The great Professor Tim Noakes, a top-class sports scientist, sportsman and doctor from South Africa, has written an excellent narrative review of what is effectively the history of sports science. It makes reassuring reading if you have type 1 diabetes and want to do your physical activity in a fat-adapted state. He has meticulously explained the steps of thought that led to the idea that carbohydrates are the superior fuel.

We read it all the time in online articles, and it is still ingrained in most of our minds. It is where the idea that you need carbs for energy comes from. And with type 1, your specialist will likely advise that you need carbs for energy – we hear this a lot, and we also hear that we need to stock up on carbs before exercise to stuff the glycogen stores to their maximum capacity (around 2,000 calories for both muscle and liver). There are also many protocols that drive our desire for performance, based on the belief that glucose is the superior fuel.

How Did This All Begin?

One of the early observations of the role of metabolism in sport was that carbohydrates and fat provided most of the energy, and protein less so. It was observed that the more muscle glycogen there was, the longer you would perform before becoming exhausted. With the widespread use of muscle biopsy needles in the 1960s, it became possible to sample muscle during exercise, enabling real-time assessment of glycogen content.

There is absolutely no doubt about the findings; the studies have been replicated many times. If you examine a graph of time to exhaustion against the muscle glycogen store at the start of exercise, you see a very straight line, demonstrating that the more glycogen an athlete has at the start of exercise, the greater their endurance. If I were an athlete looking to get an edge, I would be completely invested in this. And this was the case – many sports gurus were feted for their protocols to boost glycogen stores in muscle. And many gold medals were won. It was widely accepted that glycogen stacking gets you medals because glucose is readily generated from glycogen.

Indeed, as of 2025, the US Anti-Doping Association's guidance on fuelling in sport boldly states that carbohydrates are the master fuel. It then goes on to say that "it is well known that dietary carbohydrate, even compared to protein and fat, is the most efficiently broken down and metabolised form of energy for the body." And why would you not believe an organisation whose aim is to promote drug-free maximum performance?

In addition, glucose is the only fuel available in anaerobic exercise. You may recall that mitochondria require oxygen to function; therefore, they cannot function anaerobically. And the system is clever, as one would expect. The pyruvate that normally goes to the mitochondria is shunted towards lactic acid production, which is an excellent muscle fuel in itself, especially for the heart. We can really only perform anaerobically for a minute or so, by which time the breathing has caught up, and the mitochondria can function again when they have an oxygen supply. Any excess lactic acid is reconverted to glucose by a pathway called the Cori cycle and redirected to the mitochondria.

If you exercise as a sugar burner, sooner or later, the muscle glycogen gets critically low. You will reach exhaustion. It's called "hitting the wall" in running and "bonking" in cycling. But a series of experiments on various aspects of the glucose-burning pathway, looking at ATP production in muscle fibres depleted of glycogen, have shown that the sensation of exhaustion does not correlate with energy loss at the level of the muscle cell. The energy currency of the cell, ATP, remains high in exhaustion. And of course, this is obvious when you think about it. A complete loss of energy would cause rigor mortis if there were no ATP, as the muscle fibres would be unable to function. It doesn't happen. And that highlights the problem of looking at things in isolation. We should be studying the whole human, rather than isolating the muscle cell.

Tim Noakes' idea is that there is a central governor in the brain which senses energy and de-recruits muscle fibres in response to low blood glucose, not low muscle glycogen. He postulates that there are two "glucose pools". The large glucose pool is the glycogen in the muscle, which is the one that traditional practitioners of sports medicine concentrate on. And a small glucose pool, consisting of glucose in the blood stream plus the glycogen in the liver. It is the small glucose pool that signals to the brain.

During prolonged hard exercise, the main performance risk isn't "muscle glycogen running out," but the small glucose pool glycogen in the liver pool dropping towards low blood glucose (often discussed as "exercise-induced hypoglycaemia"), which triggers central (brain) protective mechanisms that force you to slow down. In hypoglycaemia, the brain sends a signal to de-recruit muscle fibres which will, of course, degrade performance and make one feel weak.

To overcome this problem of liver glycogen deficit, one has to consume glucose, which will compensate for the lack of liver glycogen when it has been consumed during glucose-burning metabolism. The glucose that we eat to restore the brain glucose levels, does not initially contribute to the increase liver glycogen stores but raises blood glucose directly.

At cessation of exercise, the liver glycogen stores then recover, and all is well again. In a keto adapted state, because most muscle fuelling is from fatty acids, little glucose is needed to restore blood glucose, which for people with type 1 diabetes is well known. We only need a few grams of glucose to rescue hypos, not tens of grams.

Sugar-Burning vs Fat-Burning in Sports

In addition, glucose is the only fuel that can directly support ATP production in anaerobic exercise. You may recall that mitochondria require oxygen to function; therefore, they cannot function anaerobically. And the system is clever, as one would expect. The pyruvate that normally goes to the mitochondria is shunted towards lactate production, which is an excellent muscle fuel in itself, especially for the heart. We can really only perform anaerobically for a minute or so, by which time the breathing has caught up, and the mitochondria can function again when they have an oxygen supply. Any excess lactate is reconverted to glucose by a pathway called the Cori cycle in the liver and redirected to the mitochondria.

If you exercise as a sugar burner, sooner or later the muscle glycogen gets critically low. You will reach exhaustion. It is called hitting the wall in running, and "bonking" in cycling. However, a series of experiments on the glucose-burning pathway, looking at ATP production in glycogen-depleted muscle fibres, have shown that the sensation of exhaustion does not correlate with energy loss at the level of the muscle cell. The energy currency of the cell, ATP, remains high in exhaustion. This is obvious when you think about it: a complete loss of energy would cause rigor mortis if there were no ATP, as the muscle fibres would be unable to function. This does not happen – and that highlights the problem of looking at things in isolation. We should be studying the whole human, rather than isolating the muscle cell.

Tim Noakes' idea is that there is a central governor in the brain which senses energy and de-recruits muscle fibres. This response is due to low blood glucose caused by a reduction in liver glycogen, not muscle glycogen. If the brain sends a signal to de-recruit muscle fibres, it will, of course, degrade performance and make one feel weak. To overcome this problem of liver glycogen deficit, consuming glucose raises blood sugar to compensate for the glycogen used during glucose-burning metabolism. Glucose does not increase glycogen stores but raises blood glucose. At cessation of exercise, the glycogen stores recover, and all is well again.

So, if you want to use glucose for your sport, you will do well, and there is a lot of science to back this up. If you work to this model of fuelling for exercise, you will need to follow the many sport-specific protocols I have mentioned. If you are a sugar burner, you will need more insulin at rest, and need active insulin management for your sport. If you have type 1 diabetes, you will need to be prepared to eat glucose for endurance and adjust your insulin dosing down.

Where does this leave people like me, who are not fuelling with glucose but doing fat-burning – and therefore keto – fat-fuelled exercise? It makes metabolic sense to reduce insulin and carbohydrates in someone who can't produce insulin. But can this be made to work in sport and physical activity? Is there any evidence for the sense of fitness and vitality I have experienced on this adventure? Can this approach sustain a steady riding pace without exhaustion, even though the majority of the evidence points overwhelmingly towards fuelling with carbohydrates?

But I was pleased to find that people are researching fat burning. The breakthrough paper for me is the research on the crossover point for fat burners. There is a well-known idea in sports science called the "crossover point". It describes how the body changes its fuel during exercise. During easy exercise, the body mainly uses fat for energy. As exercise becomes harder, the body gradually switches to using carbohydrates (glucose).

Fat Adaptation: Evidence and Benefits

Traditionally, sports scientists believe four things:

1. When you reach around 60% of your maximum effort (VO max – or maximal oxygen uptake), you start using more carbohydrate than fat. This is the crossover point.
2. Everyone has a level of exercise where they burn the most fat. This is called FatMax and usually occurs at low intensities.
3. At very hard exercise (above 85% VO max), fat burning becomes very low, so carbohydrates become almost the only fuel.
4. Eating a high-carb diet gives the best performance because it fills up your glycogen stores, especially with carb-loading before events.

The fourth idea has been repeated for so long that it is treated as a fact, but newer research shows that things are not so simple. Recent studies on people who follow a low-carb, high-fat (LCHF or ketogenic) diet show something different:

1. In LCHF-adapted athletes, the crossover point shifts to over 80% VO_2 max, compared with 60% in traditional diets.
2. These athletes can reach much higher rates of fat burning – more than 1.5 g/min, instead of the previously quoted 0.3–0.6 g/min.
3. Even during very hard exercise, like repeated 800-metre intervals at more than 85% VO_2 max, they still burn huge amounts of fat. In fact, the highest fat-burning rates ever recorded were in these LCHF-adapted athletes.

This challenges the old belief about carbohydrates in high-intensity exercise, and for people with type 1 diabetes, this is reassuring. It shows that:

- We can still perform at a very high level.
- We do not need to load up on large amounts of carbs.
- We can avoid the complicated routines of pre-, during-, and post-exercise fuelling.

- Performance can match traditional carb-fuelled athletes.

Empowered Physical Activity

These findings are a breakthrough for people with type 1 diabetes, and bring into question the prevailing doctrine that carbohydrates must be the predominant oxidised fuel during high-intensity exercise. The key determinant that made this possible was choosing subjects who were adapted to burn fat. In the past, shortcuts to ketosis without suitable preparation have not shown the same results; you need to have been on a ketogenic diet for around four weeks to get the benefits. Fat adaptation is the key.

Furthermore, some researchers recently found that 30% of middle-aged, competitive athletes without type1 diabetes had prediabetic glucose values while on a high-carb diet, and that this was reversed when they switched to a very low-carb diet. This is further evidence for people with type 1 diabetes that a low-carb approach to physical activity makes sense scientifically – and we know about the inflammatory effects of higher-than-optimal glucose and insulin.

A ketogenic diet does not require the ingestion of glucose or any carbohydrate for energy in sport. However, as I have demonstrated in the early part of this adventure, getting it right every time can be a challenge. Hypo treatment should always be available, and if your long-distance sports involve a mix of anaerobic and aerobic activity, a glucose supplement might be needed. But the benefits of a ketogenic diet in type 1 diabetes are clear: reduced insulin requirements lead to smoother glucose control and the availability of a full range of fuel sources.

I have always believed that people with type 1 can do anything they want – climb Everest, sail the seven seas, and do extreme and not-so-extreme sports – the same as those without the condition. However, it is becoming clear to me that if I want to do this repeatedly and into old age, a ketogenic diet and an understanding of insulin for all the foundations of health are the best way to achieve that.

Chapter 26

Total Miles: 748

Day 11 – Eggenstein-Leopoldshafen to Kehl, 60 miles

"Jack Sprat could eat no fat, His wife could eat no lean. And so between them both, you see, They licked the platter clean."
– Old English Rhyme

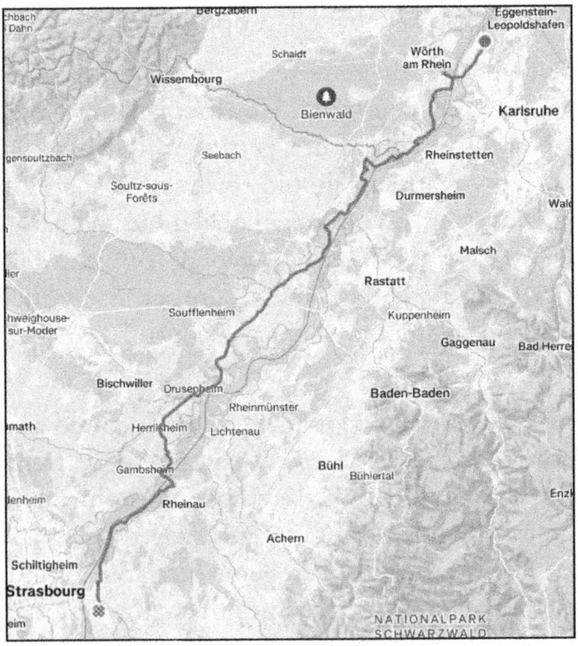

If I wanted a coasting day, then this was it. For some reason, I woke early and checked the CGM, then went back to sleep for a couple of hours. The route was going to be slightly under my target distance of 60 miles a day, and the weather looked fair. Psychologically, it is interesting how my daily distance travelled is becoming an issue. Both of my longer rides have been tough: Day 1 with a 77-mile start and some punishing climbs when I had expected 67, and the 90-mile buster yesterday, what with the ferry not running, the rain, and the late finish. It is the lateness of the finishes that really punishes. On arrival, there is still a fair bit to do before I can relax, and by the time I get round to diarising the trip, it is then too late to do anything else.

This day was a regional holiday: Corpus Christi. It marked the 60th day after Jesus' crucifixion and seems to be well observed here in southern Germany. There was no breakfast available at the hotel, and no shops were open. It was not a problem for me; I would fast it out and see what I could find. So, I injected my six units of Tresiba and no rapid just then. I was heading close to the Lidl supermarket I cycled past yesterday, and took a detour to it around a massive retail park. There, I spied the "Golden Arches", and that was my only option. McDonald's is never usually on my radar, but I was limited in my choices and starting to fear that fuel station food was going to be all I could get for the day. A Big Mac double burger with no bun made a convenient and nutritious meal, and I was on my way.

I thought the protein was about right for the day, but felt that a bit of rapid-acting insulin would be prudent. There is always the possibility of having less insulin on board when on an optimised insulin strategy. It is a concept that does not apply to the usual high-carb diet, where insulin is consistently high and often elevated above needed levels – that is why people yo-yo on the glucose rollercoaster. I do not get such a problem when I take little insulin. It is still a novelty to think about too little insulin, and I do feel excited about this, as it means that my level of insulin is near optimum; it is better to top up in a timely way with insulin than do an emergency top-up with glucose.

I was thankfully soon off the busy road and onto the quieter trails of the Rhine route. I noticed the route signs were good and helpful; clearly, the head of the local state traffic department is a cyclist. The roads around here were excellent for biking, and I was finding this in many parts of the Rhine route: smooth, often tarmacked or metalled cycle tracks away from traffic, and even where we had to blend into a road, there was nearly always a cycle lane. Not needing to share the road with motor vehicles is a rarity to a Brit like me, and a real treat. The sheer number of different cycle tracks in this region is mind-boggling; I counted twelve at one junction. The obvious route is not necessarily the right one, and map scrutiny is needed: zoom in, pan out, and get the general direction. And I remember that the sun is always in the south at midday, so I generally follow that southwards.

I soon got into my rhythm and sped along. The sun was coming out, and with a short ride in prospect, it was going to be a good one. Such was the ease of the day that I managed an actual stop by the river in a large grassy space occupied by a burger van and some chairs. It was perfect in the warm sun, and I was able to take a relaxing break. There was a small queue around the van, and the owner was a craggy-faced, large and brusque, but polite, man who knew his purpose: to sell product and make money. He was organised and efficient. I tried my best German, which was not a lot, but I felt I was expected to try. His English was not good either, so we got by with some added pointing.

In addition to the sparkling water, I ordered a Coke Zero; I needed a change of taste and did not want coffee in the sun. It was a very sweet taste, but as a rare digression from my regimen, it was acceptable. He was also selling small bottles of cold beer – around seven grams of carbs – straight out of the fridge. I like beer, but rarely drink it these days; it has quite a lot of carbs, and lagers also contain wheat.

Coeliac disease – a wheat allergy – I do not have, but coeliac disease is several times more likely in people with type 1 diabetes; they might be linked in some ways. Even though my pancreas is not producing insulin, I think it is prudent not to make a habit of taking something linked to type 1 diabetes. It cannot get much worse with respect to the diabetes itself, but might it have other subtle effects that we are not measuring? I do not know, but personally, I am steering clear – however, sometimes in a similar situation, after a day's exercise with friends, I might have a beer. It is risk versus reward.

Another interesting fact I have learned about wheat is that it contains phytic acid. A grain or legume seed contains phytic acid. What phytic acid does is effectively act as a magnet for the metals zinc, calcium and iron; it is also a source of phosphorus. A sprouting seed responding to heat and moisture has two immediate objectives: put out a root for water and nutrients, and put up some leaves to act as solar panels for energy. Once this has been achieved, the plant is self-sustaining.

In the meantime, the starch in the seed is the energy supply, and the wheat germ, containing phytic acid and other nutrients, is the source of those elements needed to support the development of the early plant. Phytic acid releases metals during this process. In the human intestine, however, it tends to act as a magnet that hangs on rather than releases its metal elements. One study has shown that eating zinc-rich oysters with bread reduces zinc absorption to almost zero. It is something to consider if you eat pulses and grains; the timing of eating other foods might be important.

I found a lovely seat facing the river, and took in the sun's rays. The river in these parts has many lakes and tributaries that flow into it. I learned that in the 19th century, an army general decided to improve the river's navigability by straightening and deepening it – and so it was that the Rhine today has changed from its original course. With such a wide and fast-flowing river, I never would have thought it possible to engineer on such a scale 200 years ago. But there is no intervention in nature without upsetting the balance; I heard that after this feat of engineering, work was needed to cope with flooding in the wet season, as all that diverted water, having a clear, straight run, hits an unexpected downstream bottleneck.

I think it is all now in harmony, but it does go to show how changing a fine balance – in this case, the course of a river – will alter the environment. Change one variable, and there are consequences; not necessarily negative, but altering any system leads to knock-on effects. It is exactly this in type 1 diabetes: we must replace our missing insulin, but we do it imperfectly.

Off I went along a delightful rural route. The sun was shining, and I was making good time. It was easy to feel good. I was just following the river and the signs to Strasbourg, and the sat nav – today it was Google Maps again – for once, agreed with me. Now that was a rarity! I coasted into a large village with a decorative roundabout, which was not typical for Germany – it must have been a local thing. Then, I spotted a shop. It was called a boulangerie. Then another, a charcuterie. Boulangerie? Charcuterie? I had strayed into France. There were no borders and had been no notification, but it was a weekday after 2 pm, and the shops were open. Corpus Christi was not observed here. How lucky was that?

The charcuterie did not stand a chance: chicken drumsticks, cured meats, and something called fromage de tête, which was a terrine with jellified meat chunks – bits of a pig's head, I guessed. It had no carbs and looked good, so it was something I could munch on en route. It was perfect timing, and I spent a happy fifteen minutes sitting on a bench consuming about half of what I had bought, then set off on my way, feeling good.

It is amazing how French this tiny village was: the décor, the street lighting (it always amazes me how individual street lighting is in French villages), and the decorated roundabouts. There was even a lady in a mint-green Citroen 2CV pootling along the cobblestone street. Yes, definitely France; no blending of styles across a border. Unmistakably, Germany is one metre that way. Unmistakably, France is right next to it.

Just up the road, I topped up with water, some meat and cheese at a Lidl. I also bought some dark chocolate with nuts – and for some bizarre reason, I bought some cream. I felt like I needed it, and I was getting fed up with cheese. To date, my diet on the roads was meat- and cheese-heavy; far too much processed meat for my liking. I usually eat a wider variety of foods, so I decided I must add some variety. I had a few squares of dark chocolate, expecting to burn them off on the ride.

My glucose after the ride had nudged up to eight, and I needed an insulin correction. In addition, the chocolate added to my carb intake – but not by much: perhaps six grams. I absentmindedly took a couple of units of rapid insulin to cover the chocolate; I really do not know why. I was not thinking about insulin, but something else; a couple of units would have been fine if I were in an office all day. Things like this error happen sometimes – other times, I cannot even remember if I have injected or not.

The cream, I know, pushes my glucose up. I seem to reach a higher plateau than desirable when I take a lot of cream, in the high single figures (multiply by 18 to calculate mg/dL). But this time, being fit and having good insulin sensitivity, that small insulin correction cut in very quickly, and then I found myself chasing a possible hypo indication, with a vertical down arrow on the CGM. Some glucose tablets were needed.

I avoided an actual hypo, and never had symptoms; I was responding to the trend on the graph. I carried on riding. The gradient on the CGM seemed too steep on this occasion. Often, I ignore the CGM and ride to the start of the hypo sensation, but I think I was more alert because of the indulgence of lunch and the lapse in concentration regarding my insulin. And why I indulged in cream is anyone's guess. I suppose there are occasions when being squeaky-clean gets too much, and you just have to give in. I can imagine the food puritans tutting…

I took the opportunity of a sunny break and booked my evening's accommodation, which was under two hours away – but the time had rolled on, what with the break by the river and this one. My estimated time of arrival had slipped from 16:00 to 18:00. In addition, I had chosen to extend my journey to take me out of

Strasbourg and on to a small town on the German side of the Rhine close by. An hour later, I was heading out of France and back into Germany. There was now a brisk wind from the south, and it was time to get the head down and dig in. But it was no effort really, just a change of gear, a bit slower, and a bit more pressure on the pedals. I was quite fit now, and physical effort was not something I needed to worry about.

The last couple of hours were a delightful ride along a mixture of roads, cycle paths and gravel tracks along the Rhine. There were a few fishermen out braving the wind and the increasingly cloudy sky. It was cool, and I needed to keep pedalling and wear a long-sleeved top. It was an uneventful and relaxed arrival at a delightful boutique hotel in the town of Kehl, which is a small, pretty town in the Black Forest, and a popular tourist destination. It was complete luck for me to choose this place to stay, tucked away just off the centre of town.

The hotel had secure bike parking called a Velo Box, which was essentially a locked, heavy door off the street leading to their small garden. It was uncovered, but the bike would be safe for the night. To be honest, I never felt the need to be careful with parking any more than normal; I always lock up and turn off the lights, but that is a habit. To quote the saying from Arab countries, "Trust in Allah, but always tie up your camel." It works. Plus, my bike is old, scratched, and not a magnet for any tempted criminals looking to turn a profit – that is freeing in itself.

After getting all the admin out of the way, I took myself to the bar to indulge in a bottle of sparkling water. The water was drunk in minutes; I ordered a second straight away as I felt dehydrated. Best to listen to the body and drink to thirst – I needed all of that water. But on the trip, I had not felt weak or dehydrated. When I felt thirsty, I paid attention. I could almost feel the water being absorbed.

I went up to my room and got on with my own admin: charged up the batteries, checked the food diary, recorded the events of the day, sent out some pics on Instagram, made sure insulin had been recorded, and wrote a diary entry ready for this book. Having showered and washed my clothes, I spent a bit of time checking the weather. I had had a good sunny day that day, but clouds were brewing in the afternoon; it was not looking as good tomorrow. With wall-to-wall rain on every weather app I could find, it was likely to be correct. I had calculated at least a seven-hour ride to get to Basel as my intended destination – but that was okay, as today was 10 miles less, and I was feeling good.

I turned off the phone, unfazed. I am used to the weather now, and tomorrow I will be in Switzerland briefly, before heading back into Germany. I can see my progress on the map and have reached well over halfway. It is all looking good.

For some reason, I never recorded the meal I ate in a restaurant that night, but I did note that I took a couple of units of rapid, in addition to the now-usual six units of Tresiba. I think it was lamb cutlets with a few vegetables. It did raise the glucose, but I was pleased to see a good level when I woke.

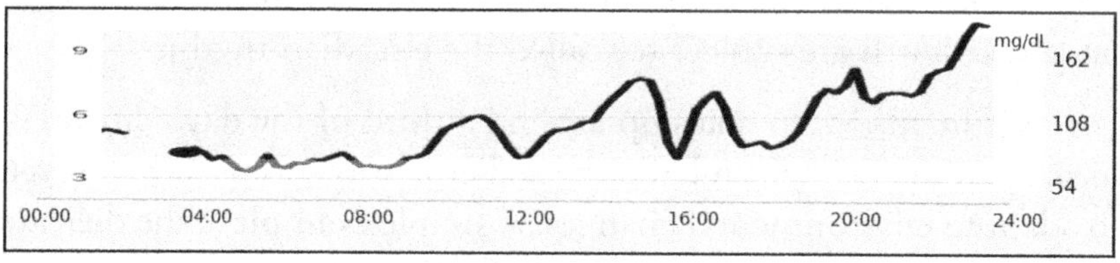

Chapter 27
Foundations of Health: Circadian Rhythms and Sleep, Keeping the Body Synchronised with Nature

Like a circle in a spiral, like a wheel within a wheel, never ending or beginning on an ever-spinning reel
– Windmills of Your Mind, The Thomas Crown Affair

A psychiatrist friend of mine once told me that when he asked patients, "If there's one thing we could change today, what would that be?" the most common answer was that they would like to sleep better. This chapter is about the 24-hour rhythm that all organisms on planet Earth are subject to, called the circadian rhythm.

For us humans, sleep takes up around a third of the day. Circadian means "around a day" (in Latin, circa diem). Organisms have evolved to adapt to environmental changes. A simple example is the delicate leaf of the mimosa plant. It opens during the day and closes at night to reduce water loss from evaporation. However, if you expose a mimosa plant to constant darkness over several days, it continues to open and close its leaves on a 24-hour cycle. That implies the presence of a built-in clock that has evolved to prepare the plant for morning light. Even bacteria have been shown to exhibit daily variation in activity.

A significant study of this in humans was conducted by Michel Siffre, a French scientist who lived in a cave for 60 days in 1962, and repeated the experiment in 2000 for 73 days. He had no contact with the outside world and remained in a dimly lit environment.

His body clock adopted a free-running 25-hour cycle in the absence of sunlight or other time cues. Each day, he woke approximately one hour later than the day before. Over 24 days, he effectively lost a whole day because he had not entrained his circadian rhythm with the day-night cycle and was thus unable to reset to 24 hours. People who are blind, through damaged or absent eyes, adopt a different rhythm from those with a functioning visual pathway. This has practical implications. For instance, if you try to synchronise your lunchtime eating to a 24-hour clock, but your circadian rhythm is out of phase, your body may not be optimally prepared to process food.

If we look at human behaviours, it has long been known that different physiological or cognitive functions are more, or less, effective at certain times. For instance, most people sleep between 11 pm and 7 am. You are likely to make your best decisions in the middle of the morning and again in the middle of the afternoon. You are more likely to crash a car at 04:30 am or shortly after lunch. The postprandial dip that people talk about, which follows a meal, is largely due to the body clock rather than eating itself – it is just that the alerting signal from your body clock is not very strong at that time of day.

Body systems have rhythms. Body clocks are primarily controlled by light, secondarily by temperature, and thirdly by food. These are known as zeitgebers (German for "time-givers"). Many cellular processes, such as cell division, occur at specific times of the day or night. Skin cells, for instance, divide at night. This is likely because dividing during the day, when exposed to ultraviolet (UV) radiation, could increase the risk of mutations that can promote skin cancer. The body is prepared for the rising of the sun; it does not wait for the sun to come up before it reacts.

If you do something that shifts your body clock, this can disrupt natural physiological processes. Different body systems operate differently at different times, and this has implications for the timing of medical interventions. For example, light therapy for seasonal affective disorder – a mood disorder linked to the changing seasons

– is far more effective when given in the morning than at night, by a factor of around two. The same applies to chemotherapy. Administering chemotherapeutic agents at specific times in the 24-hour cycle results in varying levels of effectiveness and side effects.

So how is this organised? Current interpretations of the science suggest that there is a master clock in the middle of the brain connected to secondary clocks in every cell throughout the body. If you took cells from, say, the liver (secondary clocks) and placed them in a Petri dish, they would show a 25-hour cycle. Even under constant light, they would maintain this rhythm. The master clock brings them back to a 24-hour cycle. It is located in an area called the suprachiasmatic nucleus (SCN), deep in the brain. Left to its own devices, the SCN would also adopt a 25-hour cycle. Resetting it to 24 hours begins when a light signal enters the eye in the morning. This light sets the master clock and synchronises the secondary clocks. Without light, it does not reset.

The retina has non-visual receptors in addition to the light receptors (photoreceptors). These respond to blue-green light, but rather than sending a visual signal to the brain, they send an instruction to the master clock in the SCN. Melanopsin is the pigment found in these photoreceptors. This blue-green range of wavelengths is present in natural daylight. It is present in most artificial lights and is prominent in harsh blue-white lights, including high-intensity LEDs. This is the wavelength that affects your circadian clock. People who have had a stroke and can't see because the visual part of their brain is damaged can still reset their body clocks if the SCN is intact.

Sleep Drive

This brings us to the next point. Exposure to artificial light late at night delays the body clock. It is biologically unnatural and unphysiological. That is not good for us, as it disrupts the natural timing of sleep and metabolism. Pre-industrial night lighting was relatively dim. For example, candlelight is low in intensity and relatively deficient in blue wavelengths.

It is not just about colour and wavelength; it is also about brightness and the timing of light exposure. Humans have evolved over hundreds of thousands of years. It is only in the past century that we have had access to bright artificial lighting. We are the only species that deliberately expose ourselves to bright light at night, which disrupts our circadian biology. People who do night shifts tend to have shorter life expectancy than those who work during the day.

Eating out of sync with your circadian clock is also associated with impaired metabolism. Many IT device manufacturers now include features that restrict blue-green light in the evening. Light can shift the body clock by more than an hour in the morning, helping to synchronise it to the natural day-night cycle. The effect of light diminishes throughout the morning, and by around noon, its phase-shifting effect is much weaker. Morning light is therefore critical.

As the day progresses towards the sleep period, the circadian clock gradually drifts later, contributing to the natural evening delay in alertness. The circadian clock then recovers during the dawn and early morning hours, aligning with the day-light cycle.

Out-of-sync phase shifts of the body clock due to poor light management are cumulative; if the clock is not reset each morning, this phase delay disrupts metabolic regulation as secondary cellular clocks fail to synchronise with the master clock. What this means is that, even when you want to go to sleep, the other circadian drivers may still be trying to keep you awake. Jet lag is a good example of a desynchronised circadian clock. The worst thing you can do at night is check your email on your laptop without a blue-green light filter activated. Otherwise, it will cause a circadian phase delay and may make it harder to fall asleep.

The circadian shift is one part of a sleep theory called the Two-Process Model, which explains how our body regulates sleep timing. Circadian drivers for sleep are called Process C. The second component of this model is the homeostatic sleep drive known as Process S. You might think of Process S as a sleep-promoting substance that accumulates during wakefulness, induces sleep when it reaches a particular level, and then dissipates during sleep, reaching a low concentration by morning. The chemical most commonly associated with this process is adenosine, which builds up in various brain regions and promotes sleepiness. During sleep, adenosine levels are lower.

However, Process S does not fully explain our experience. We do not feel increasingly sleepy throughout the day in a linear fashion; we can remain fully alert throughout the day, but still experience predictable dips in alertness, such as the early-afternoon dip. This is because Process C, or the circadian alerting signal, counters the homeostatic drive, Process S.

Our adaptive sleep drive is also shaped by lifestyle choices, such as phone use, screen time or late-night exercise. An understanding of these habits allows us to make informed decisions, even if we occasionally choose to "take a hit" and disrupt our rhythm temporarily – we then have the tools to recover the situation.

Chronotype

Another essential concept is chronotype: are you an owl, a lark or a hummingbird? This trait is genetically determined – it is hardwired. If you are someone who functions well in the morning and goes to bed early, you should embrace that. Attempts to work against your chronotype are generally unsuccessful. The remainder fall somewhere between the two types and show characteristics of both on a sliding scale. You do not need to test; most of us just know. From an evolutionary perspective, it makes sense for members of a group to have staggered periods of alertness so that someone is always awake to keep watch. It would not necessarily be safe for an entire tribe to sleep simultaneously.

Another important concept is biphasic sleep. There is considerable historical evidence suggesting that people living in pre-industrial societies naturally adopt biphasic sleep. This means going to bed at, say, 9 or 10 pm, waking around 2 am, staying awake for an hour or two, then going back to sleep. This may have been evolutionarily advantageous, allowing people to tend to fire or animals. Cultures that practise siestas, such as in Mediterranean countries, demonstrate biphasic sleep patterns. Many of us might fall into this pattern if modern work schedules did not so tightly regulate our lives. The expectation that eight hours of uninterrupted sleep is "normal" is a relatively recent idea. Fragmented sleep is, in fact, quite common. Many people wake in the night and believe they have a sleep disorder, when, in reality, this is a normal physiological pattern. A quiet activity before returning to bed may be all that is needed.

For anyone raising teenagers, it is important to understand that as adolescence progresses, the circadian rhythm becomes increasingly delayed. Teenagers naturally want to go to bed later and wake up later. This is not simply rebellion; it is a biological development. In that sense, we are running schools for adults, not for the pupils.

This biological delay in teenagers overlays their inherent chronotype of being an owl, lark or hummingbird. Added to this is the common habit of using screens late at night, which further delays the body clock. If a teenager goes to bed very late and then misses the early morning light, they may not receive the necessary signal to reset their master clock. One marker of the end of adolescence is the circadian clock's return to a more conventional timing.

In summary, sleep is one of many circadian phenomena regulated by the body's master clock, whose signals actively promote wakefulness. The vital phase response to light is most sensitive at the beginning and end of the day, and bright morning light, alongside darkness at night, helps stabilise body rhythms.

The circadian cycle affects a wide range of biological systems. For example, there are thought to be many hundreds of circadian-controlled genes and systems, including the immune system, gene transcription, insulin regulation, cortisol levels, body temperature, and sleep patterns. The role of the central clock is to synchronise all these systems so that they interact efficiently and healthily. Core body temperature is a helpful indicator of your position in the 24-

hour cycle. If someone is disconnected from environmental cues, kept in constant darkness or light, they adopt a free-running 25-hour cycle.

Melatonin

Melatonin is a hormone best known for its role in sleep. It helps synchronise peripheral clocks and participates in a feedback loop that stabilises the master clock (the SCN). If taken at the right time, melatonin supplements can shift the circadian rhythm. It is a chronobiotic – it shifts the body clock's timing. It also increases hand and foot temperature, which lowers the core body temperature. It is not a sedative. Like morning light, melatonin creates a phase shift, so knowing your circadian phase is useful, especially after travel or disrupted routines.

Melatonin is secreted by the pineal gland in response to darkness. It is also produced in mitochondria for its antioxidant functions, but outside the brain it does not affect circadian rhythms. It is a question of nuance; this same molecule can have many actions. Melatonin affects insulin in the following ways:

- At night, it reduces insulin secretion (conserving energy use during sleep).
- It may increase insulin resistance slightly – this is protective against hypoglycaemia.
- Poor sleep and melatonin imbalance (chronodisruption) are linked to increased insulin resistance and poor blood sugar control.

Circadian Rhythms and Insulin

Although we usually think of insulin release as occurring when we eat, it is also strongly influenced by the time of day. Insulin itself has a circadian rhythm. People are naturally more sensitive to insulin in the first part of the day and more resistant later in the day. This suggests that eating earlier is biologically easier for the body – but not so early that it clashes with the temporary reduction in insulin sensitivity caused by the dawn-effect hormones, such as cortisol and GH.

For people with type 1 diabetes, this becomes a compromise. Cortisol rises in the early morning as part of the wake-up process, temporarily decreasing insulin sensitivity, an effect that fades about 90 minutes after waking. This can make early breakfast insulin doses tricky, as mentioned in an earlier chapter. At the same time, fasting for longer periods – such as 16 hours – can support metabolic health. People with type 1 have to blend these facts with their own routines and lifestyle. It is rarely perfect science; it is practical living.

When everything is working well, insulin rises and falls through the day in a steady rhythm. This helps the body absorb glucose when needed and store extra energy safely. When this rhythm is disrupted – by irregular eating, constant snacking, or eating late at night – blood sugar becomes harder to manage. Over time, these mismatches can contribute to insulin resistance and increase the risk of metabolic problems, including type 2 diabetes.

Constant snacking is especially disruptive because it interferes with another hormone called leptin. Leptin follows its own circadian rhythm. It rises at night to reduce hunger and support fasting during sleep.

Insulin also works best earlier in the day. When insulin is high at night – because of late meals or late snacking – it blunts the normal leptin signal and confuses the brain about the body's energy stores. Eating late in the evening, especially high-carb or high-fat meals, pushes up insulin at a time when tissues are naturally less responsive. This encourages fat storage and increases the risk of insulin resistance.

Over time, the brain becomes less sensitive to leptin's "we have enough energy" message. This is leptin resistance, which often develops alongside, or before, insulin resistance. You can have type 1, type 2, or both, and leptin resistance plays a part in each of these conditions if insulin is higher than optimal. Leptin regulates appetite, weight, fertility, and even bone health, but its main job is energy balance.

Eating when the body is preparing for sleep makes digestion harder. Digestion is an inflammatory process, and the gut needs rest at night. Heavy late meals often sit uncomfortably because the body is trying to cool down for sleep. Protein digestion generates heat, which works against this cooling. From the perspective of both leptin and insulin, eating too close to bedtime creates confusion. The insulin spike after a late meal interferes with leptin's signalling to the hypothalamus. The brain receives a mixed message and assumes energy levels are low, so it encourages eating. Poor light habits – especially bright light late at night or missing morning light – further weaken leptin signalling.

For people prone to late-night eating, shifting the main meal earlier in the day makes a real difference. Even something like a Big Mac eaten at midday causes less weight gain than the same meal eaten late at night. The point is not the food choice but the timing (chrononutrition). Our biology runs on a clock. Modern metabolic problems often arise from a combination of poor lighting, late meals, inappropriate food choices, leptin resistance, alongside other lifestyle factors.

In addition to leptin and insulin, many other hormones also follow 24-hour rhythms. Cortisol rises before dawn, GH pulses early in sleep, and catecholamines like norepinephrine affect appetite and feeding behaviour. Cholesterol production also peaks at night. This reflects the circadian system's coordinated regulation of both metabolism and daily physiological patterns.

In type 1 diabetes, insulin is injected rather than produced internally, so its timing is no longer automatically linked to the body's natural rhythms. This creates challenges. But, as we have seen throughout this chapter, lifestyle habits – light, food timing, sleep and movement – can help bring the rest of the system back into alignment.

Understanding and Improving Sleep

Many people struggle with sleep. The mechanisms behind it are not overly complicated, but several factors must align to ensure good sleep quality. If you look at sleep research, you will encounter hypnograms, which show brain activity across sleep cycles. The brain switches between three states: wakefulness, rapid eye movement (REM) sleep, and non-rapid eye movement (NREM) sleep. A complete sleep cycle lasts approximately 90 to 110 minutes and repeats several times throughout the night. The process generally follows this order:

NREM Stage 1: The transition from wakefulness to sleep, lasting a few minutes.

Stage 2: A period of light sleep where heart rate and breathing slow down and body temperature drops.

Stage 3: This is the deep or slow-wave sleep stage, when most brain repair and memory consolidation occur, especially for semantic memory (e.g., remembering where you bought your bicycle), as opposed to procedural memory (e.g., how to ride it).

You then enter the first REM stage, characterised by rapid eye movements, increased brain activity (similar to being awake), temporary muscle paralysis, and vivid dreams. REM sleep is when dreaming occurs. During this stage, the body is paralysed (except for the heart and lungs) as a protective mechanism, which stops us from acting out our dreams physically.

Most deep sleep happens early in the night and decreases with each cycle – the opposite of REM sleep. It is normal to wake briefly after each cycle – most people roll over and go back to sleep. People who believe they sleep poorly often become anxious after waking during the first cycle, which, ironically, keeps them awake.

Sleep is vital. Laboratory studies show that rats, and likely most mammals, die if deprived of sleep entirely, though the exact cause remains unclear. Other factors also influence sleep. Alcohol reduces consciousness but wears off during the night, making waking more likely – especially during REM stages. Meanwhile, caffeine blocks adenosine receptors (Process S) and remains in the body for several hours. When caffeine wears off, adenosine can then promote sleep. That same adenosine can be repeatedly blocked by caffeine binding to it, thereby keeping us alert. Caffeine does not degrade adenosine;

it only blocks its action. Some sources recommend avoiding caffeine after midday to help with sleep. People differ in their ability to metabolise caffeine, and this can be assessed through genetic testing. Stimulants such as caffeine, chocolate and certain prescription drugs may reduce sleep drive.

Late-night exercise also affects sleep by increasing alertness and core body temperature, especially if it is intense. Avoiding mental stimulation, anxiety or late meals can all help restore balance. Blue light phase-shifts melatonin in the wrong direction and delays sleep. Late meals interfere with natural body cooling and leptin signalling, which can disrupt sleep.

Many people simply spend too long in bed. If you need seven hours of sleep but go to bed at 10 pm and rise at 8 am, you are spending ten hours in bed, three of which may be spent tossing and turning – and you will come to associate your bed with poor sleep.

If you struggle with sleep, ask: is there sufficient homeostatic sleep pressure? Has adenosine built up? Are you reducing wakefulness appropriately before bed? If you visit a sleep clinic, one of the first things they will assess is whether you are spending too much time in bed. Trying to "catch up" by sleeping in can worsen the problem.

Optimising Sleep Practices: Sleep Hygiene

There are many factors that contribute to a good night's sleep:

- Has your body clock shifted?
- Are you exposing yourself to light in the morning?
- Are you avoiding light – especially blue light – at night?
- Are you reducing your homeostatic sleep drive with caffeine, exercise or late-night eating? Are falling alcohol levels affecting your sleep?
- Are you respecting your chronotype (owl, lark or hummingbird)?
- Are you spending more time in bed than you need for sleep?

To try to mitigate poor sleep, if you wake up and can't sleep after 20 minutes, get out of bed and do something quiet in dim light. And avoid stimulating activities or electronic devices.

In some situations, sleep disruption is more persistent. For example, long-term alcohol use or a serious head injury can significantly impair sleep regulation. In such cases, sleep hygiene becomes even more important. One of the most common causes of relapse in people recovering from alcohol dependence is the inability to sleep.

Sleep is a complex but essential part of our circadian biology. Understanding its interaction with light, hormones, temperature, behaviour and metabolism allows us to optimise our routines for better health, especially in the context of conditions such as type 1 diabetes.

Chapter 28
Total miles: 818

Day 12 – Kehl to Neuenburg, 70 miles

"Do the best you can until you know better. Then when you know better, do better."
– Maya Angelou

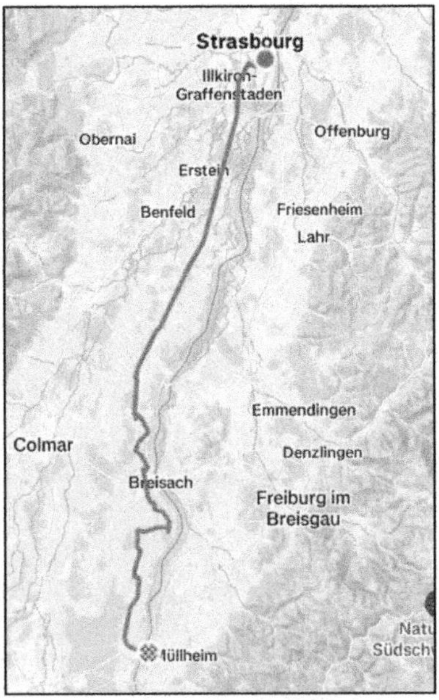

There is no way around this. Today looks rainy, and it doesn't look like I can avoid it: wall-to-wall rain, according to my usually reliable

XC weather app. It often gets timings wrong, and I am hoping it has this time; a glance at the rain radar is not hopeful – but do I see a sliver of a rain-free area around Basel? Two other apps are predicting rain as well; however, Darren Betts on the BBC weather app, who is meant to be a reliable weather forecaster, mentioned that the rain belt was slowly drifting east. Still, it did not seem like I was going to be able to avoid a drenching.

Additionally, the temperature was only expected to reach 12 degrees Celsius at best. After yesterday's lovely weather, except for the wind, the day was shaping up to be another "dig in and get the job done" kind of day. The three-day forecast looked less than ideal for cycling, and it had been a challenge at times to carry camping gear without using it but I am used to it, and have adapted my plans to suit the conditions. Adventures are all about adaptation.

I was on Day 12, with nine to go. This was the third quarter of the trip, a time when the novelty of the first quarter has worn off, and anticipation of the end has not begun. But it felt significant to be over halfway, and I had coped with everything so far. I was feeling fit, and my mindset was positive; I relished the challenges of the day.

I set up my route the night before, checking both Google Maps and Bikemap, and settling on Google Maps. The only reason for this is that Google Maps is more likely to "have a go" when I lose my track. It had taken me on at least one wild ride over disused rail tracks to a hidden lorry park, but it got me there in the end. It looked like a straightforward ride close to the riverbank, crossing from side to side over bridges when the path changed sides. I double-checked that I was not dependent on a ferry to cross the river. I was learning, one mistake at a time, although there seemed to be a few alternatives in that stretch of the Rhine – I had options if it all went wrong.

I would cross into Strasbourg and spend some time in France that day. My guidebook suggested Basel as a destination, but I thought it too big an ask at over 80 miles, and in my experience, I would probably add 10% to that with detours and retracing missed signposts. Plus, arriving in a city sends the satnav into overdrive when it has too many choices. It somehow wants to take the quietest route, and often, I just want the quickest.

That morning, I took advantage of the inclusive breakfast provided. I managed some cucumber and scrambled eggs, but indulged with added processed keto items: bacon, Edam cheese and a slice of mortadella pork loaf. I added a couple of units for that meal, and it was all good. As I ate, I pondered my day. My glucose tracking was looking good and I was getting good results with my split-dose, long-acting insulin and small rapid doses at mealtimes. How far was I going to cycle that day? I was well ahead of schedule in terms of distance. I had planned for 60 miles a day and was averaging 65, so a shorter distance today would be okay if I needed to bail out. I decided to delay my final decision; I would ride in the wet all morning and then assess the situation in the afternoon.

So, that was the plan: get a reasonable distance and appraise the progress, nothing more complicated than that. But after all of that anticipation of rain and preparation to keep things dry, I set off in fine weather! That was the first thing I did not need to worry about. Everything was packed in waterproof bags, and rain would not have been an issue, but to be dry was a bonus – and an incentive to make progress.

I was, as usual, ache-free and set off as if it were the first day; another bonus of the low-inflammation keto diet. I had come to expect pain-free rides now – what a luxury that is at my age! I cycled over the impressive white and curving double suspension bridge for pedestrians and cyclists into France, called Passerelle des Deux Rives. I would be cycling in France for most of the day. I did not go into Strasbourg, but skirted the centre to the south. I would have liked to take a look; I was told last night it was worth it. But I knew I was close.

Strasbourg is the formal home of the European Union, and within a mile of the centre, there is a dramatic change in the cycling infrastructure; I found myself riding on perfect cycleways – beautiful, smooth tarmac, signs everywhere, and smooth, curved transitions onto pavements. No right angles here. Of course, it was a vainglorious demonstration of European culture and a show for visiting overseas dignitaries. For someone like me, more at home on narrow roads and cycle paths that stop abruptly when things get dangerous (like at roundabouts), it was like Utopia.

I was starting to enjoy whizzing around with well-groomed bright young things on the latest electric bikes, looking self-conscious about how cool they looked, but it was short-lived. Once out of the "Bureaucrat's Enclave", I noticed that the generous funding had run out. About a couple of miles out, it was back to normal – still excellent, but more rough and ready. Nevertheless, I managed to get through the residential and light-industrial back streets of suburban Strasbourg with few map errors. I had to keep panning out and zooming in to ensure I was not about to be led a merry dance around suburban streets. Sometimes, it is better to just power through on the main roads to make progress – and make progress, I did.

The saviour of this day was the Rhône and Rhine Canal, a flat, smooth and linear route going on for miles parallel to the River Rhine, with few deviations other than to criss-cross the sides to remain on the path. It was a treat not to need the satnav and get some serious miles in. I was now cycling briskly along it. It was remote, with a hard-compacted gravel surface and only a handful of cyclists on the route.

My usual rolling sound, a tarmac hum, became a high-pitched crunch as the path rolled by beneath my wheels. I could tell when I was approaching a village or town by the number of dog walkers; they never go more than a mile out of town. I can tell when a fast-food outlet is just up ahead in parts of Britain, and now I know it is the same on the continent too: litter appears on the roadside about a mile out when drivers/cyclists/walkers have finished their meals and discarded their waste.

I continued for two hours before taking a coffee break by the canal. "Pillboxes", heavy concrete buildings featuring holes for machine guns, remained from the Second World War. Along the canal, two of these structures were strategically placed to defend it. I stopped and took a look around. They were sunk deep into the earth, but there was no way into them; the ladders had been removed, and the entry point was full of logs and debris. The building was probably French, as we were on that side of the border, but it was also quite stylishly sculpted for a building with such a grim purpose; it had an almost comical eyebrow-like brim above the slit for the guns. I wondered if it had ever been used.

I used the flat surfaces I found there to have a brew-up and listen to the very loud birdsong in this peaceful, quiet place; it is rare to get a moment without the intrusion of an internal-combustion or jet engine. The volume of the birdsong was unbelievable and so clear – a joy. A family of swans passed by with their newly hatched cygnets. I went to take a picture, and mum and dad quickly rounded them up and kept them close.

The clouds were gathering from the west (from my right, as I was heading south), and it seemed that yet another frontal system was making its way in from the Atlantic via the flat land of France. It had clearly picked up a lot of moisture, and soon the skies were filled with high-level grey cloud. It would lose height as it passed and likely dump its rain, so I needed to press on.

I stopped again at Breisach, having briefly crossed back into Germany, to check progress and book accommodation ahead. I was not going to make Basel, and wanted to avoid Swiss prices and stay in either France or Germany. I bought some fresh salmon and cucumber for my meal.

I decided to eat; listening to my body, it told me I needed food. I took a bite of soft, creamy St. Albray cheese. It was zero carbs and 25 g of protein. I would use all of that up on the final ride to my stopover. I did not need any rapid-acting insulin. Indeed, my levels had been nudging slowly downward all day. That would indicate I had slightly too much insulin, or had more insulin sensitivity; I did not know, but was not worried about it and did not need to check the meter regularly. I was confident my strategy was working well –

besides, a gentle hypo, if it did happen, would be easy to feel and correct while continuing to ride.

Occasionally, I still find this freedom a novelty, but I have become used to it. Indeed, 10 years ago on the North Sea Cycle Route, I would have been piling in the carbs and checking the meter. I would have been in Germany chomping away steadily on chocolate – not the 90% cocoa I eat for a treat nowadays, but full-on, high-carb local chocolate, mostly four or five bars a day, with nuts or rice added.

I was not worried about the ups and downs of glucose; after all, I could only test very occasionally with a finger-prick meter, so most of the time I was not aware of my glucose level unless it reached hypo level. It was not all that bad at the time – perhaps 12–15 mmol/L (216–270 mg/dL), then down to hypo level most days, but, overall, reasonable by the standards I set myself back then.

In those days, I did not really consider optimised insulin; it was all about glucose optimisation. If only I had known then that insulin was not a free ride and came with consequences, I would have approached things very differently. As they say, you can't alter the past – but when you know better, *do* better!

I had always relied on physical activity in a misguided attempt to compensate for poor glucose control; after all, as the story goes, both high glucose and lack of exercise can cause heart disease. Few standard clinicians would mention insulin as a culprit. My strategy, given my poor glucose management, was to mitigate the risk by exercising. I was a fully trained and up-to-date doctor, but no one was talking about the dangers of excess insulin. It was considered a free ride. We were not given that information – if it even existed.

I remember going to a talk on insulin initiation in type 2 diabetes by a local consultant. It was not long after my own diagnosis, so I was very keen to learn. The consultant almost bragged about the insulin doses he used in some of his type 2 patients – up to 300 units per day, a whole pen full!

For someone like me, with no functioning pancreas using 20 units a day, he was clearly addressing insulin resistance, but if one is insulin-resistant, adding more to steamroll the body into submission now seems a doomed and thoughtless strategy. To think that people are getting that right now, as I write, is alarming.

A quick review on Booking.com of available places threw up a hotel in Germany about 15 miles away, perfect for the day's ride and with an early enough finish to relax a bit. I had to do a diversion for repair works after finding myself in a wood with a lot of tree debris on the path. There, I picked up another front puncture; not a pinch but a thorn, which I located when sweeping the inside of the tyre. I have cut my finger sometimes doing this, but this time it was incident-free and a pair of pliers efficiently extracted the offending spur. I was well prepared. This time, it was a routine five-minute fix, and I was back on my way.

In an hour, I completed my day's ride in steady rain. I was so used to it now, that it barely registered. When I finally crossed the bridge into town, although I was wet, I was pleased with the progress of the day. The psychological boost from my earlier canal route was welcome.

I was staying in a family-run hotel with an eclectic mix of buildings and garden artefacts – gnomes, a children's playground, fountains and sculptures. It was more like a grand home than a corporate one, with none of the over-studied design elements marking out a corporate identity. This was a one-off. The receptionist escorted me to a locked garage for my bike, and my stay was easy and comfortable.

My window view included a park with a prominent, red-block tower about 30 metres high, called the Wuhrlochpark. It had square windows in which every other brick was left out, a bit like a tall, slim Jenga tower. Completed in 2022, the area translates to "The Park of the Old Weir Basin". It began life as a working part of the town's defence and industry. A simple weir was built on the stream to slow the water and divert part of it into channels that powered mills, fed workshops, and helped protect the lower town from flooding. Over time the basin, hollowed out by centuries of controlled water flow, became part of the landscape itself. Now it hosts an observation tower of rusted Corten steel and red stone bricks, linking the walled town on the hill with the countryside and park below.

As I climbed the stairs, I glimpsed the Rhine and its surroundings from all sides. It was pleasant and gentle, but not dramatic. The twilight was falling, and I headed back in the cool drizzle to my hotel. I was feeling upbeat today, and made my way eagerly to the restaurant for a large plate of fresh pork hocks, a fresh salad and some water.

I took my usual six units of Tresiba, and a couple of units for the meat. It was getting a bit late; my leptin levels would be raised and complaining, and my poor old intestine would have to keep going until that meal was digested. Then it would be ready for sleep. I already was.

It had been a perfect day to make progress after the sapping day before; I was headed for St. Moritz on time, and my progress map showed that I was indeed moving towards my goal. I was in southern Germany, on the Swiss border. Tomorrow, I would stop heading south for a couple of days and head east toward Lake Bodensee and the end of the navigable Rhine.

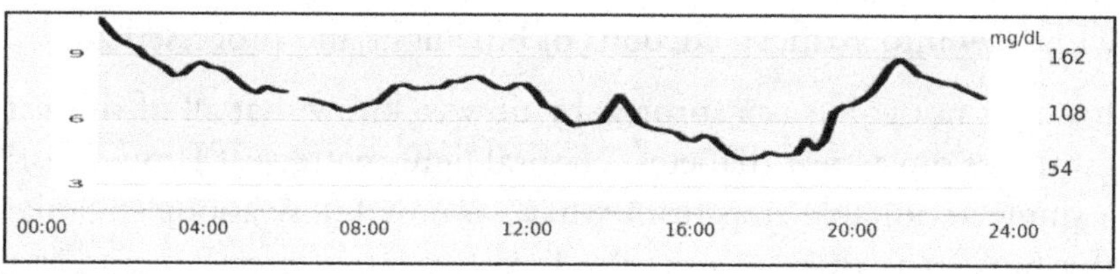

Chapter 29
Foundations of Health: Our Lived Environment

"Some old-fashioned things like fresh air and sunshine are hard to beat."
– Laura Ingalls Wilder

The previous chapters have highlighted how a holistic approach to our type 1 diabetes can be leveraged to improve insulin use and glucose control: our diet, physical activity, and sleep quality. The world we inhabit daily – our lived environment – affects us, too.

How do we spend most of our waking hours, indoors or outside? If we are outside, are we walking through woodland, along rivers and ridgelines, or threading between office blocks and car parks? Do we shift our behaviour in winter when the light fades early and the temperatures bite? Do we brace ourselves and adapt, or do we withdraw into artificial cocoons of blue light and processed air?

It might not come as a surprise by now to know that all of this can influence our type 1 diabetes. Natural light matters. If I could distil a single actionable step from what we now know about circadian rhythms, it is this: go outside. It is free, it is effective, and it is immediate.

Yet, somewhere along the way, modern life has quietly ushered us away from this natural balm. We have traded sunlight for strip lights. Dawn and dusk have become sideshows in our focused, rush-hour routines. We surround ourselves with LEDs at midnight and wonder why we can't sleep.

Modern Lifestyles, the Circadian Rhythm, and Forest Bathing

Our evolutionary physiology has not changed with our modern living habits; it still runs on cues from the natural world, especially light. The timing, intensity and spectrum of light we receive each day directly impact our circadian rhythm, melatonin secretion, mitochondrial function, insulin sensitivity, and inflammatory balance.

In short, light calibrates us. When we miss that calibration, the fallout is not just theoretical, it is hormonal, metabolic, and real. And that is not all. Nature itself appears to calm the nervous system. A growing body of evidence tells us that being in a natural environment, particularly one with trees, water and open space, reduces the very hormones that make blood sugar harder to manage. Cortisol, adrenaline, noradrenaline – these are reduced when we immerse ourselves in what the Japanese call Shinrin-yoku, or "forest bathing".

This is not simply a poetic turn of phrase. It is a structured, evidence-backed practice: walking slowly and mindfully in a wooded area, allowing the sights, sounds and smells to anchor us. The outcomes are measurable. Studies have shown that Shinrin-yoku:

- Reduces blood pressure and heart rate
- Enhances parasympathetic activity (rest and digest) while downregulating sympathetic activity (fight or flight)
- Improves sleep quality
- Reduces symptoms of depression, anxiety, anger and fatigue, while increasing feelings of vitality

Interestingly, similar effects have been documented in urban green spaces, like city parks, suggesting that proximity to nature, even in modest doses, has a biological impact.

Perhaps the most famous Western example of this kind of thinking comes from a retrospective study of surgical patients in Pennsylvania between 1972 and 1981. Postoperative recovery following gallbladder surgery was significantly faster in patients whose hospital room windows overlooked a natural scene – trees, grass and sky – than in those facing a brick wall. Fewer analgesics were required. Nurses wrote fewer negative notes in charts. Healing improved, likely due to the combination of reduced stress and increased exposure to natural light and scenery.

Why? Perhaps because nature does more than decorate our environment. It heals us at the cellular level.

The Body Takes Cues From Nature

Even beyond Earth's atmosphere, our bodies are still looking for their natural cues. Astronauts, who spend weeks and months in microgravity, face unique physiological stressors. They orbit Earth every 90 minutes – one sunrise and sunset per hour. The absence of gravitational load, the disrupted circadian rhythm, and the persistent exposure to artificial lighting all take a toll. One condition in particular, spaceflight-associated neuro-ocular syndrome (SANS), leads to optic disc swelling, visual distortion, and retinal changes. Mitochondrial dysfunction is now being considered as a contributing mechanism.

Exposure to red and near-infrared (NIR) light – wavelengths that are naturally present in sunlight – are being investigated for their potential to support mitochondrial function during long-duration spaceflight. These light frequencies promote mitochondrial respiration, reduce oxidative stress, and improve cellular repair processes. The implications for life here on Earth are obvious. We have access to these potentially healing wavelengths every morning and evening – yet we block them out with sunglasses, shelter behind double-glazed windows, or sleep through their arrival.

The Light Spectrum

Electromagnetic radiation has many uses, from communication (Wi-Fi, mobile phones) to heating (microwaves), medical imaging, and therapeutic interventions such as radiotherapy and laser surgery. Laser light, for example, is used in treating diabetic retinopathy.

The light that humans see is the visible part of the electromagnetic spectrum. Most of the wavelengths of the electromagnetic spectrum are invisible to us, but we can still sense non-visible light. What we can see – red to violet light – is only a narrow band of electromagnetic radiation, between roughly 400 and 700 nanometres (nm).

The full solar spectrum reaching Earth ranges from about 250 to over 4000 nm, with visible light only accounting for a small portion. Light longer than red (infrared) and shorter than violet (ultraviolet) is invisible but biologically active. The majority of the photoreceptors in the retina respond to certain wavelengths, which we interpret as colour and light.

Other animals perceive different parts of this spectrum. For example, snakes such as pit vipers, and some pythons and boas possess specialised infrared-sensitive pit organs that allow them to "see" the heat signatures of their prey. Similarly, many birds, insects, and some fish can detect ultraviolet (UV) light. Bees use UV patterns on flowers as visual guides for locating nectar, while birds may use UV cues in mate selection and navigation. These adaptations reflect how profoundly different wavelengths of electromagnetic radiation can shape physiology and behaviour across species.

Our exposure to natural light has been altered by the technologies we rely on daily. Artificial light sources – LEDs, fluorescent lighting, and screens – often emit a narrow band of visible light, typically rich in blue wavelengths and lacking the broader spectrum of natural sunlight, particularly in the NIR and UV ranges. We spend a lot of our lives indoors, under lighting that excludes large sections of the natural electromagnetic spectrum, especially NIR. Modern low emissivity, or Low E, glass also blocks certain infrared (IR) wavelengths from entering buildings. This reduction in spectral exposure may have biological consequences that are only beginning to be understood.

IR radiation, particularly NIR, accounts for over 50% of the solar energy that reaches Earth. This light penetrates deeply into the skin and even the underlying tissues. Because of its tissue penetration, NIR has the potential to influence a substantial proportion of cells in the body. In general, longer wavelengths of light penetrate biological tissues more deeply than shorter wavelengths. NIR light (650–1200 nm) can penetrate deeper into tissue without producing noticeable heat. It can influence cellular activity, contributing to changes in cell behaviour. And even non-heating levels of IR can have significant biological effects.

Melatonin, Health, and Resilience

One important molecule influenced by NIR light is melatonin. Often called the "hormone of darkness", melatonin is associated with sleep and is produced in the pineal gland. The previous chapter taught us how it phase-shifts our circadian rhythm towards sleep. It is suppressed by blue-green light, so exposure to this wavelength later in the day can reduce our capacity to sleep.

However, less well known is that melatonin is also produced locally within cells outside the brain, particularly in mitochondria, and throughout the body. This intracellular production is not circadian rhythm-dependent, and primarily functions as an antioxidant.

Melatonin is synthesised from tryptophan, an essential amino acid that must be obtained through the diet. Tryptophan is first converted into 5-hydroxytryptophan (5-HTP), then to serotonin, and finally to melatonin. This process is influenced by light exposure and the availability of cofactors such as vitamin B6, magnesium and zinc. The gut microbiome may influence this pathway, as certain microbes can metabolise tryptophan into serotonin and melatonin precursors, adding another layer of dietary impact. Tryptophan is found in foods such as chicken, eggs, cheese, fish, tofu and seeds.

Red and NIR light may enhance melatonin production in mitochondria, improving cellular energy production and survival. Unlike classic antioxidants like vitamin C, which neutralise one or two reactive oxygen species (ROS), one molecule of melatonin can scavenge up to ten ROS or reactive nitrogen species (RNS), thanks to its unique cascade reaction.

Cellular melatonin deficiency, seen in mitochondrially compromised tissues, leads to dysfunction. For example, studies have shown that in neurodegenerative diseases such as Alzheimer's and Parkinson's, mitochondrial damage correlates with lower local melatonin production, contributing to increased oxidative stress and neuronal degeneration.

In oncology research, cancerous tissues often show a marked reduction in mitochondrial melatonin. This is thought to result from a metabolic shift away from oxidative phosphorylation towards glucose metabolism as the fuel source – a phenomenon known as the Warburg effect. These findings underscore the role of melatonin not just as a sleep regulator but as a key component of cellular health and resilience.

In summary, exposure to NIR from natural sunlight may support mitochondrial health by enhancing melatonin synthesis directly within cells. Artificial lighting, in contrast, lacks this wavelength and may contribute to mitochondrial dysfunction over time. This represents a subtle, yet significant, divergence from the light environment under which human physiology evolved.

We know a great deal about the effects of invisible light at the red end of the spectrum, but what about the violet end? UV light, especially UV-A and UV-B, also plays an important biological role. It is well known that UV light can penetrate the skin and cause damage if exposure is excessive or mistimed; sunburn is a common example. UV exposure at appropriate times, especially in the morning, acts as a reset mechanism.

UV-A light, in addition to blue-green light, reaching the skin and retina about an hour after sunrise, affects serotonin and dopamine activity, and may also influence thyroid hormones. These neurotransmitters not only affect mood and alertness, but also lay the groundwork for melatonin synthesis later in the day. Importantly, most artificial indoor lighting and glass windows block UV-A, meaning we miss out on this entraining signal unless we go outside.

UV-B light, meanwhile, is essential for the production of vitamin D in the skin. When the sun is more than 30 degrees above the horizon – typically between 11 am and 4 pm in summer in the UK – UV-B radiation triggers a photochemical reaction that converts 7-dehydrocholesterol in the skin into vitamin D3. Of course, these times will vary quite a bit depending on where you are in the world.

Vitamin D3 is then converted in the liver into its storage form, 25-hydroxyvitamin D, and later activated in the kidneys into calcitriol, the active hormonal form that regulates calcium and phosphate metabolism, immune function, and even gene expression.

We may also get another inactive form of vitamin D, D2, from plants. The active form is relatively constant, while the storage form varies with the seasons, being higher in the summer. Blood tests typically measure the storage form, which does not reflect the circulating biological form.

Vitamin D and Type 1 Diabetes

In the UK and similar latitudes, the window for vitamin D synthesis is generally limited to the months from March to October. The amount of skin exposed and the time of day are key variables, among others.

Apps and solar-tracking tools can help estimate vitamin D synthesis potential, but the principle is clear: more exposure yields more endogenous, or natural, vitamin D, up to a plateau that lies within the bounds of safe sun exposure. Under conditions of high UV and with substantial skin surface exposed, up to 20,000 IU can be synthesised per day from natural light.

During winter, UV-B lamps and/ or supplementation may be necessary. UV light never occurs on its own in nature, so a UV-B/A lamp should ideally be used with full-spectrum light – for example, with the window open, outdoors, or alongside a NIR panel – as some research suggests NIR may help counterbalance oxidative stress from UV exposure alone.

Current UK guidelines recommending 400 IU per day are generally considered insufficient for maintaining optimal vitamin D status. Many experts suggest taking 2,000–3,000 IU of vitamin D3 per day, especially during the winter months. The quality of supplements varies, so it is important to check available options carefully.

Vitamin D also interacts with other fat-soluble vitamins, particularly vitamin A, as adequate vitamin A is needed for proper vitamin D signalling. An additional factor to consider is metabolic context. In people with high insulin levels or higher body fat, vitamin D can become sequestered in adipose tissue, reducing its bioavailability.

High-carb diets, which can contribute to higher insulin and increased body fat, may also indirectly lower vitamin D status. This highlights the potential benefits of metabolic flexibility and fat-adapted states, where vitamin D can circulate more freely. In this way, a ketogenic or low-carbohydrate diet may help support vitamin D availability and regulation.

Historically, the consequences of vitamin D deficiency were profound. Rickets, a disease that causes soft, deformed bones, was once common in northern cities of the UK, where there was limited sunlight and heavy industrial smoke. This was seen in areas such as Glasgow, in Scotland, during a period of mass factory employment. Children raised in dense, sunless tenement housing lacked sufficient UV exposure and also had poor, vitamin D-deficient diets; their bones bowed under their weight.

The link between sunlight and bone development led to the addition of vitamin D to staple foods. Surgeons attempted to correct the deformities by physically straightening bones, an intervention that laid the foundation of the speciality we now call orthopaedics. The term itself is derived from the Greek roots: "ortho" meaning straight, and "paed" meaning child. It proved far better to treat the cause of rickets than the symptom.

Today, rickets operations are effectively historical. In the same way, it is preferable to manage insulin over glucose in type 1 diabetes.

How Environment Shapes Our Health

Understanding our lived environment in this way reveals a powerful, often-overlooked lever for health, particularly for those with type 1 diabetes. From forest bathing to full-spectrum light exposure, and from mitochondrial melatonin synthesis to UV-driven vitamin D production, environmental inputs clearly shape internal physiology. Our modern departure from the natural cycles of light and dark, activity and rest, may contribute to some of our present metabolic challenges.

By consciously realigning our behaviours with natural rhythms – seeking outdoor light, limiting artificial light at night, and nourishing our cells through activity and targeted nutrition – we not only honour our evolutionary biology but may also dramatically improve our ability to manage insulin, regulate inflammation, and protect long-term health.

Chapter 30
Total Miles: 879.5

Day 13 – Neueburg to Waldshut, 61.5 miles

"When we experience adventure, we find ourselves in the present moment and savour all the beauty that life has to offer."
– Unknown

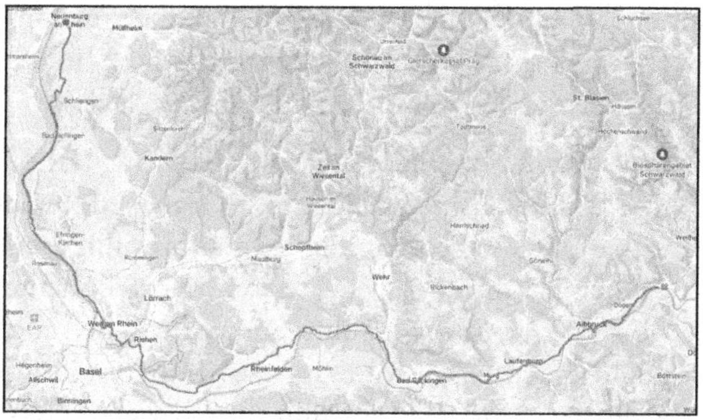

I have had plenty of time to reflect on my learning; the main requirement of this adventure, learning about optimised insulin, was beginning to be met. There is so much detail in this vast subject that I could only scratch the surface, but I felt I now had a solid grounding that allowed me to start putting it into practice.

A quick recap might help at this point: insulin is a hormone central to the body's energy management, and it responds to much more than just carbohydrates in the diet. Wherever there is metabolism, insulin is present – either active or less active. High insulin levels are anabolic and promote fat storage. The body cannot burn fat when it is storing it.

On the other hand, low insulin levels facilitate fat burning, making fuels such as fatty acids and ketone bodies available. Different tissues have different requirements regarding their fuels, so low insulin levels enable tissues to choose their preferred fuel source.

Natural insulin has a very short duration, and is found primarily in the circulation around its target tissues in the abdomen. Synthetic insulin, by contrast, has a longer duration and, because it is injected into the skin, tends to act more in the muscles and less in the liver.

As a result, more insulin is needed at mealtimes to achieve the same effect as natural insulin. This makes multi-fuelling more difficult, because insulin inhibits fat burning. Ketogenic diets reduce the need for insulin, and physical activity improves insulin sensitivity. Taking care of our circadian rhythms can also help reduce insulin levels, as can exposure to natural light and the outdoors. Mindset plays a similar role; reducing stress lowers blood glucose levels.

Looking back, I think I have been chasing the wrong target, glucose, over the years. It is insulin that needs to be managed, in addition. I now believe that glucose control follows good insulin management and not the other way around. Glucose control can be achieved with a very high-carb diet, but the insulin required will be much higher. Of course, tight glucose control helps to avoid complications, but achieving it through optimised insulin, in my view, offers the best overall health.

One person I met on an optimised insulin course told me he had used various insulin pumps for 20 years, but it was only when he focused on optimising his insulin that he achieved his best glucose control, and felt better in the process.

This adventure is exposing me to all of the foundations of health; it has been fascinating to feel the effects of variation from day to day.

I have started to build a radar map with five arms, each representing one foundation of health, with lines going from the centre outwards, where I can rate a foundation of health along a "ladder" of ten. I rate each "spoke" daily, based on how well I am optimising my insulin. The aim is to reach tens across all spokes, but often something will be lagging – sometimes food, other days mindset or sleep.

It is a helpful visual representation of how I am doing, and if something feels off, I can often pinpoint where the problem lies. It is also enabling me to embed the concept of optimised insulin into my daily routine, and after a few weeks, it is becoming second nature. You can create your own using an Excel spreadsheet graph.

Today was shaping up well. Sleep was good, but I woke early and did not get back to sleep, so the circadian rhythm rating was a 5. Physical activity was a 10 every day, and nutrition varied. It is ketogenic, but the food quality I chose was not always ideal; overall, it will rate between 6 and 10. Mindset was also varied, but I felt good in this respect today, even though some days were a challenge. And, of course, my environment would rate nearly 10 for the three weeks – plenty of natural light and green spaces, and time to switch off and meditate. In many ways, it is as good as it gets.

When I finish my challenge, it will change as I spend more time indoors in a conference setting, sitting down mostly, but even in this situation, there will be opportunities to exercise outside – and I can get back to my preferred two-meals-a-day option, etc. We have to adapt to our environment, but now we have the knowledge and tools to help do that.

Today's breakfast of scrambled eggs was supplemented by bacon and cucumber, a boiled egg, a small amount of cured meat and a slice of cheese. I should have left the cured meat, but it seems cultural in these parts. Overall, it was a good energy infusion to start the day. With lowish glucose, I was not going to overdo it with insulin; I put in a unit of rapid and my usual six units of Tresiba. It was a good choice, as it turned out.

I had started to look forward to an early breakfast. Normally, when not cycling for six hours, I skip it and have a late lunch. I try to get 16–18 hours between my last meal of the day and my first; I manage it most days, but I cannot say I am squeaky clean every day. When it is raining and I cannot get out or settle to anything, I want to eat. It is nothing to do with nutrition and everything to do with boredom, and these boredom-meals are never satiating; I barely even notice I have eaten them – my stomach does not seem to register it, or at least does not send the right message to my brain.

To counter this negative scenario, I have learned to stop what I am doing for 15 minutes and switch to something completely different. It usually works. It is not a sugar craving – any keto food will do, but it is not needed for energy either. I also notice I rarely chew this food or appreciate the taste and texture like I do when eating mindfully, it is just shovelled down, like a pelican. Those who struggle with cravings and addiction to ultra-processed food will probably recognise this.

If I am occupied, I can go a whole day without food and not even want it. On the whole, I find fasting gets easier with practice; I rarely feel hungry when I break my fast, but I am ready to eat and, of course, I need to eat to get the calories in.

Too much protein in one go will almost certainly cause glucose challenges, especially if it is the last meal of the day. In winter, there is less opportunity for exercise unless I do indoor core work or go for a walk. If it is cold and dark, that is a big ask. So, I usually have two meals a day, with a 16–18- hour fast and a final meal no later than 8 pm.

Today, I set off under a cool, light breeze and grey skies – which has become the defining weather of this trip. It is a straightforward run to Basel. The satnav went into a bit of a tizzy, but it is not unusual, and I would miss cursing it if it were perfect. I was on a track between the river and a motorway, and it could not decide which it preferred. At one point, I was apparently on the motorway, then seconds later, I was on a gravel track. I checked visually, and yes, this was a gravel track!

I panned out the map, found a straightforward route and turned off the screen to enjoy the view. Low cloud merged with the fast-flowing river, its banks submerged under the water, and the bushes that were normally on land, but were now on the flood plain, bent in the current. Half-submerged branches headed downstream, following the main current. People were out photographing the scene; it must have been an unusually heavy rainfall this year. Even a few cormorants were drying their wings on the banks. The path remained flat, with cornfields and arable crops nearby. Hills began appearing to the east, which was to be my route in a few hours' time.

Still cold, I stopped at a café in the northern suburbs of Basel to warm up. There was just me, a local man, and a young woman standing behind a fixed-odds betting machine. A baker dropped off a few loaves, and the TV played daytime telly. I sorted my route and checked for accommodation. My next target was Bad Säckingen, then Waldshut by evening; it would be the perfect stop to keep my distance target. If I managed this, I would have three days to spare – they were my buffer days to ensure I reached St. Moritz on time.

Having cursed Google Maps earlier, it retaliated, directing me down towards the river, which would have been fine, if it had been the Rhine route – but it was not. Tarmac gave way to gravel, then to a grassy, single muddy track, slippery and narrow. My tyres were near their limit. After a tense ride, I met a steep, winding stairway under a rail tunnel curving up to the road around a fast-flowing and noisy tributary stream. I was sure it was not part of EV15.

The stairs were narrow, slick with wet, and perilous. I tried to haul the whole bike and luggage up in one go, but one pannier caught a step and suddenly detached. It slid down the bank, luckily caught by a bush, otherwise it would have plummeted into the stream. I removed everything else from the bike and continued taking the bike and luggage in stages. Then, aghast, I noticed my phone had come off its mount and was missing. My heart sank. I backtracked and found it teetering precariously on the edge of a step next to the stream. It was a lucky break. I grabbed it, zipped it in my jacket and pushed on.

After discovering and rejoining the proper road route, I followed four older e-bikers for a few miles into the town centre. A Woolworths store greeted me, a brand long gone in the UK. The Woolworths in Bad Säckingen was, as I remembered from home, offering Pick 'n' Mix sweets and random household goods. I grabbed a gas cylinder to fuel my morning coffee ritual. It was time for foraging: for some reason, I craved cucumber. Fruit was off-limits due to carbs, and nuts were possible but I found they generally made my joints ache. I found a Bio Laden supermarket, which is a common sight here, and found my cucumber. I ate half of it with smoked salmon – luxury food in a now sunny square.

Back on the road, I noticed my glucose had been creeping up. I had needed a unit that morning and another for this meal, 20 g of protein, one unit at rest. Something was changing in my body. The food foundation of health was okay; could it be one of the others? Sleep had been reasonably good, and physical activity was excellent – but a lot in a relatively short space of time. My mindset was good, and I was getting plenty of daylight. I probably needed rest. But I felt good otherwise, and the glucose was only nudging up slowly, so there was no crisis – it was not in the category of concern. With a foundations of health approach, I can be more nuanced in my response to glucose, rather than assume it is a diet/insulin mismatch; it might not be the diet at all.

It was mid-afternoon, and I wanted to push on. A three-day break was in reach and I wanted to bank the time. If the glucose rise was due to tiredness from too much physical activity, I would recover then. Waldshut was reachable, and Booking.com had found me a basic, cheap place with no meals but safe bike storage.

By early evening, low clouds gave way to heavy rain. I was soaked and cold. I deployed another Sainsbury's sandwich bag for my phone, but meanwhile, water had seeped into my handlebar bag – money, passport, charger, spare phone. I moved it all to a dry pannier. My bike was plastered in mud; the chain was caked in grit, and the brakes made a grinding sound as the fine gravel stuck to the rim and acted as a grinding paste when I braked. I would clean it tomorrow.

After a warm shower, admin, and hanging out my kit, I headed to a rustic restaurant. I had sirloin steak and salad: 250 g of steak. My blood glucose was 6 mmol/L (108 mg/dL). Two units would have covered the macros, but I took four. My experience told me that I needed more. Ketones were at 1 mmol/L, a good level for me. Some with type 1 hit 3 mmol/L of ketones, but 0.6 mmol/L is typical for me and I was happy with 1 mmol/L.

My glucose slowly dropped to 3.1 mmol/L (54 mg/dL) overnight. The Libre alarm went off and I awoke. I had no symptoms, but the trend was nudging down. I took 9 g of glucose tablets in anticipation – so much for adding a couple of units for the protein based on "experience"!

By morning, it was 5.4 mmol/L (97mg/dL). Fingerpick tests for my calibration experiment read 6.2mmol/L (112mg/dL) (Keto Mojo) and 5.8 mmol/L (104 mg/dL) (Wavesense). I noticed that the Freestyle Libre was reading at least 0.4 mmol/L (7.2 mg/dL) lower than the others. Did that mean my actual asymptomatic, Freestyle-defined "hypo" was not a hypo at all? Maybe it was really over 3.5mmol/L (61mg/dL) and not 3.1mmol/L (55 mg/dL)?

I should have stuck to managing symptoms rather than the numbers. CGMs are brilliant, but they are a tool with flaws. Nothing is perfect in type 1 diabetes – but that event reminded me of the need to use common sense once in a while.

Onwards: tomorrow I would be in Konstanz, which is at one end of the navigable Rhine. I had not seen a Rhinekilometer marker post for a while, but if I did spot one in Konstanz, it would say "0".

Last year, I motorcycled to this spot in hot sun, and camped on the lake's west side. This year, I decided to take the east bank; my guidebook told me it is the most pleasant route and I wanted to visit the Zeppelin Airship Museum, which is located there.

The good news was that sun had been forecast. Even though I am British and we constantly moan about the weather, we never let it beat us; if we did, we would never do anything. We can get all four seasons in one day there sometimes. They say that in the UK, it is cloudy for three-quarters of the year – the rest of the time, it rains! It is not true; we can go a few weeks with glorious sunny days without rain, and it is wonderful, but when that happens, we tend to start panicking about drought. The weather always gives us something to talk about…

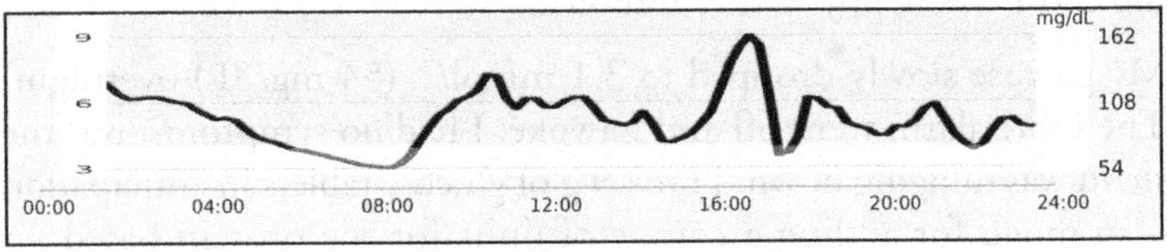

Chapter 31
Foundations of Health: Mindset

Mindset, Brain Chemistry, and Type 1 Diabetes

Living with type 1 diabetes means being on call every moment of every day. There is no pause button while we deal with other crises in our lives. This constant background load affects our mood, our reactions, our thinking, and even how the brain handles fuel. Understanding these processes removes the mystery and helps us respond with confidence rather than frustration.

This chapter brings together two linked ideas: how the brain's chemistry is shaped by diet, glucose and insulin, and how our mindset and behaviour influence life with type 1 diabetes.

Glutamate and GABA: The Brain's Balancing Act

The brain relies on two major chemical messengers to regulate its activity. Glutamate is the main excitatory signal, the accelerator that drives learning, movement, alertness, memory and decision-making. GABA is the main inhibitory signal, the brake that prevents overactivity, supports calm thinking, and allows proper sleep.

Too much glutamate or too little GABA creates a state of overstimulation. Many people recognise this as anxiety, irritability, difficulty settling, or a sense of being "wired and tired". The balance between glutamate and GABA matters far more than the level of either one alone.

Glutamate is produced inside neurons (nerve cells), primarily from glucose metabolism. GABA is made directly from glutamate by an enzyme called glutamate decarboxylase (GAD). This conversion depends on a stable metabolic environment. Disruptions in fuel supply or insulin signalling may influence this balance.

How Diet Shapes Glutamate and GABA

The type of fuel available to the brain influences how much glutamate and GABA we produce and how well we recycle them.

High Carbohydrate Intake

Glucose enters the brain through GLUT3 transporters in neurons and GLUT1 transporters in astrocytes (support cells that help maintain neurons), largely independent of insulin. Glucose availability influences glutamate production.

This system works well when glucose is steady. However, significant glucose fluctuations and high insulin levels can stress these systems and may alter neurotransmitter balance.

Insulin affects the brain through the phosphatidylinositol 3-kinase (PI3K) pathway, a major signalling system that regulates energy handling. PI3K regulation involves insulin and is discussed in a later chapter. Sustained high insulin levels may alter PI3K signalling and could influence downstream metabolic processes, including aspects of the glutamate-glutamine cycle. Astrocytes may struggle to clear glutamate efficiently when ATP production becomes erratic, especially during glucose dips.

Low blood glucose exaggerates this problem. When glucose falls, energy availability to neurons and astrocytes also falls. Glutamate clearance can become impaired. Cellular signalling pathways, including PI3K, may be affected. In more severe cases, glutamate may accumulate. As a result, people may feel confused, argumentative, emotional or disoriented, and afterwards, a period of fog or headache is common. These are normal biological responses to an energy shortage in the brain.

Ketogenic or Low Carbohydrate Intake

A ketogenic or low-carb diet changes the brain's fuel supply. Ketones enter neurons easily via MCT transporters and alter the citric acid cycle metabolism. They can support GAD activity, potentially increasing GABA levels. They may also stabilise mitochondrial function and create a more consistent ATP supply, helping glutamate recycling through astrocytes. Because insulin exposure is lower and steadier, this can help regulate PI3K signalling, supporting a healthier balance between glutamate and GABA. Many people notice a calmer mind, better sleep, fewer episodes of irritability, and fewer symptoms after mild hypos. This is consistent with what we know about glutamate, GABA and PI3K.

Why This Matters in Type 1 Diabetes

Type 1 diabetes naturally involves glucose swings, insulin changes, and periods of metabolic stress. All of these influence the brain. High carb intake combined with variable insulin dosing can influence glutamate activity, exacerbate the effects of hypoglycaemia, and contribute to irritability, anxiety and cognitive fatigue. A ketogenic or reduced carbohydrate intake tends to stabilise fuel supply and improve the brain's inhibitory control through GABA.

Mindset in Type 1 Diabetes

Even with stable fuel and good habits, mindset plays a major role. Type 1 diabetes requires constant monitoring, frequent decisions, and readiness for the unexpected. This background pressure can affect motivation, mood and behaviour.

The Limbic System

Much of our emotional regulation sits in the limbic system in the brain, which includes the amygdala, hippocampus, hypothalamus and cingulate gyrus. This system links intellectual thought with automatic bodily responses; it reacts to glucose swings, hypoglycaemia, insulin changes, stress, sleep disruption, and even environmental cues, among others.

Hypoglycaemia, in particular, can confuse limbic signalling. The mood changes around impending and actual hypos can appear to an observer as rude or inappropriate behaviour. Many people with type 1 recognise the social anxiety that follows such events, especially in public or professional settings.

Acute Mood Symptoms

Immediate mood symptoms are more often linked to hypoglycaemia than anything else. People describe confusion, shimmering vision, hunger, irritability, sleepiness, anxiety, or the urge to withdraw. Some experience nightmares or aggression. These typically occur between 3 and 4 mmol/L, though some feel them at lower glucose levels.

High glucose typically causes slower, more prolonged symptoms, such as tiredness, foggy thinking, slower reactions and reduced concentration.

People who reduce carbohydrate intake often experience fewer glucose swings, which reduces these acute symptoms. One study found six times fewer hypos in people consuming around 75 g of carbohydrate per day.

Diabetes Stress and Self-Efficacy

A questionnaire of young adults with type 1 diabetes found a clear pattern. Fear of hypos and fear of complications were associated with reduced quality of life. Self-efficacy – the belief in one's ability to cope – improved it.

Self-efficacy is not self-esteem; it is the confidence that one can take action when needed and influence outcomes. It supports motivation, wellbeing, and long-term consistency. Strong self-efficacy protects against burnout. Hope functions similarly. In children, higher levels of hope were linked to better glucose testing habits and as a result, better HbA1c. Taking responsibility and feeling capable improves mental wellbeing.

Burnout and Language

Burnout occurs when someone is overwhelmed. They may stop testing, delay putting on a new sensor, guess insulin doses, or fall into irregular eating patterns. None of this reflects a lack of care, only a high burden of work. Language shapes this experience. Some clinical terms feel judgemental. Better alternatives include "management" instead of "control", and "values" instead of "tests".

Avoiding labels such as "good diabetic" or "non-compliant" helps people stay engaged without shame. Numbers do not define anyone. Understanding the foundations of health, including mindset and metabolic stability, leads to more sustainable progress.

Eating Disorders and Insulin Manipulation

Eating disorders occur more often, or more severely, in people with type 1 diabetes. Insulin manipulation can take many forms, from taking extra insulin to enable "cheat-eating", to omitting insulin for weight control. Up to 40% of young people may experience this at some point.

The daily pressure of matching insulin to food and the experience of weight changes at diagnosis can influence body image. Binge eating, bulimia, anorexia, and chaotic patterns of restriction and overconsumption have all been reported.

A ketogenic approach is often labelled restrictive, yet many people find it reduces chaotic eating, stabilises glucose, and makes insulin decisions simpler. Phrases like "you need a treat" or "you must eat carbs for energy" may reflect bias rather than evidence.

Recognising food addiction is important. People often say they feel "addicted" to sugar or carbs. These patterns are coping strategies, not character flaws.

Mindfulness and Practical Support

Mindfulness, breathing exercises and paying conscious attention to the present moment can significantly reduce stress. These practices engage the parasympathetic nervous system, reduce cortisol, and help people respond rather than react. This can soften the emotional spikes that come with glucose swings and decision fatigue.

Even small amounts of outdoor activity, movement or relaxation techniques support mental steadiness. These are practical tools, not theoretical ones.

Depression

Depression is two to three times more common in people with type 1 diabetes, with long-term studies showing higher rates of psychiatric symptoms in those individuals during adolescence and adulthood. Depressive symptoms are associated with higher HbA1c and more DKA episodes.

Depression may involve both psychological and metabolic mechanisms. Signs include apathy, insomnia, loss of interest, irritability, poor concentration or unexplained changes in glucose patterns. Early recognition and treatment are important.

Staying Proactive

Type 1 diabetes is demanding, but it is manageable with the right tools and understanding. Recognising emotional and glucose-related patterns is the first step. Establishing routines around food, sleep, activity, and reflection supports stability. Self-efficacy grows with small, consistent wins. Seeking help is practical, not a weakness.

Mindset is not fixed; it can shift. Even small improvements matter. With knowledge, clarity, and a consistent approach, people can live well with type 1 diabetes.

Chapter 32
Total Miles: 935

Day 14 – Waldshut to Konstanz, 56 miles

"A pessimist sees the difficulty in every opportunity; an optimist sees the opportunity in every difficulty."
– Winston Churchill

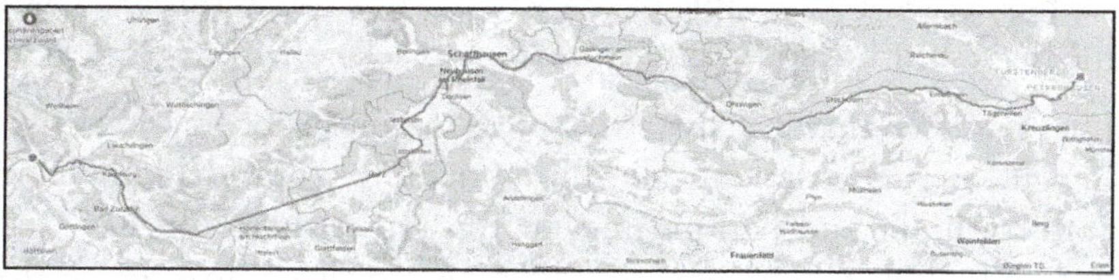

Today is meant to be the final day of heading east before crossing the expanse of the Bodensee by ferry and beginning the turn south, following the lakeside, and eventually climbing into the hills on the approach to St. Moritz. This persistent weather front had lingered longer than expected, stubborn and unpredictable – which suggested the low-pressure system was likely being blocked by a strong high-pressure ridge over eastern Europe, possibly centred over Russia.

The weather forecast had been a moving target for days, with any promises of sunshine being constantly pushed back, like a mirage on the horizon that kept retreating. I had prepared as thoroughly as I could, sealing essentials in plastic bags, taking extra care with anything electronic, and waterproofing the phone. I carried a big, heavy-duty charger with enough power capacity to recharge the phone four times. It was fully charged but for reasons unknown, the phone would not take the charge; it sat there, stubbornly stuck at 20%, which was not going to last long – not with all the tasks I was relying on it for.

The usual morning rituals unfolded: calibrating the glucometer and the ketone meter. By now, I was used to putting on wet shoes, and the waterproof jacket had become less of a weather item and more of a standard part of the uniform.

I had booked a room at a hostel last night, and there was no catering. Breakfast was makeshift and uninspired – a few slices of salami and half a cucumber left over from the day before. It was all I had to hand but it seemed about right. The shops were closed, as was typical for early morning in rural Germany, especially on a Sunday. I settled on my standard six units of Tresiba long-acting insulin, supplemented by a couple of units of rapid-acting insulin to cover the makeshift breakfast, and two strong black coffees.

I have noticed that if I have two coffees in quick succession, it raises my glucose – not dramatically, but noticeably – but I had my hand coffee grinder and had ground far too much. It would have felt wasteful, almost rude, not to indulge in the ritual, so I set up the Jetboil stove right there in my room.

My glucose had dropped overnight to a mild, asymptomatic 3 mmol/L (54 mg/dL), but had rebounded nicely to 6 mmol/L (108 mg/dL) by the time I was up and moving. Sleep had not been particularly refreshing. I awoke feeling heavy-limbed and unmotivated, my body registering fatigue despite what should have been enough rest. I was not feeling it today, and that was part of the reason I used a couple of units of rapid insulin – a kind of sixth sense. I was keen to set off, regardless; momentum, I find, often trumps lack of enthusiasm.

By this stage, I was well into the southern reaches of the Black Forest – that relaxing landscape of rolling green hills thick with trees, through which the Rhine lazily meanders, matching the winding rhythm of the roads. The houses here were beginning to show alpine character, with steep pitched roofs, tiled and fitted with built-in snow catchers. They had heavy wooden shutters, flower boxes brimming with colour, and charming little details such as drainage chains instead of downpipes, which gently guided rainwater to the ground.

My poor bike, however, was not enjoying the scenery. It was spattered with mud – not just the tyres or frame but the brakes, derailleur and drivetrain, all coated in a cake of damp grit. The previous night, I had taken the panniers into the shower to rinse them off, and had dealt with the worst of the muck on the chain using a cleansing wipe, followed by a dose of chain oil. It was not perfect but it would have to do.

A couple of links were starting to seize; I could feel them catching rhythmically through the pedals as they skipped and resisted over the smaller, rear cogs. I gave the chain a waggle of encouragement. It would certainly survive the journey, but preserving it for as long as possible was a matter of mechanical respect. One has to look after machinery with as much care as the body. I was a few days away from a stopover in Lindau, where I could give everything the attention it deserved.

I plugged in the phone once more. There was still no charge; the screen flickered, briefly came to life, then powered down again. I tried a second cable, but there was still nothing. I had no choice but to use the backup phone – an older iPhone model – but that, too, was out of power. It was not the start I had hoped for. I had been looking forward to documenting this stage of the journey in full: GPS tracking, Strava logging and CGM readings, all powered by battery. Now, with just 20% charge left, it felt like everything was on a knife-edge.

Without CGM, I needed to fall back on traditional finger-prick testing. It was not ideal, especially in the rain, where wet fingers prevent blood from forming a bead and ruin test strips. I briefly considered mapping using the fold-out paper map from the guidebook, but it was unmounted and not waterproof – impractical in these conditions. And it was Sunday. The shops were closed, so buying a new charger was out of the question. My only real hope was a café – somewhere with a plug socket and a warm seat – which I tried but there was no plug in sight. I even tried plugging my phone into my laptop and draining its battery, but nothing was working.

Outside, the wet began to seep through my gloves and into my sleeves. I gave up on power, mounted the bike and started riding, partly to get moving again, partly just to warm up. Within the hour, the last of the phone's battery had drained away. The CGM was down, the GPS gone. Manual diabetes-management mode was now fully engaged. It used to be the norm but, to my surprise, I felt a little unsettled about it.

With no digital guidance, I decided to take the direct, well-signed route along the main road straight to Konstanz. It was a trunk route but being Sunday, it was relatively quiet; it was nothing like the constant hum of traffic on a UK main road. The tarmac was smooth, the bends forgiving, and the climbs gentle. I decided to ride the 25 miles to Schaffhausen on this major road and worry about details later. I am no stranger to traffic, and the priority now was progress, not perfection.

Then, about 10 miles from Waldshut, I turned right without thinking, following a familiar green cycle-route sign to Schaffhausen – having forgotten I was supposed to avoid exactly that.

At the junction was a tiny village. On the left, I spotted a small tabak-laden corner shop selling newspapers, soft drinks, snacks, cigarettes and other essentials. As I cycled past, I saw something unexpected through the window – a rack of phone accessories on the back wall. I doubled back, propped up the bike outside and stepped in. Using a mix of halting German, English, hand gestures and goodwill, I explained my situation.

As luck would have it, right there on the counter were small, bright-green charging packs, the Chimpy brand. Swiss-made, rental-based; you usually return them for a deposit minus a €3 usage fee. They were not high capacity, maybe a third of what my "brick" carried, but, crucially, they were fully charged.

I bought one immediately, then a hundred metres later turned around and bought another for insurance. If one failed, the other would cover me. Together, they would see me through the day – each pack gave one-and-a-half full charges. They were lightweight, about the same size as my phone, with a short cable that looped over the top, tucking the pack neatly behind. They were perfect; I now rarely go anywhere without one.

That moment of finding a battery by pure chance reminded me of a common adage: "Be ready when your opportunity arrives!" The real challenge is recognising the opportunity. That unexpected find in that tiny shop, on a Sunday, in an unassuming village, transformed the day. Suddenly, I was operational again – with CGM data, a functioning map, GPS for guidance, Strava for tracking, and a live ketone monitor.

I checked the CGM: glucose was rising, hitting 9 mmol/L (148 mg/dL). It was not stabilising; it was climbing. That was unusual. I checked the continuous ketone meter. It had risen from 0.5 mmol/L to 3 mmol/L. What did this mean? With no carbs in the meal, glucose was rising because of a lack of insulin – possibly a *relative* lack, triggered by adrenaline or cortisol. But still, I had not given enough insulin to suppress the glucose, so it climbed, unchecked. And what causes ketones? Fat burning! And what allows fat burning? Low insulin!

Insufficient insulin is not something you see often in conventional type 1 diabetes management. We are always taught to watch for *too much* insulin. "Insulin on board" is usually about hypoglycaemia. But here we had the opposite: too little. It was not optimal, but it did suggest I was very close to optimal – just slightly under. I was about to hit the road again for another push to Schaffhausen, and I did not want any drama, but clearly I needed to top up the insulin to prevent further rise. I have plenty of hormones that raise glucose levels, but insulin is the only one that lowers them.

What happened next was the most powerful demonstration – if ever one was needed – of insulin's effect on ketosis. I took a single unit, with a cautious calculation of insulin sensitivity of 2.5, aiming to bring glucose down from 9 mmol/L (148 mg/dL) to 6.5 mmol/L (117 mg/dL), and hoping Tresiba would smooth out the rest. That happened as predicted: the ketone level dropped sharply from 3 mmol/L to 0.5 mmol/L. This was insulin regulating the level of ketones.

From an earlier chapter, we know that ketones can self-regulate by stimulating beta cells to secrete insulin. I could not do that – but I could inject it. This ketone drop was an example of that effect in action. Few people wear continuous ketone meters, so it is rarely seen. We are all used to taking correction doses for high glucose, and we often assume it is due to a mismatch of carbs and insulin. But how many times is it actually due to insufficient insulin?

In any event, this was reassurance that there is no risk of DKA if we correct glucose early and use insulin to suppress further ketosis. What a demonstration of metabolism in action! I have made a presentation slide of this very moment, and use it often; it shows that if you have enough insulin, diabetic ketoacidosis is simply not going to happen. Yes, there are clinical exceptions, but for 99.9% of cases, this single graph puts an end to the woolly thinking around nutritional ketosis and diabetic ketoacidosis.

I pressed on for Schaffhausen, this time sticking with the road. The route had no real climbs, its curves flattened for cars and its surface like velvet – no frustrating zigzags, no right-angle crossings to rejoin the cycle path. I occasionally spotted the bike track disappearing into the wooded hills to my right, but that was not for today; I did not have it in me.

Schaffhausen is the site of the famous Rheinfall, Europe's largest waterfall by volume. I had intended to visit it but Google Maps sent me wandering in circles around the town centre. I eventually gave up on technology and reverted to something more reliable: the local road signs.

I ended up on the opposite bank of the river from where I wanted to be, but still got a decent view, standing on a wall looking across a railway line near a station. As expected, the attraction was thoroughly touristy. Small, colourful boats took visitors into the mist and spray, everyone wearing bright, waterproof jackets. They spent a few minutes near the base of the falls before drifting back to make room for the next group. It probably would have been fun, especially with the recent rain swelling the river to full power, but the last thing I needed was another soaking.

Instead, I headed for warmth. I found a local bar that doubled as a café. No one inside spoke much English but I managed well enough with gestures and my slowly improving, though still basic, German. It was a friendly, local place. I wrapped up in extra layers and sat on the small covered terrace outside, sheltered from the drizzle, and watched the slow pace of a Sunday morning unfold. After finishing my coffee, I booked a hotel in Konstanz. The rest of the day's ride would be completed in under 60 miles. It was mildly hilly in parts, but not especially testing. Still, my legs were feeling it; I was not flying along, like previous days.

Glucose was still high, hovering around 10 mmol/L (160 mg/dL), and I was not responding to insulin in the same way; a single unit would drop me only 2–3 mmol/L (36-54 mg/dL), which was different from the response on Day 1, when a unit at that glucose level sent me crashing into a hypo. My food intake had not changed. I was relying on meat and cheese – not in large quantities, so there was not much carbohydrate or even gluconeogenic protein to push glucose up. And yet, I needed more insulin today than on any other day of the trip. I had a slight headache, the kind that hints at dehydration or the start of something like an infection.

I drank a litre of water and continued dosing insulin, adding another unit, then another, just to keep things under control. It was strange. I was working hard today, and the data showed it; I was pushing through, but with what felt like twice the usual effort. I had to make single-unit corrections more often, and even then, I was not seeing the usual drop in glucose. Was I coming down with something? I was not sure.

By now, I had covered nearly 900 miles without a break. At 800 miles, I had felt strong – fresh, even. The cumulative strain was probably showing. I was not falling apart, but I had to draw on reserves I had not needed before. It was one of those rides where you do everything right, everything the same, and still the results are different. Today, my type 1 was not cooperating; maybe it was stress hormones, maybe something else, I could only guess. What I did know was that this was a day to keep my head down and get the job done, trusting that tomorrow would be better.

Two kilometres outside Shaffhausen, I rejoined the EuroVelo Rhine cycle route. The junction was a jumble of signage, twelve directions at once, but my route was clear. I followed it through a recently flooded section. Inflatable barriers had been laid down to protect the path, and the route continued along the Rhine, coated in fine, slick sediment from the previous night's overflow; it made for slippery riding over the next few kilometres. The river to my left surged downstream. It was brown and swollen with silt and rain, carrying whole trees with it, their roots ripped from the banks upstream.

I climbed a gentle incline into the picture-book village of Stein am Rhein, which revealed itself as one of those delightful surprises you stumble upon without planning. The village is famous for its beautifully preserved, half-timbered medieval buildings, many with elaborately painted facades showing fruit bowls, flowers, horses and carts, and even playful cartoon figures. I had never heard of it, never researched it – but it was clearly a magnet for visitors.

Situated at the western edge of the Untersee, where the lake connects with the Bodensee via the Rhine, Stein am Rhein grew around a monastery and thrived as a fishing village. Today, its prosperity comes from tourism, but it is no less charming for it. The cobbled square was wet and uneven, making the short ride through it a minor challenge. I paused to refill my water and grab a few snacks before pushing on. I was so close to Konstanz, I could almost feel it.

Back on the bike, into the countryside, I continued winding through farmland and low, forested hills. It was pleasant, though I was too focused on progress to fully absorb my surroundings. I glanced at the ketone meter. It had dropped from 2 mmol/L earlier to 0.6 mmol/L for most of the last stretch. That was telling: it was the insulin. The higher doses I had had today reduced my ketone levels but I was still in the multi-fuelling range.

I pedalled the final miles through damp woods and quiet roads, powered not just by my legs but by resolve. Eventually, the vast blue expanse of the Bodensee appeared through the lifting cloud. I had made it. I checked into a hotel about a mile from the ferry port. Tomorrow, I would begin the next chapter – turning south along the eastern bank of the Bodensee and continuing to St. Moritz. But first, I went to find food.

I spotted a restaurant but, of course, it was Sunday and they were closing early. I was not in the mood to search far. Supper became a continuation of lunch: leftover salami and cheese. I was not especially hungry, so it was enough. It was not ideal, but adequate. A warm meal would have been nicer. I brewed a camping-stove coffee in the hotel room, knowing it might delay sleep but needing something warm; hot water did not appeal that night.

I now have a clear understanding of the foundations of health that I use as a framework to manage my type 1 diabetes – not strict rules but guiding principles. Today, as on every day of this journey, I rated my performance against each of those foundations.

Starting with sleep, I noted it had been decent – not great, but respectable. I still felt tired on waking, suggesting residual fatigue. I gave it an 8 out of 10.

Food, though ketogenic and functional, was not inspiring; no real variety, warmth or joy. It did the job required, but little more than that. I rated it a 5.

Physical activity dropped below the usual nine or ten. I felt every mile, every incline, every effort. I was not underperforming, but it took more from me than expected. I gave it a 7.

Mindset was not negative, but it was a day for digging in. I was not riding on enthusiasm, just doing what needed to be done. Adaptable and steady, but without much spark. I rated it a 6.

Environment, by contrast, was exceptional. Despite grey skies, rain and chill, I had cycled through some of the most beautiful countryside I have seen. Hills, rivers, medieval villages, painted buildings and wide-open spaces – even without sunshine, it was remarkable. I gave it an 8.

I plotted these numbers on a radar map, a visualisation I have come to appreciate; it shows how well I have supported myself across the core areas of health, and how that relates to insulin use and glucose stability.

One key detail: glucose control does not appear on the map. That is deliberate. Glucose is an *outcome*, not a root; if I get the foundations right – sleep, food, activity, mindset, environment – the glucose tends to follow. It is a reflection of internal balance.

Despite the challenges, I had stayed in range about 90% of the time today. Yes, glucose was higher at points, and I used more insulin than usual, but that does not mean I overused it. My personal rule is simple: use as much as necessary, but as little as possible. That does not mean underdosing or avoiding corrections; it means being strategic. If more insulin is needed to meet the day's demands, so be it – but use it with intent.

I suspected what I needed was a rest. Not just a night's sleep, but a proper break. I would see how things felt in a few days. The body adapts, but it also whispers when it needs recovery. I have learned to listen.

And so, the day ended – not triumphant, but complete. I took my usual six units of Tresiba, my nightly anchor, and settled in. I was now just seven days from my final destination and, remarkably, still ahead of schedule.

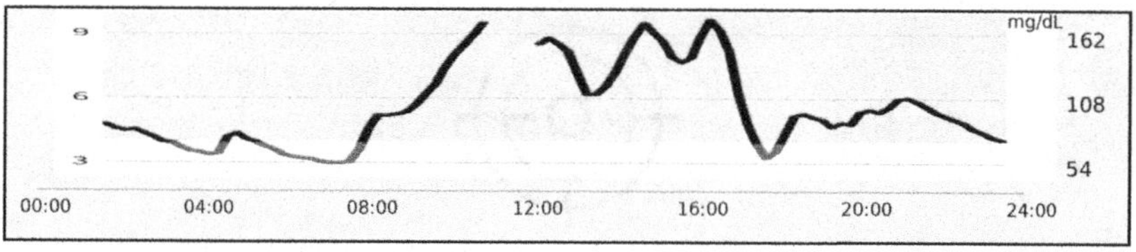
mg/dL
162
108
54
9
6
3
00:00
04:00
08:00
12:00
16:00
20:00
24:00

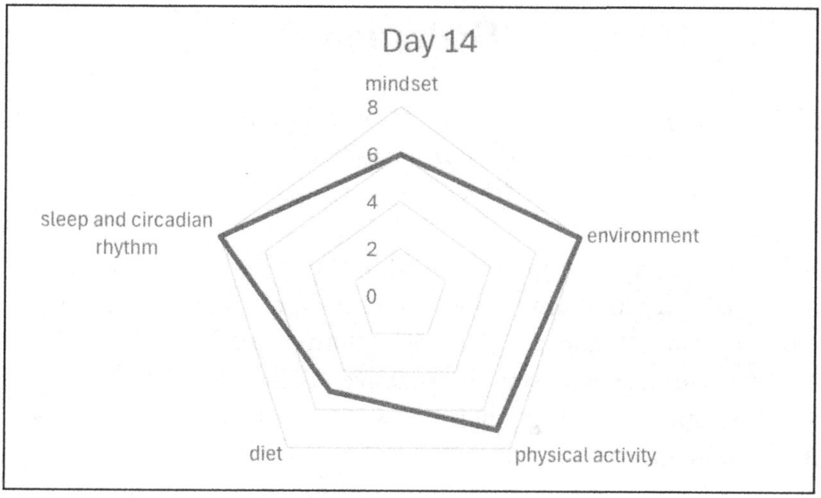
Day 14
mindset
8
6
4
2
0
environment
physical activity
diet
sleep and circadian rhythm

Chapter 33
Hydration

"Water is life's matter and matrix, mother and medium. There is no life without water."
– Albert Szent-Gyorgyi

When I was growing up, we played in the fields on farmland. Even in hot weather, the farm labourers who were out in the sun all day only drank about a litre and a half of fluids. Usually, it was water or cold tea, because that was the practice at the time. I followed the same practice, drinking when I was thirsty; I knew no other way. And it seemed to work fine.

Hydration is a topic that everyone has a firm opinion about. Over the years, we have all heard endless advice about drinking enough water. It is a frequent theme in health conversations. Everywhere you look, someone is telling you exactly how much to drink for a certain distance or on hot days, or which fluid is best. And then there is maybe the strangest idea of all – overhydration to "detox". People seem to like the idea that flushing things with water, like hosing down the patio, must also work inside the body.

But evidence suggests that the human body has evolved to use resources carefully, including water. Healthy urine is usually straw-coloured. When you are underhydrated, it gets darker; when you are overhydrated, it turns almost clear. Over the years in clinics, I have noticed that urine samples are becoming paler. Maybe we are overdoing it.

What are the current recommendations? What should we actually do when hydrating? Of course, fluids are not only for thirst – we drink tea, coffee and alcohol socially.

Where Does Our Water Come From?

There are two main places: what we drink and what our bodies make. The water our cells make is called metabolic water, and it is produced during cellular respiration. When mitochondria make energy, they produce water and carbon dioxide. Oxygen accepts electrons and joins with hydrogen ions to form water. To put numbers on it, when metabolised, 100 g of fat produces about 100 ml of water; 100 g of protein produces about 42 ml; and 100 g of carbohydrate produces about 60 ml. Humans get around 10% of their daily water requirements from their metabolism, and more when exercising, when some of it might even contribute to sweat.

We lose water through urination, breathing, sweating and bowel movements. Stool is about one-third water. Urine also removes nitrogen waste as urea. One interesting idea I found was that the water produced by metabolising protein approximately matches the water needed to excrete the urea produced from that protein. Birds and reptiles do even better – they excrete uric acid, which uses less water. In fact, birds actually gain water from protein metabolism, and some desert animals survive entirely on metabolic water.

Hydration and Heart Health

Water and sodium balance are essential for the cardiovascular system. The brain's osmoreceptors (salt concentration sensors) sense when cells shrink from lack of water, and that triggers thirst. They also release antidiuretic hormone (ADH) to reduce urine production.

When blood volume drops, other receptors send signals that activate hormones such as renin, angiotensin II, and aldosterone, which help the body retain sodium and water. All of this helps keep blood pressure stable, especially in the brain.

These hormones often activate even before you drink anything, in anticipation of fluid loss or dehydration. Some scientists think that problems with this so-called renin–angiotensin system may be linked to diseases like hypertension, obesity, diabetes, and even cancer.

Salt retention is partly controlled by insulin. Too much insulin means too much salt is held in the body, raising blood pressure. Certainly, many blood-pressure-lowering medications target the renin-angiotensin system. Reducing salt helps, but it is really treating a symptom of too much insulin, which is linked to both major types of diabetes. When you reduce insulin, you help reduce salt retention.

Water and Metabolism

Water also affects appetite and metabolism. Drinking water can stretch the stomach and make you feel full. A 2016 study showed that people who drank water before meals ate 22% fewer calories. Cold water can increase thermogenesis – the body uses energy to warm the cold water, which slightly raises metabolism. A 2003 study showed a temporary 30% rise in metabolic rate after healthy adults drank about two cups of water at 71°F (22°C).

How Much Should We Drink?

The "eight glasses a day" rule is too simple. Actual need depends on age, health, activity, sweat, and more. Most people can just trust their thirst. The National Academies suggest 2.7 litres per day for women and 3.7 litres for men, with 80% from drinks and 20% from food – just over two litres and three litres of actual fluid.

My best advice? Drink when you are thirsty! Sometimes we miss cues and become tired or hungry, but it is worth prioritising hydration first. Or carry out a "urological investigation", by looking at your pee. Pale yellow is ideal; dark means drink more; clear means overhydration (and frequent bathroom breaks).

I once watched a TV programme in which an interviewer spoke with bushmen who had been trained in the South African army. They worked in the Kalahari Desert in 40°C heat, wearing full combat gear. They were given two litres of water for the entire day – and they were fine. They just drank when they were thirsty. They did not look ill, at least not on TV. And someone in combat readiness would need to stay alert. These days, drinking only when thirsty seems like a "radical" idea.

Dehydration

To understand dehydration, it helps to imagine a 70 kg person. With about 55% body water, they carry roughly 38.5 litres of water. Every 1% of body weight lost is about 0.7 litres gone. Hydration is assessed clinically by observing physical cues to estimate the degree of dehydration.

- Mild dehydration (1–2% body weight loss, about 0.7–1.4 L in a 70 kg person): Thirst, darker urine, mild tiredness, dry mouth.
- Moderate dehydration (3–4% body weight loss, about 2.1–2.8 L): Headache, dizziness, irritability, faster heartbeat, dry skin.
- Severe dehydration (5–6% body weight loss or more, about 3.5–4.2 L): Weakness, confusion, very little sweating.

To see how extreme dehydration can get, look at Formula 1 drivers. In hot conditions, they can lose 2–4 kg of sweat, and in places like Singapore, sometimes the full 4 kg. That is around 5–6% of body weight – right in the range for severe dehydration. Yet they still perform at the highest level, at least for the duration of a race. The body is remarkable in extreme environments and seems designed to survive.

Overhydration

This leads us to overhydration – something we impose on ourselves. It is unnatural. More people in endurance events like marathons have died from drinking too much than too little.

This problem partly stems from a 1969 exercise physiology paper that was later misinterpreted, leading to the recommendation that athletes replace 100% of their predicted sweat loss during a race. The American College of Sports Medicine even suggested drinking up to 1,200 ml per hour. But many studies show this does not improve performance and can cause stomach problems.

We produce water from the combustion of glucose and fat. Glycogen also stores water (carbohydrate), which is released during its use. So, not all water loss needs to be replaced by drinking water. Burning fuel produces water (metabolic water). A marathon runner who finishes at the same weight they started may actually be overhydrated by up to two litres.

A dangerous form of overhydration can cause low blood sodium levels, where cells swell with water, especially in the brain, increasing pressure. Symptoms include confusion, lethargy, seizures and coma. Common causes include drinking to prevent dehydration, psychogenic over-drinking, certain drugs, and SIADH (a condition where the body releases too much antidiuretic hormone, or ADH).

So where do I stand? Pretty much where I began. I drink when I am thirsty; I listen to my body. I do not believe we need to drown ourselves in water to be healthy. The body evolved in conditions of scarcity; it knows what to do. We just need to listen.

Cutting carbohydrates has helped me understand my body in a way I could not before. This adventure was originally called "Silence the Chainsaw and Hear the Birds Sing", which fits perfectly with hydration.

Water Memory, Magnetic Effects, and the Moon

The French immunologist, Jacques Benveniste's work appeared to suggest that biological effects remained even after extreme dilution. Because these dilutions could go beyond the point at which any molecules of the original substance were likely to remain, some saw this as support for homeopathy's proposed mechanism. The claim was highly controversial. Some dismissed it without fully investigating.

Subsequent research examined changes in water under magnetic fields, stirring or dilution. Some studies showed changes in hydrogen bonding or surface tension, others found nothing. The debate goes on. The truth is, we still do not know everything about water.

We all know the Moon moves oceans, but does it move us? After all, we are 60% water. Does the tide affect humans? According to current science, no. The gravitational difference between your head and your feet is tiny compared to the gravity acting on oceans. Our internal fluids are influenced by blood pressure, movement and cell activity, not the Moon.

Are there subtle effects that might exist, but we can't yet measure? Possibly – there is so much to discover. Remember, the microbiome did not officially "exist" until recently.

Chapter 34
Total Miles: 979

Day 15 – Konstanz to Lindau, 32 miles

"Change is the law of life and those who look only to the past or present are certain to miss the future."
– John F. Kennedy

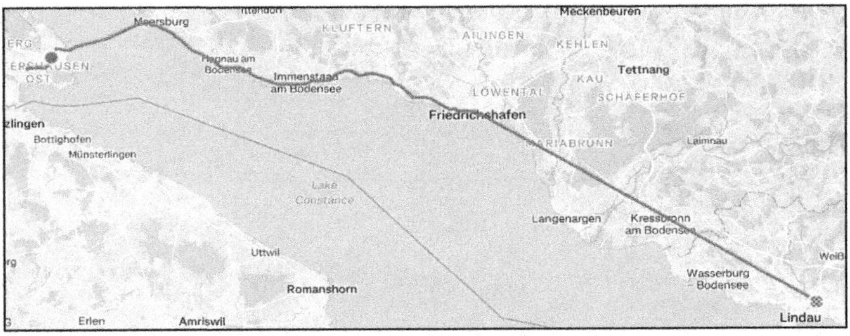

I was not intending to cycle today. The forecast was gloomy, with rain all day, but the next three days looked dry – until an anticipated further deterioration. However, feeling fired up, I was keen to press on. On the last two days of the adventure, there would be the challenge of hills, and I might have to have a rethink if the Albula Pass was closed across the Alps, but as of today, it was expected to open in four days' time. So, if I pressed on with longer distances, it would be closed; I needed to be patient.

But I also decided I needed a ride out today. The town of Konstanz looked nice, but the weather was cool and wet, and it was not a place to hang around. The rain was easing, so I decided to press on to the south of Bodensee. I wandered down to the ferry terminal, which was a slight downhill to the edge of the lake. Top survival tip: if you need to find a river or any body of water, follow the downhill!

I was going to arrive in St. Moritz three days early, based on progress so far. I was feeling fit enough overall, and the bike had proven itself to be up for the job; it was unlikely to encounter any greater punishment than it already had. So, after the day's effort, I decided I would take a rest. I intended to spend three days in Lindau, the last town in Germany on the border with Austria. To get to Switzerland, I would need to pass through Austria and Liechtenstein on the first day of the final push to St. Moritz.

I also decided to abandon camping. The weather had dampened the desire, and I needed dry places and electricity to record everything. I could, of course, do this from a tent, but camping in the damp and wet is a skill in itself, and is fine if there is no alternative. The discipline needed to keep everything dry was not something I wanted to contend with now.

I planned to ship back the excess bags of camping gear before I headed out on the final days of riding; the last three days would be the most gruelling in terms of gradient since the first two days after leaving Stroud, so it was a perfect time to take a break to let my body relax and properly nourish itself.

I opted to stay in Lindau, a trivial 27 miles away, with fairly flat roads. The Zeppelin Museum in Friedrichshafen, which I planned to visit, was about halfway along; it is dedicated to the first golden era of flight, in the 1920s, when experimentation was maturing into commercial viability, and airships led the way in air travel.

Breakfast was okay, with eggs, cucumber, jellied meat, and a small piece of cheese. For the last two or three days, glucose levels had been trickier to control, but it was all relative. Doing roughly the same thing on each of those days had required more vigilance with the rapid-acting insulin. I might just have been tired, but it coincided with a much less rigorous diet; I was nibbling cured meats and cheese, and they did not feel healthy – more just a fuelling substance. I had tried mixing it up with some fish and veg but had not eaten out for two nights, instead using up the remnants of the day's food. This is the difference between fuel and food. And all of those additives in cured meats cannot be good.

I had six days to correct this and would put it to good use tomorrow. I did not think alcohol was that healthy either. Alcohol is more toxic than sugar, and I had been having small amounts on some nights when eating out. I would also stop this for the next few days; I did not feel that this was puritanical or suffering, just a reset.

It was even more challenging to get the glucose level down that morning. I normally liked to get started after eating breakfast, but 45 minutes of standing on the ferry across the north end of Bodensee meant the protein was not being metabolised, and glucose was building up from its breakdown into glucose. I had taken a unit for breakfast and took another one on the ferry, plus two more single units en route. My reading nudged 10 mmol/L (180 mg/dL) but soon came down with the effort of cycling, and remained good all day. I really did not have to bother with diabetes for the rest of that day.

For most of the history of insulin use in type 1 diabetes, diet was more restricted than it is now. Over the years, the carbohydrate content has shifted to reflect more closely the general population's diet. Beginning at 10–20% of total energy intake, it ballooned to 55–60%.

Carbohydrate counting and insulin dose adjustment have been the mainstays of type 1 practice for decades. In the 1970s, when the new guidelines to prevent heart disease were introduced, the carb content of the diet went up – and it kept going. The idea was that because type 1s have three or four times more heart attacks than those without, a diet designed to prevent heart attacks in people without type 1, recommending low-fat intake, was acceptable for type 1s too.

Did you spot the flaw? Type 1s have no ability to be so accurate and sensitive with insulin, so the increase in carbohydrates is a big ask, if we are aiming for good glucose control. The wonderful and freedom-giving pen could not cope either; nor could the modern rapid insulins designed specifically to get around the problem of high carbs.

The mean HbA1c in England and Wales is 70 mmol/mol, or 8.6% – which is, let's face it, a disaster. The tragedy is that it is avoidable. And still widely practised.

When we discovered the cause, insulin deficiency, daily life and longer-term survival improved for everyone. And yet, we still revert, even today, to managing the *symptom*, glucose, rather than the *cause*, insulin. It can work, but I do not think that should be the aim; we need to understand how treating the cause can be optimised, and then all of the symptoms will improve. You can treat the pain of an abscess and also medicate to lower the temperature, but this alone will not heal the cause. It is best to drain the abscess, which involves using the appropriate treatment directed at the root cause.

I headed into Friedrichshafen, roughly following the road that hugs Bodensee, having decided on a leisurely, slower-paced cycle ride. However, I soon got into a brisker speed as I went – trying to ride slowly was stressful. I parked up at the Zeppelin Museum.

In this part of Germany, the birth of airships began. For something built over a century ago, the scale and engineering confidence were immense. These ships of the air were simply huge and offered a high level of luxury attainable only by the very few. Inside, the actual body was built with luxury dining, seating and bunk areas, as well as vast viewing galleries. It must have been the equivalent of space travel today.

But the best exhibit by far was the *Gaylord Gladiator*. It was not an airship at all, but a car built just after I was born. It represented the ambition and optimism of the jet age and space age we had entered at that time. The design was influenced by the great US brands, and indeed this car had a Chevy eight-cylinder engine and a scalloped side panel painted off-white, à la Ford Mustang, setting off a black body. It had a huge downward and rear-slanting chrome grille, to mimic a jet intake. The bonnet and boot were as long as each other, with a two-person aircraft-style cockpit in the middle. All the mandatory dials, plus more, peppered the wooden dash, and the chrome and leather trim set it all off. The rear ended in exaggerated fins and a large, corrugated chrome rear panel sprouted twin exhausts. The wheels were spoked with knock-off hubcaps and whitewall tyres. If it comes up for sale, I am selling everything – it might buy me the spare tyre.

While it was still spitting with rain, I holed up in a café and checked for accommodation in Lindau. I would easily make it. The rain had finally eased, but resumed again for the last hour. I took the route following the south road by Bodensee towards Lindau. My Strava map failed to record anything on that short ride and produced only a straight line in an obviously embarrassed attempt to cover up its error.

After a few miles, the road ahead was flooded under an underpass. It was about two feet deep, and I could not guarantee there would not be any potholes lurking beneath the surface. All of my electrical equipment was wrapped up in the waterproof rear panniers, but they would be half-submerged if I went for it. I could have taken them off and carried them to the other side, but I opted to add a ten-mile detour; I had time that day, and on this stretch of the journey, after all that distance, it was no big deal.

I soon made short work of the remaining uneventful miles, with no view of the lake because of the mist. I headed for a small hotel a couple of miles from the centre. It was on a hill and I had a balcony with, I was told, a distant lake view, which I hoped I would see tomorrow.

It would be a strange experience relaxing for three days; I was definitely in "go" mode. The next three days of rest would be a good time to take stock and regroup after the focused dash to get the miles in while I remained injury-free and healthy.

I also needed to do some work on the bike. It needed the head bearings tightened. I had noticed it a couple of days ago on a smooth stretch of road: just the tiniest amount of "give". I decided to service it. If I did nothing, it would easily do the distance, but I needed to look after all of my resources, and the bike was an essential tool right now. Plus, it is a good feeling when mechanical things are working perfectly.

I was not at all surprised that the heads needed adjustment; they had taken the brunt of all the kerbs, tree roots and uneven surfaces on the journey, plus the weight of the camping luggage. Remarkably, the bike had withstood the punishment. I was in awe of those aluminium rear frame tubes, which were no wider than my little finger, and pleased I chose it over my touring bike. The ride feel was excellent, and even under load, it gave the impression that all my effort was going straight to the rear wheel; this is not the case on all bikes. Whoever designed this bike had me in mind.

I finished the day with the leftovers (again!), including some tuna, cucumber, a bit of pork slice and some Emmental. My diabetes control was good, as I gave myself six units of Tresiba and a couple of units of rapid-acting insulin. The glucose level stayed steady through the night. Tomorrow was a rest day. It would require some thought. Should I reduce my insulin dose when I rest, or keep the same dose?

My spider map looked good today. I gave nutrition a 5 (having had a good breakfast but poor daily food, tins and packets). Exercise was a 10 – no issues. Sleep was good. I gave it a 9. And environment and mindset were rated 10.

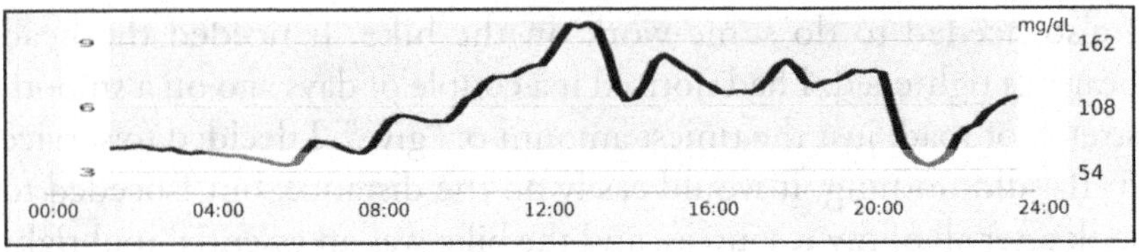
mg/dL
162
108
54
00:00
04:00
08:00
12:00
16:00
20:00
24:00

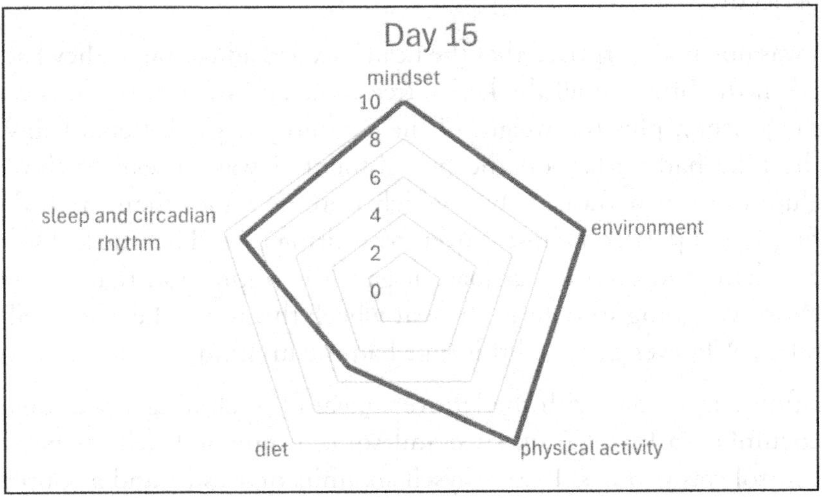
Day 15
mindset
10
8
6
4
2
0
environment
physical activity
diet
sleep and circadian rhythm

Chapter 35
Cholesterol and Lipids

A high-fat diet, such as the ketogenic diet used in optimised insulin for type 1 diabetes, is often a cause of concern. It is typically associated with heart disease, but this is a matter of debate and depends largely on the metabolic context. We know from earlier chapters that the relationship between saturated fat and heart disease is more complex than once thought, but cholesterol remains a great concern for many. This chapter aims to explain cholesterol and its transport, and how metabolic conditions influence heart health.

Cholesterol is a fatty, wax-like substance found in foods that come from animals, and is also produced by our own bodies. It belongs to a family of molecules called sterols, defined by a characteristic ring structure. The word "chole" relates to bile, because cholesterol is used to make bile acids in the liver. Cholesterol is not "fat" in the way we normally use the word – fat has a different chemical structure.

People often talk about cholesterol as "good" or "bad", but that is an oversimplification. It is neither. A cholesterol molecule in "good" cholesterol looks and behaves in exactly the same way as cholesterol in a "bad" cholesterol carrier (see below). What matters is how it behaves in the body.

Cholesterol is essential. Every cell in the body uses it to keep its outer membrane strong yet flexible. It helps form the protective coating around nerves, allowing electrical signals to travel along them, and serves as the base material for hormones such as cortisol, oestrogen and testosterone.

Cholesterol is often treated as a fixed number – a result on a blood test that is either "good" or "bad". In reality, cholesterol is not static; like glucose, insulin and cortisol, it follows a circadian rhythm that is controlled by the body's internal clock. This circadian rhythm influences how cholesterol is made, moved and cleared. These patterns exist even when we are not eating – food matters, but timing matters too. Most cholesterol in the blood is made in the liver, and this process peaks at night, usually between midnight and the early morning hours. Cholesterol is constantly recycled. As tissues break down and rebuild, cholesterol moves around to where it is needed. Neutrophils, for example (white blood cells that help fight infection), only live a day or two. We make and break down billions of these cells each day, and every one of them contains cholesterol. This is a reminder that cholesterol metabolism is dynamic and finely tuned, supporting cell regeneration, removal and repair.

Cholesterol measured in the blood represents it being transported to tissues to take part in essential cellular processes. About 70% of cholesterol comes from our own internal production (the "endogenous" pathway), and about 30% from food in a typical mixed diet (the "exogenous" pathway). Vegans consume zero cholesterol, yet still have cholesterol in their blood because the body makes it. If we do not eat cholesterol, the liver makes more to meet demand. The liver acts as the body's reservoir, adjusting production to keep levels steady, while the brain makes its own supply. Cells are quite independent. Every nucleated cell can make cholesterol for itself if needed, which shows how important this substance is.

The pathway for making cholesterol is complicated, involving many steps and enzymes. Each of those steps produces molecules that can also be used to make other important biologically active compounds. Cholesterol, and the pathway that produces it, gives rise to many vital substances, including:

- Steroid hormones
- Vitamin D
- Coenzyme Q10
- Bile acids

Cells also protect themselves from having too much free (biologically active) cholesterol. They can "lock it away" by turning it into an ester, or they can push it out of the cell, where it is collected and processed.

Interestingly, the brain contains about 20% of the body's cholesterol, making it the most cholesterol-rich organ. Due to the protective blood-brain barrier (BBB), the brain is largely isolated from the rest of the body's cholesterol traffic. A small amount may pass through the BBB, but the overwhelming majority of brain cholesterol is synthesised locally within the brain.

Because cholesterol does not readily cross the blood-brain barrier, circulating LDL and HDL – complex lipid transport systems that carry cholesterol around the body – have minimal direct influence on brain cholesterol levels. Instead, the brain maintains a tightly regulated, self-contained cholesterol system that supports synapse formation, myelin maintenance (a protective coating around the nerves), and neuronal signalling.

Brain cholesterol synthesis and turnover follow circadian rhythms, coordinated with sleep-wake cycles. Cholesterol synthesis in the brain is highest during sleep, peaking during slow-wave (deep) sleep and declining during waking hours, reflecting subtle circadian variation. This rhythm aligns with periods of brain repair, such as myelin sheath maintenance, membrane repair and new growth, so that during sleep, the brain effectively services its lipid infrastructure.

Much of this cholesterol resides in glial cells – non-neuronal cells that support the neurons structurally and metabolically. A lot of it is found in the myelin sheaths, which improve electrical signal transmission, as well as insulating nerve fibres.

Brain cholesterol turnover is extremely slow. While plasma cholesterol might be turned over within days, cholesterol in the brain may persist for anywhere from six months to five years. The disposal of surplus cholesterol relies on specialised transporters: lipoproteins, which carry it to the liver for further processing.

Lipoproteins: The Transport System

Cholesterol cannot travel in the blood by itself because it is not water-soluble. Instead, the body packages it inside lipoproteins, which are small particles made of lipids and proteins. They act like delivery vehicles, carrying cholesterol, fat-soluble vitamins and triglycerides (fat) around the body. The main lipoproteins are:

- Chylomicrons
- VLDL (very low-density lipoprotein)
- IDL (intermediate-density lipoprotein)
- LDL (low-density lipoprotein)
- HDL (high-density lipoprotein)

Lipoproteins change composition as they deliver their triglyceride loads. When they carry a lot of triglycerides, they are larger and less dense. As these triglycerides are dropped off to tissues – mainly muscle and fat cells – the particles become smaller and denser. Proteins on the surface of lipoproteins help them dock with cells, allowing the particles or their contents to be taken up for use in tissue growth, repair and energy production.

HDL is often called "good cholesterol", but it is really a lipoprotein that helps remove excess cholesterol from tissues and carry it back to the liver. Cholesterol is not LDL or HDL; there is a big difference. LDL and HDL carry cholesterol in the body for delivery and removal, while HDL cholesterol is the amount of cholesterol in an HDL lipoprotein. Other fat-soluble substances in LDL, like triglycerides or some vitamins, could in principle also be measured.

Lipoproteins are transport particles, not cholesterol itself; they carry varying amounts of cholesterol depending on the body's needs.

Apolipoproteins: The Tags That Direct Traffic

Every lipoprotein has apolipoproteins (protein tags that act as address labels) on its surface. Think of these as ID tags that tell the body:

- Where the particle should go
- Which receptors should accept it

- What it is supposed to carry

The most important tags are:

- ApoB-48 → found on chylomicrons (dietary fat from the gut)
- ApoB-100 → found on VLDL, IDL and LDL

Receptors that recognise ApoB-100 are found throughout the body, with the highest concentration in the liver. These receptors remove LDL particles from the bloodstream so their cholesterol can be used or recycled by cells. LDL receptor activity follows a circadian rhythm and tends to be lower at night.

LDL

LDL's job is to carry cholesterol from the liver to tissues that need it. It is not "bad" by itself. In a calm, lower-insulin environment, LDL is cleared efficiently, delivering cholesterol where it is needed for structure and repair.

Small, Dense LDL

LDL becomes a problem only when:

- It stays in the bloodstream too long
- It becomes oxidised
- It enters inflamed vessel walls

When triglycerides are high and insulin levels are elevated, limiting fat uptake into tissues, LDL stays in circulation longer and becomes small and dense. At this point, it is easier for it to get trapped in the walls of arteries and become oxidised. This small, dense LDL (sdLDL) is more strongly associated with heart disease – unlike the larger, fluffy LDL that tends to be seen in people eating fewer carbohydrates.

Statins lower overall LDL levels, but primarily reduce larger, fluffy LDL, which is less harmful to arteries. They have limited effect on sdLDL unless insulin and triglycerides improve.

LDL cholesterol tends to rise overnight, peak in the early morning, and fall during the day. This circadian variation is typically around 5–10%. For most people, this change is modest, but it can be larger in diabetes, insulin resistance or disrupted sleep. This also means morning fasting blood tests often show higher LDL levels.

HDL: The Return Journey

HDL is made mainly in the liver and intestines, starting as a thin, nearly empty disc with just enough structure to travel through the bloodstream. HDL has a circadian rhythm; it is usually lowest overnight and highest during the day. As a result, the LDL-to-HDL ratio is often worst in the early morning. After synthesis in the liver and intestine, HDL begins its round-trip journey:

1. Cholesterol Efflux – Collecting Waste

HDL collects excess cholesterol from:

- Cells
- Foam cells in artery walls (immune cells)
- Other lipoproteins

This pickup is helped by special transporters on cells that push cholesterol out for removal.

2. Cholesterol Esterification – Packing the Cargo

Once HDL collects free cholesterol, an enzyme called LCAT converts it into a tightly packed, chemically inert "ester", allowing HDL to grow from a flat disc into a sphere. This helps HDL collect even more cholesterol.

3. Travel Back to the Liver

Loaded HDL travels through the bloodstream towards the liver.

4. Uptake Into the Liver

The liver takes cholesterol from HDL using a special receptor called SR-BI, which selectively pulls in the cholesterol but leaves the HDL particle behind to be reused.

5. Bile Acid Creation

The liver turns much of the cholesterol into bile acids, needed for fat digestion.

6. Excretion

Around half of the cholesterol in bile acids is reabsorbed, but some cholesterol leaves the body in the stool.

This whole loop is called reverse cholesterol transport.

How Diet Shapes Lipoprotein Patterns

High-Carb Diet

A diet high in carbs – particularly refined types – raises:

- Insulin
- Triglycerides
- Small, dense LDL

and lowers:

- HDL

This happens because excess carbs are turned into fat in the liver, overwhelming the system. In a high-carb diet, excess carbs can be turned into saturated fat, which then affects cholesterol and lipoproteins. Several decades ago, starchy foods were known as "fattening foods".

Low-Carb or Ketogenic Diet

On a low-carb diet:

- Insulin is low
- Triglycerides are low
- HDL rises
- LDL tends to be larger, lighter, and less harmful to arteries

The liver is not overwhelmed, and fat flows smoothly through its intended pathways.

The importance of this change in lipid profiles with diet is significant. Most, if not all, of the existing medical data on lipids and heart disease comes from a high-carb, high-insulin, fat-storing metabolism. A ketogenic diet, by contrast, is a low-carb, low-insulin, fat-burning metabolism, in which lipids behave differently.

We need to take care when extrapolating data from one diet to another until more data on each diet is available. Current evidence suggests that a ketogenic diet does not appear to promote heart disease. In certain anecdotal cases, it might even do the opposite – but it is too early to draw firm conclusions on this claim.

Why Coronary Arteries Get Damaged

First of all, the images you see of coronary arteries getting blocked like limescale in a pipe bear little resemblance to how artery disease actually develops. This part will help you understand why.

Our arteries are lined with a thin, protective layer called the endothelium. When this lining is healthy, blood flows smoothly and nothing sticks to the walls. But when the endothelium becomes stressed, inflamed and more permeable, this is where trouble begins.

Many everyday factors can stress the endothelium. High blood pressure pushes and stretches the vessel wall. Smoking adds toxins that injure the lining. Lack of exercise, poor sleep, and chronic inflammation weaken it. Emotional stress releases adrenaline (epinephrine), which the heart is highly sensitive to because of its abundant beta-adrenergic receptors. This increases heart rate and force or contraction, which adds strain to the coronary arteries – especially at bends and branches where blood flow is already rougher.

Glucose and insulin also play a major role. When glucose stays high for too long, it sticks to proteins, promotes inflammation (remember AGEs from the section on inflammation?), and makes the endothelium stiff and less protective. High insulin levels, common in insulin resistance, increase inflammation and change how blood vessels behave. Over time, these processes make the endothelium leaky, and contribute to fibrosis and hardening of the arteries.

Once the lining leaks, sdLDL cholesterol can slip inside the vessel wall more easily. Here, LDL can become oxidised, triggering inflammatory "danger signals". White blood cells rush in to help, swallowing the oxidised fat, but they can't adequately process the excess lipid, and so they become swollen foam cells, packed with oily droplets and debris. These foam cells collect into fatty streaks – the first stage of artery disease.

It is important to understand that cholesterol is not the original cause of the damage; it shows up because the vessel wall has already been injured by other stresses. A helpful way to think about this is the firefighter analogy. Cholesterol is like firefighters at a burning building: they are found at the scene, but they did not start the fire. The "fire" is the inflammation and damage caused by high blood pressure, high glucose, high insulin, toxins, stress and other factors. Cholesterol appears at the site of injury as part of normal lipid transport, but in the process, it can build up and become part of the problem.

So why do the coronary arteries suffer more than others? Because they are squeezed with every heartbeat, are highly sensitive to adrenaline exposure, have complex twists and branches, and sit inside an organ that uses huge amounts of oxygen, promoting oxidative stress. These pressures make the coronary arteries particularly vulnerable to injury and plaque formation.

Genetics and Cholesterol

Some people inherit genes that make them produce more LDL or clear it more slowly. HDL levels also have a genetic component. Familial hypercholesterolaemia is an example in which LDL receptors do not function properly or are absent. For everyone else, cholesterol reflects a mixture of genetics, diet, inflammation, insulin levels, and energy balance.

Bringing It All Together

Cholesterol is a key structural and signalling molecule which follows a circadian rhythm of production in the body. Problems arise not simply because cholesterol exists, but because of the metabolic conditions in which it travels. High insulin, inflammation, and overloaded fat transport pathways create an environment where LDL gets trapped and oxidised. Low insulin, stable blood glucose, and a natural fat-burning metabolism create an environment in which LDL and HDL are less likely to become dysfunctional.

Understanding this helps us approach cholesterol with greater clarity.

Chapter 36
Total Miles: 979

Days 16, 17 & 18 – Lindau

"The secret of change is to focus all your energy not on fighting the old, but on building the new."
– Socrates

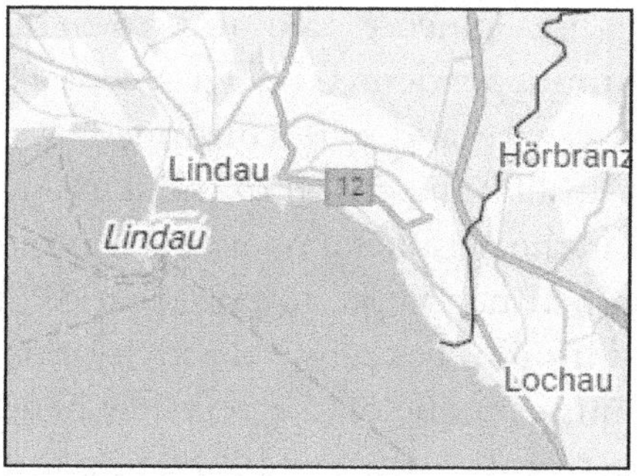

I was by now habituated to early starts, as the sun rises very early on these near-midsummer mornings, and I was awake at 6 am.

It was finally an actual sunny morning. The lake was just visible in the distance as I wandered onto the balcony and brewed a coffee using the camping stove. It was a generous balcony and overlooked a well-tended lawn that belonged to the three-storey, modest residence. I had no immediate neighbours, and it was lovely and quiet. The view extended to houses along the shoreline, about a mile away. I decided to stay for three nights and knew I would be comfortable here. Although the room was way over-generous for my immediate needs, I would sprawl out and fill up the space, no doubt.

The Jetboil did its usual rapid boil, and a rich black coffee was prepared through the syringe-like AeroPress. It has been a good companion in the mornings, and a quality morning coffee time has allowed me to focus and gather my thoughts. I took a few idle paces up and down the short balcony and gazed at the snow-capped Alps beckoning me in the south; I could not wait to get stuck into them. But there were matters more pressing: I had to decide what to do about today's insulin.

I was now on a reliable six units twice a day of Tresiba, and a few units here and there of Novorapid. The big question was: should I go low or high on this sedentary day? I had to decide how much the physical activity foundation of health had contributed to my insulin requirements.

Physical activity uses glucose and improves insulin sensitivity through the insulin-dependent GLUT4 receptors. Insulin is busy during physical activity and gets consumed; we call it "insulin sensitivity". Also, insulin injected into the skin – as we with type 1 do – is mobilised in the peripheral tissue, such as muscles, more than internally (remember the arterial to portal ratio?), so muscles get a lot of the injected insulin. For physical activity, this characteristic of injected insulin must be one of the very few benefits of type 1 in exercise over non-type 1s – the insulin getting to the muscle more than the liver – and I'll take it!

What I needed to decide was: how much physical activity would I do on these down days? I was planning on a bit of walking to look around the area and search for boxes to send my camping gear back; I might use the bike, but overall, it was planned to be a typical non-adventure day of perhaps an hour or two of light-to-moderate activity. Obviously, I wanted to maintain good blood glucose levels.

My options for insulin dosing fell into three categories: take the usual sedentary dose as I was doing before the trip; take the dose I have used on this trip based on the assumption that I have some insulin sensitivity because of my effort; or take something in between. So, it would be either six, eight, or seven units of Tresiba twice a day… Choices, choices!

Honestly, there is not much difference – up to four units over 24 hours. With my level of insulin sensitivity index, usually one unit to 2.5 mmol/L (44 mg/dL) – a 10 mmol/L (180 mg/dL) allowance. With something like a basal or long-acting insulin, that would be slowly metabolised over 24 hours, as it works so slowly, we were talking about 0.4 mmol/L per hour, which is easily managed by the glucose-raising counter-hormones like adrenaline. So, there we had it: I would go for my usual sedentary dose of eight units of Tresiba twice a day.

The next question was, should I have breakfast? Well, it was paid for, and there were keto options. The correct answer would have been: "No, I don't need it on days like this", but human nature and "free" food meant I succumbed to my weak will. It was good – scrambled egg and bacon, plus a nice roast of coffee. There was also some Emmental cheese. Emmental was originally produced in the Emme valley, just to the southwest of here; however, Emmental is not a fully protected brand, so I guessed this cheese was original in name only.

It was time for some tourist activities. A quick Wikipedia search told me that this town's coat of arms includes the Linden tree (Elm), which gave the town its name. It is a pretty, medieval town built around an island, now fully accessible via a causeway. The gardens are a tourist attraction, and the harbour boasts the only lighthouse in Bavaria – an impressive claim for a landlocked state! The southern end of town borders Austria, and it is a short distance to Liechtenstein and Switzerland. Over time, it has flipped from being an imperial free city under the Holy Roman Empire, to an Austrian town, then German; it was briefly French after the Second World War, and is now German again. Nothing is constant, so it is ironic that the town is built on Lake Constance.

I took a meandering walk downhill to the old town, and it was as lovely as the guidebook described. And the warm sunny day made this part of the trip feel like a proper holiday. Having taken the mandatory pictures of the lighthouse, I headed to the shops for some supplies. My cycling shoelaces were kaput, and I also needed some parcel tape and a tape measure for posting some gear back. I sourced a couple of boxes from the supermarket, then I was on my way in the heat, uphill, to my residence. It was nice to be in lightweight trainer-style shoes instead of soggy cycling shoes, and the warmth made all the difference.

Now that I had time to spare, this was an opportunity to take stock of the trip and tot up the distance. Being so busy logging various data in the mornings, I had had no time to look at it; I would do so during this three-day break. I must be getting close to my 1,000-mile mark. My various sources – Strava, Bikemap and Google Maps – told me I had now completed 979 miles, yet I still had well over 100 miles to go.

I was well on track and should complete the 1,000-mile challenge on the first day of my journey's resumption – and I had six days before I needed to be in St Moritz. Happy days! I was looking forward to the three days of rest and recuperation; it would be good not to have to check a couple of maps, work out the route and check for river crossings to ensure that none of the "bridges" were ferries. It would be brave indeed to cross the River Rhine by boat here – it is a fast-flowing torrent, as it descends from its source in the Alps just a couple of hundred miles away.

I decided to spend the rest of the afternoon on the balcony. I had topped up with asparagus, butter, salmon and cucumber, and some meat that was jellified and slightly tinged with the flavour of vinegar. It was on the deli counter, so I had no idea of its macros. I felt obliged to buy asparagus – or Spargel as it is called in German. My Duolingo German language app, which I used every day for three months (to no avail in the end – I am still rubbish at German!), was full of phrases that included it, so I had to try it out in the market. Cooked to perfection on my camping stove, with copious amounts of butter and salt, it was food fit for the gods.

It was a big ask for me to sit in the sun on a balcony and simply take in the view; I was adapted to being active. Forcing myself to rest for an hour, I idly glanced at my CGM. The decision about Tresiba seemed right; my glucose trace was much smoother today. That extra couple of units of insulin appeared to have done the trick. I also suspected that, by making this adjustment, I might be stimulating glucose-raising hormones to support a normal glucose level. Is that a good thing? I like to think that harmony requires balance, so it is probably beneficial – but perhaps that is the wrong way to look at it. The maxim "as much insulin as needed but as little as possible", means just that – as much as needed. It will vary. Were those extra two units more than needed, and then the counter-hormones were activated to protect against a hypo? It can feel like a balancing act. But it was working, and I never had a hypo, so I guessed it was a good calculation.

I think back to the glucose-fuelling algorithms I used to follow before I discovered the ketogenic diet. I mostly had too much insulin on board, then compensated by consuming more carbs. There was no balance there, just constant corrections for excess insulin. Now I understand insulin, I can adjust doses, adding or subtracting as needed, and good control follows. And that, at least for me, is liberating. It means I can work within a tight range and micromanage when necessary.

Most of the time, though, I can forget about glucose control altogether, knowing that good insulin management means glucose will follow. This has been a recurring theme throughout my trip: minimising insulin almost always leads to better glucose control – but getting glucose right for its own sake does not necessarily optimise insulin. Glucose is a symptom of type 1; insulin is the cause. And insulin is not a free ride – that is why I have flipped the problem on its head.

I had plenty of spare time, so I decided to look at some other data I had captured. The Strava app was open and I took a peek at the heart rate zones I had been riding in. I have never been the world's biggest fan of tracking data, but I admit it can be useful when training for something. I have done it all in the past – Fitbit, Oura ring, and now continuous glucose monitors. I have decided that the latter is enough for now. It is a daily commitment, and a serious one at that; everything else feels like fluff.

These days, it seems that even just preparing for a sport takes extra time: setting up devices, downloading data, stretching, hydrating, coordinating clothing and shoe colours, choosing the right shades for your mood, setting up music and so on. I am old school; I just go out and run/move. Most people's warm-up routines resemble my maximum effort! But I never seem to get injured despite my less-than-serious preparation – then again, I was not training to compete, only to survive.

However, for this trip, I needed to collect data, so I thought, why not add a heart rate monitor? It would serve as a proxy for power. Not that I was big on power – I averaged 125–150 watts, whereas proper cyclists generate two or three times that. While researching, I found that you can now buy cycling pedals that accurately measure the effort required to pedal and convert it to power. Heart rates can only estimate this, but at twice the price of my entire bike when it was new, and considering that I was merely pottering along the Rhine – nowhere near a "King of the Mountains" challenge – I opted for the heart rate monitor instead.

Incredibly, despite the ritual of putting it on and removing it for the past fortnight, today was the first time I had looked at the results.

So, what are heart rate zones?

Heart rate zones for running include:

- Zone 1 (warm-up): 50–60% max heart rate
- Zone 2 (endurance): 60–70%, suitable for low-intensity endurance where conversation is still possible
- Zone 3: 70–80%, around half-marathon pace, where you can speak in short sentences or the occasional word
- Zone 4 (gasping): 80–90%, interval workout zone
- Zone 5 (done in)

Training in different zones is said to improve overall fitness.

The science of heart rate zones is complicated. Maximum heart rate is often estimated as 220 minus age, but nowadays it is marketed as an oversimplification. There are many gurus who make a reputation on their own interpretation of sports science. There is something called the Gellish equation (207 minus 0.7 x age) or, if that is not precise enough, the Tanaka formula (208 minus 0.7 x age); take your pick – there are plenty to choose from.

The numbers, however, have questionable accuracy, as sex, age, fitness level, dehydration, altitude, time of day and natural individual variation can skew them by + or - 20%. For me, a calculation of the formulas produced a max heart rate of 161.5 for Gellish, 162.5 for Tanaka, and 155 for 220 minus age – and with a +/-20% error, that meant my actual range could be anywhere between 125 and 192.5 bpm. Practically meaningless!

But, for the purpose of science, I made an exception for this trip and, looking at my heart rate data, it appeared that I had spent most of my time in zones 1–3, which seemed about right.

Curious, I searched for comparisons and came across a paper about Team Novo Nordisk, a professional cycling team composed entirely of athletes with type 1 diabetes. Founded in 2005 as "Team Type 1", the team was renamed "Team Novo Nordisk" in 2013. They had achieved some success at their level.

What caught my eye was a 2020 study they published while they were still using insulin pens for glucose management. The study, published in BMJ Open Diabetes Research and Care, examined glucose control in 16 male cyclists training for nine consecutive days. The average duration of type 1 diabetes among them was 11 years, and their total daily insulin use was 24–28 units per day.

Interestingly, most used once-daily basal insulin and, despite an average of 11 years with type 1, their HbA1c was 7% (48 mmol/mol). Their training sessions lasted 2–6 hours per day, covering 35–113 miles daily – the same distances as me, although they were obviously faster. Their bikes were undoubtedly new, lightweight and high-tech, and probably cost more than £500, and they were not hauling 20 kg of luggage like I was.

Their macronutrient intake aligned with the glucose-fuelling philosophy common in sport:

- Carbohydrates: 63% ± 8%
- Protein: 15% ± 3%
- Fat: 22% ± 8%

Each day, a registered dietitian and team physician provided printed dietary plans for their meals – luxury!

By contrast, my macros were:

- Carbohydrates: 6%
- Protein: 26%
- Fat: 68%

Their in-ride nutrient consumption accounted for 12–25% of their total daily energy intake. I, on the other hand, barely ate anything while riding. The insulin requirements reflected the dietary difference. My daily insulin use was 16–18 units, compared to their 24–28 units. They spent 76% of the time in range; I was getting 89%. Their outlying results were high glucose; mine were lower glucose but asymptomatic for hypo. I was also twice their age, on average.

The discussion section of the Novo Nordisk paper highlighted a higher prevalence of nocturnal hypoglycaemia in their athletes. If this occurred, they were more than three times as likely to experience hypoglycaemia the next day, and had a twofold risk of low glucose levels during cycling. I have never worried about or experienced any of these effects; low-insulin states, by comparison, protect me from this issue.

The research team noted that "these findings highlight the need for additional pre-bed[time] carbohydrates and/or insulin dose reduction strategies around physical exercise training to minimize potential aberrations in glucose throughout the nocturnal period."

Fair enough, if you are a carb-loader… I used to worry about these same things when I was carb-loading, and I sometimes avoided long-term strenuous physical activity precisely because of those risks. Now, I can pedal away with the rest of them, without any concerns about nighttime hypos. So, I believe this optimised insulin paradigm has real potential; I have clinically outperformed the pros at their own game on this trip – though I won't be winning any medals for it.

The discussion in the paper goes on: "The potential long-lasting insulin-sensitising effects of endurance cycling illustrate the need for intensive monitoring of riders and dynamic, individualised glycaemic management strategies. These data provide a foundation for developing individualised nutritional, physiological and therapeutic strategies that may assist in improving exercise performance through glycaemic optimisation in elite cyclists with type 1 diabetes."

Put into English, this means: there is plenty of potential there for more research (done by us type 1s), and more tech. Or you could just optimise your insulin and enjoy your sport. We know that fat burning and keto-adaptation do not impair endurance performance or cause hypoglycaemia late into the night – and it is so much easier to do.

I can only conclude that some people prefer complexity to simplicity. Perhaps that is the trouble: some people might actually enjoy complicating things if they can. And if you believe in the supremacy of glucose as a fuel, you have little choice. I think the evidence in favour of keto as a logical choice in type 1, with no loss of performance, has been presented in the chapter on physical activity.

To be fair, at the very pinnacle of the elite level, a hybrid approach might be necessary, but the elite level applies to only a tiny fraction of people living with type 1 – and the training-zone heart rates of these athletes in this study were not at this level.

I was getting restless from all the sitting around, so I headed out for a long walk, and picked up some salmon and cucumber. I also tried a Greek yoghurt, having had elevated glucose with other brands earlier. This particular brand, as it turned out, did not cause a blip on my CGM – such is the fickleness of managing food and type 1. For my evening Tresiba basal dose, I stuck with my usual (non-trip) amount of eight units. It worked perfectly.

~ ~ ~ ~ ~

Days 17 and 18

The second and third days of rest passed by pleasantly in warm sunny weather. I had exactly the same breakfast, did my last Jetboil brew-up of the trip, and packed the stove in a large box of camping gear and other surplus-to-requirements items to ship back to the UK.

It took an age to catalogue everything for customs, and then I had to haul an unwieldy box to the post office. It was a good training aid – an awkward 12 kg box – and I managed some impressive upper-body work in the process.

There were some nice markets and a pop-up street food market down by the lake. With Lindau being only a few miles from Friedrichshafen, a blue and white airship was buzzing about in the blue skies most days.

I took this rest period to look at more data. I spent some time analysing the results of my comparison between a finger-prick ketone meter from Keto Mojo and the SiBio continuous ketone meter. There was a significant discrepancy, with the SiBio consistently under-reading; the difference was 20% on average, but far more on some occasions.

However, to me, the trends were the most interesting, not the numbers. My ketone average for the whole trip was 1.2 mmol/L, a tenth of the levels typically found in diabetic ketoacidosis. I found that I was always in the safe zone for ketones – yet more proof, if ever any more were needed, that nutritional ketosis does not cause diabetic ketoacidosis.

The three glucose monitors I had used were pretty consistent, with 0.2–0.4 mmol/L (36–72 mg/dL) errors. For me, that is manageable, but for those without hypo awareness, it could be critical. On a single occasion, the difference was 1.2 mmol/L (20 mg/dL). There was no outlier device; all were either at one end or the other, or in the middle. This will not come as a surprise to someone with type 1 diabetes – we all learn that no tech is perfect, but with increasing reliance on technology, we need improved accuracy. Sometimes, being old-school trained can provide a better understanding of technology's limits.

It is a whole new experience to relax in the afternoons, and if I were honest, I missed the routine of riding through the countryside. By late afternoon, I could not bear the sedentary pace any longer and took off on a run, and repeated it the next day. That was my happy place.

For me, running gets the imagination going, and I can get creative at these times. I do not really run for fitness as such, but being in the countryside and setting the mind free no doubt helps with my mindset. I am not naturally drawn to gym work and single-muscle block training, so I occasionally do some light weights at home, mainly using kettlebells, a chinning bar, and some bodyweight exercises. I also do some basic primal moves and use a slackline and longboard for balance.

Note the word "occasionally"; it is difficult to be motivated when you cannot see any progression. I have sometimes done a routine for weeks at a time and seen no results. But I know I should keep doing them before I wish I had, as infirmity creeps up silently on all of us, eventually. I will keep trying.

I felt much better after my run in the park, but taking time to slow down and adapt to the tranquillity of my lakeside dwelling was beneficial, too; I certainly had some excellent glucose profiles in this rest period. Others find different activities relaxing – each to their own. When I slow down my mind, other possibilities open up.

During those couple of runs, I rediscovered the joys of a mind in free-flow. I never get that on a bike. In those mind-spaces, I find time to work through things – not necessarily problems, but meditative running can help. It is more about creative thinking with me; pieces of the jigsaw that defy logical solutions begin to fall into place, and all sorts of random stuff can force its way to the front. "Does the moon affect our body water?" was one of the thoughts. Those three days were certainly a good time for the mindset foundation of health!

It was time to service the bike, tighten the headset, and clean the chain. The brakes also needed a check. The pads seemed okay, if worn down. There would be a lot of downhill cycling on the last descent to St Moritz. Last year, a rider in the Tour de Suisse shot over the edge of a hairpin bend. Braking requires a lot of anticipation, given the bike's weight and the relatively puny – but adequate – rim brakes, compared with disc brakes. Wet rims and rim brakes are not the best combination on rainy roads, and rain was forecast for the last two days of my trip.

I did a risk assessment, decided the pads were on the edge, but risked it anyway. After this break, I would be travelling light, which would make a huge difference to the handling of the bike. It would all be fine. I hoped the sunny spell would continue, but the weather pattern in in this area was thunderstorms at night. However, the Alps were beckoning, and their snow-capped peaks could be resisted no longer.

It was becoming exciting now: tomorrow I would complete the 1,000 miles and cross some national borders. Tomorrow night, I would be within a single day's ride of my destination, St Moritz. But I am going to split the distance and take two days to enjoy the mountains. My hotel for the conference is close to the bustle of the centre of town, and I am happy here in the peace of the countryside; I am going to make the best of it.

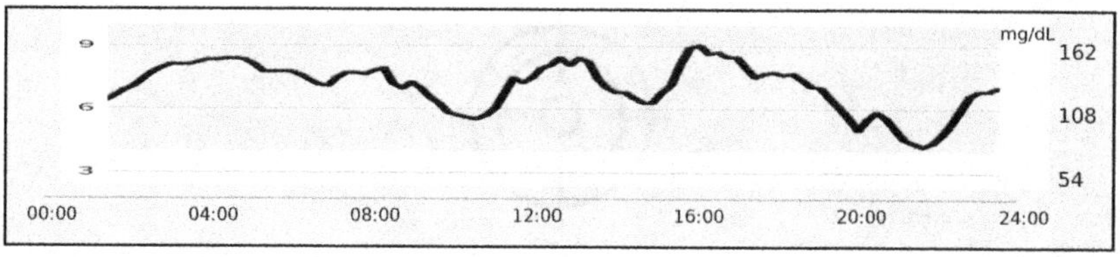
9
6
3
mg/dL
162
108
54
00:00
04:00
08:00
12:00
16:00
20:00
24:00

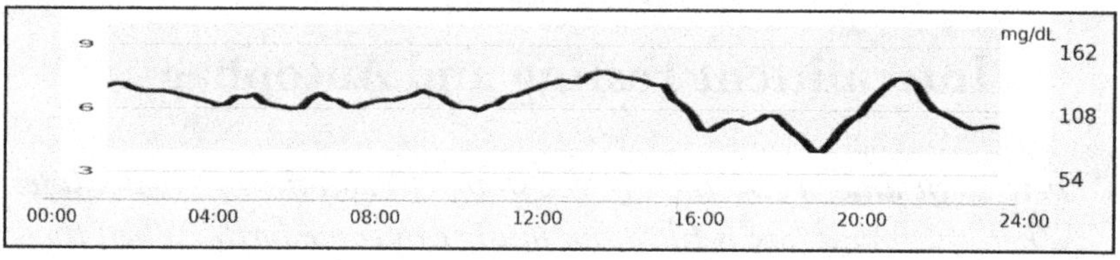
9
6
3
mg/dL
162
108
54
00:00
04:00
08:00
12:00
16:00
20:00
24:00

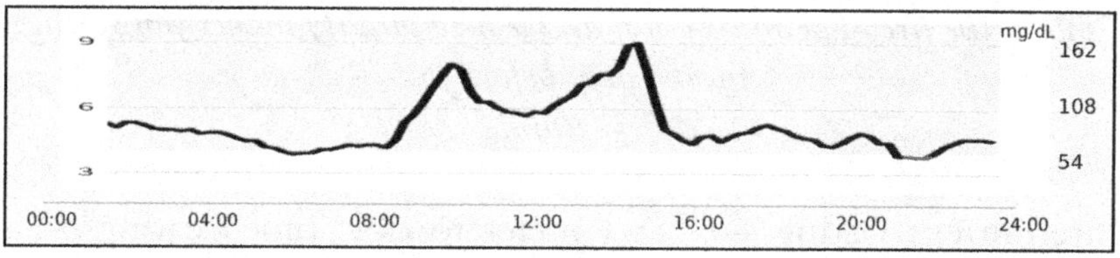
9
6
3
mg/dL
162
108
54
00:00
04:00
08:00
12:00
16:00
20:00
24:00

Chapter 37
Intermittent Fasting and Autophagy

"There is an unseen sweetness in the stomach's emptiness. We are lutes. When the sound box is filled, no music can come forth. When the brain and the belly burn from fasting, every moment a new song rises out of the fire. The mists clear, and a new vitality makes you spring up the steps before you."
– Rumi

Intermittent fasting – what I prefer to call "timed eating" – is common among people without type 1 diabetes, and people with type 1 can do it safely, too. Many religions include fasting, and most people tolerate it well.

When someone with type 1 diabetes follows a low-insulin lifestyle and sets their basal insulin correctly, choosing when to eat becomes much easier. Basal insulin keeps blood glucose steady in the background, so only small amounts of insulin are needed for meals. Glucose levels remain more stable, and during prolonged activities, only small snacks may be required. A continuous glucose monitor helps a lot.

The term "intermittent fasting" may evoke the idea of starvation, which can concern newcomers. In many religions, fasting means giving something up, even though people often still eat a little at prescribed times of day. Some physicians also conflate fasting or fat-burning with starvation, but these are not the same. Nutritional ketosis – burning fat due to low-carbohydrate intake – is generally safe in the long term. Starvation is not. Both states produce ketones, but for completely different reasons.

In nutritional ketosis, you still get enough calories and insulin, and the body runs normally. For people with type 1 diabetes who choose to follow a ketogenic lifestyle, timed eating can help keep blood glucose within a safer range. Avoiding food for certain hours of the day helps stabilise glucose.

Many people use patterns like 16:8 or 18:6, where all food is eaten in an 8- or 6-hour window. The fasting period between meals activates a beneficial cell-cleaning process called "autophagy".

The discovery of autophagy earned a Nobel Prize. Autophagy means "self-eating". Cells break down old or damaged parts and recycle them. It was once thought that autophagy occurred only during starvation, but research shows it also occurs when fed. When fed, this happens if there is a delay in food consumption; for example, getting enough calories into an 8-hour eating window, will enable sufficient autophagy.

Autophagy reduces inflammation, clears waste and maintains cellular health. It usually begins after about 16 hours without food. Three major systems inside the cell are involved: mitochondria, lysosomes, and mTOR.

Mitochondria, we know, are tiny power stations that make ATP, the biological energy molecule. They also help with stress signals, calcium balance, and the creation of hormones like melatonin.

Cells can gain or lose mitochondria depending on how active we are. When you move often, you grow more mitochondria. When you are inactive, you lose some. Old or damaged mitochondria are constantly cleared out and digested in lysosomes, which are baggy spheres inside the cell that collect waste products from the synthesis and breakdown of the cell structures, including mitochondria.

These breakdown products include amino acids, as well as lipids, sugars, and other small molecules. Lysosomes recycle them and return useful molecules to rebuild the cell. But lysosomes are more than recycling bins; they also assist mTOR, a central nutrient-sensing switch.

mTOR stands for mammalian Target of Rapamycin. Rapamycin was first discovered in bacteria from the soil on Rapa Nui (Easter Island) and later discovered to block the cellular pathway that was subsequently named "mTOR". This discovery became important for cancer therapy, transplant medicine, and ageing research.

mTOR responds mainly to amino acids:

- When amino acids are available, mTOR turns on, telling the cell to grow, repair, and make proteins.
- When amino acids are low, mTOR turns off and autophagy begins.

Here is the clever part: when mTOR turns on, lysosomes release amino acids produced from earlier protein breakdown. These amino acids then enter the cell and become building blocks for new proteins. The instructions for these proteins come from DNA, which acts like a library of recipes. All proteins – including enzymes and hormones – are made this way.

Enzymes power the chemical reactions that let cells make and use energy. Hormones guide metabolism, growth and communication. Without DNA-directed protein production, insulin would not be available, mitochondria could not make ATP, and cells could not repair themselves. So, the lysosome-mTOR-DNA choreography is vital for keeping metabolism running smoothly.

If mTOR stays active too often – such as with a high-carb diet and, hence, high insulin (a growth promoter) – it leads to excessive cell growth and insufficient recycling. Overactive mTOR has been linked with diabetes, Alzheimer's disease, obesity and cancer. This is why Rapamycin, which blocks mTOR, is used in some medical treatments, such as cancer, where it blocks cell growth.

mTOR also influences which amino acids are used for growth. During fasting, decreased mTOR activity preserves essential amino acids (the ones the body cannot make) for critical functions, while non-essential amino acids can be recycled for energy. This is likely to be one of the strategies used to enable humans survive long periods without food.

As I ride through the countryside, I sometimes imagine what eating would have been like a thousand years ago; I might have eaten bitter leaves, small fruits, fish, eggs, nuts, or the occasional animal. Food scarcity would have been normal for my ancestors. Autophagy and low mTOR activity would have kept them alive. When food is abundant, cells grow more, make more waste, and the liver has to clean it all up, which can raise inflammation. Insulin also plays a major role. Insulin affects mTOR through several chemical pathways.

One important pathway is called PI3K (phosphoinositide 3-kinase). PI3K helps cells respond to insulin. It affects how cells take in glucose, grow, and use energy. Scientists study PI3K because problems with this pathway show up in insulin resistance, metabolic disease, and even brain disorders like bipolar disorder. When insulin does not work well, PI3K signalling becomes dysregulated, disrupting the whole system.

When I first had type 1 diabetes, all I did was count carbs and take insulin; I had no idea about mTOR, PI3K, autophagy, mitochondria or any of this. It feels good to understand it now.

Cells work better with controlled fasting periods. Timed eating allows cells to recover and repair. I do not always manage it, and while travelling, I have not followed it strictly. But other foundations of health – sleep, diet, mindset and physical activity – are strong, and they help me use insulin effectively, so I can keep daily volumes "as much as necessary but as little as possible".

In two weeks, my activity will change, and I will adjust again. Everything changes: mTOR, autophagy, insulin needs, and the entire metabolic system.

Extreme Timed Eating in Practice

The ZeroFive100 project was a five-day, 100-mile run/walk challenge with zero calories consumed. Two people with type 1 diabetes (myself and a close friend) and six people without type 1 took part, and there were no problems. Everyone finished the project safely. Glucose levels remained within the normal range for the vast majority of the time, and basal insulin doses decreased over the five days.

Ketone levels in type 1 participants were almost identical to those in participants without type 1 diabetes; you could not tell the groups apart. Roughly 25,000 calories were burned – about ten times the amount of glycogen stored in the body. Fat-burning and ketone production powered the whole event. Breath testing confirmed everyone stayed in the fat-burning zone.

Ketones also have a mood-lifting effect, and this project made that very clear – everyone's mood improved each day.

The project had three key goals for type 1 diabetes, and all were met:

1. Sugar for energy is not required. Fat stores can supply fuel, and muscles can preserve glycogen during aerobic activity.
2. Glucose is not needed when taking insulin, as long as basal insulin is set correctly.
3. Nutritional ketosis did not lead to DKA.

Intermittent fasting can be a helpful tool for managing insulin sensitivity and improving metabolic health. It is safe for people with type 1 diabetes when basal levels are accurate. This extreme project helped reassure clinicians that skipping breakfast in type 1 is safe.

In real life, a 16-hour fast can easily include a night's sleep. A late breakfast then fits perfectly with the natural drop in cortisol after the dawn effect, when insulin becomes more sensitive. It makes metabolic and practical sense – not only for type 1 diabetes, but for everyone.

Chapter 38
Total miles: 1,040

Day 19 – Lindau to Chur, 61 miles (1,000 Miles at Balzers)

"On a day when the wind is perfect, the sail just needs to open, and the world is full of beauty."
– Rumi

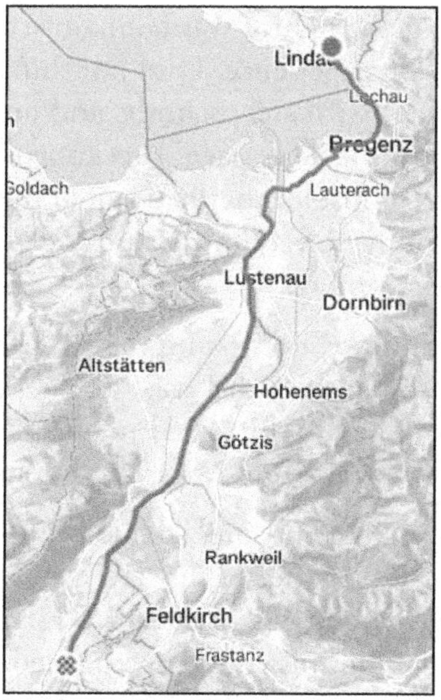

Today is the first day of the final push. I feel strong and more than up for the challenge. The rest over the past few days had done me good, and the next three would be shorter rides – there was no rush.

The first question was, "What to do with my insulin today?" I had had excellent glucose control during the rest days, after nudging up the basal by a couple of units. Should I taper it from eight to another eight this morning, then seven tonight, and six the next day? Or would that be encouraging a hypo, as I had on the first day?

The difference, of course, was that on day one, I was less fit than I was now. I had done a couple of hour-long runs in the past couple of days; but then again, that had been on eight units. The terrain today would still follow the Rhine, so it would be fairly flat. I was planning on completing 50 miles. What to do?

It is funny to me how I was agonising over four units of insulin. It would be easy to compensate for if I did go hypo, as it was only basal – two units over 12 hours was nothing.

But in my quest to get it right, I was taking my time to consider it. I could only base it on experience. I did not think this was going to be another Day One, with steep climbs and an over-enthusiastic rider setting off at a ridiculous pace. I reckoned I could do it with the normal amount of insulin that had suited my last two weeks of cycling, so I went for the lower dose: six units of Tresiba (basal) now, and another six that evening.

So, in it went. There was no turning back; I would do the fine-tuning with rapid insulin, which I was now less afraid of. My new fitness level had only slightly increased my insulin sensitivity, and I was now confident with it – and it was serving me well.

I headed down for a final and predictable breakfast of bacon, eggs and cheese, with my first coffee of the day. My AeroPress and coffee grinder were somewhere in the back of a DHL lorry on their way back to the UK; I would miss them as I headed for the hills, but I had just two nights' stay left, and I was sure I would cope.

In any case, delaying coffee is not a bad thing in principle. Glucose handling can get tricky upon waking, with cortisol and adrenaline (epinephrine). It is often recommended to us coffee lovers to wait an hour or so after waking, to allow time for this to settle down. I knew this but rarely practised it. We all have our weaknesses.

For the protein load of the breakfast and the stimulant effect of the two coffees, I added a couple of units of bolus Novorapid. This would be my last dose until I arrived in Landquart, my destination town just north of Chur in Switzerland – so I could pretty well ignore my glucose control from then on, knowing it would be okay.

I had to do a double-take on that thought: "I can pretty well ignore my glucose control from then on, knowing it would be okay." For someone with type 1 managed on a conventional diet, that would have been near-impossible.

Type 1 back then was just low expectations and the assumption that things were going to end badly at some point. Every clinic I attended either gave me approval for being a "good diabetic", based entirely on my HbA1c, or I got the long pause when they read out my HbA1c and told me to try harder. I knew I was not a "good diabetic", but had few tools offered by them with which to help myself.

I now knew, of course, that calculating carbs and injecting insulin is a flawed approach and only works for a few; mostly those whose autoimmune expression of type 1 is more forgiving. We are all different, and if three of us with type 1 were doing the same thing, we would likely get three different results.

In a Zumba class I was attending as part of a type 1 residential course, after a meal, three of us compared CGM glucose levels: two showed a reduction in glucose, while in one person, the glucose had gone up. This was for the same meal and the same level of exercise. If you have type 1, never compare yourself to others, it will end in tears. Accept your individuality and work with it.

It was an easy load-up that morning: one saddlebag and a small rucksack of clothes. The newly serviced bike felt light. I set the satnav for Chur and my evening stopover in Landquart. I needed to restrict the miles now, or I would arrive in St Moritz too early.

Chur is the gateway to the southern Alps on the eastern side, and the hills ascend from there. Tomorrow, I would have to decide which of the two mountain passes I would use, the Albulapass or the Julierpass. I had checked, and they were both open. That was a question for the future; right now, I had to be mindful and get through the day's ride. It was going to be very significant, as the 1,000 miles would be completed around lunchtime.

Today would be a flattish romp along an ever-narrowing and turbulent River Rhine, as it swelled with the meltwater from the high Alps. It was an opaque, pale aquamarine colour as it picked up the sand and debris and carried it into the Bodensee. I would be bidding farewell to the Rhine tomorrow; it would go west, and I would go southeast.

I checked both satnavs, and they agreed on my route for today's ride. I chose Google Maps, strapped on the heart rate monitor, and headed off with a sense of excited anticipation. The sky had started to cloud over the night before, and it was still cloudy with some dampness in the air – but my spirits were not dampened.

Within a mile, I was in Austria, following the southern curve of the Bodensee towards the city of Bregenz. I did not stop there, but had to thread through the streets to avoid a wild Google Maps detour that wanted to send me onto the bypass. I did not want to mess about that day, so I ignored it and used my intuition to find the cycle track along the east bank of the Rhine. The cycle tracks there were the smoothest I had encountered, and rivalled the vanity-project paths in Strasbourg. I zipped along and was pleased to have a slight backwind.

Shortly after getting up to my pace, I was passed by a cyclist, and a few seconds later by another. I gave a nodding greeting, which was not returned. It is normal round here, but it grated with me. I should have left it…

I deduced that they were enthusiasts of road cycling and appeared to be riding beautifully sculpted full-carbon fibre framed bikes and sporting expensive-looking Lycra. I guessed they were out for a pleasant day ride. I decided to take up the chase. From time to time, I conceded the lead again, and they occasionally looked back to check me out; they must have been surprised to see me hanging on. I tried to appear nonchalant, as one does, but inwardly I was spurred on to keep up.

For the next hour, I took up the challenge and stayed on their tail. I was pretty much flat out and panting. I felt ridiculously childish in my competitiveness. I managed to keep up the whole time, and eventually got a break when they turned off, presumably heading back to Bregenz, looking cool as cool.

When they were out of sight, I stopped for a breather and gulped in the air audibly. I was sweating profusely, but I had enjoyed that; it was a good challenge to hold a serious pace for a long time. I took on some water and checked the distance: 15 miles to the target and another ten to Landquart. It was just after noon, and I had plenty of time and energy left.

The sun burst through as I nudged the northerly tip of Liechtenstein. I would be riding the entire length of the eastern border before completing the rest of the journey in Switzerland. Somewhere during the chase, I had crossed from Austria into Switzerland. I would never actually go into Liechtenstein; the border ran down the centre of the River Rhine.

With the boundless energy I had that day, I kept the pressure on the riding pace and thought about how the short, restful break had done me good. I was riding parallel to the main road from St Gallen to Chur, and reflected that I had motorcycled on that road to the same keto conference in Switzerland during the previous two years.

On a motorbike, St Gallen to St Moritz is a short half-day's ride, and there were plenty of bikers enjoying it that day. I knew exactly how they felt, but I would not have swapped places. My bike was powered by a motor that was willing to keep going: me.

I soon hit the 1,000-mile mark. It was a great moment, and I felt celebratory. I took a few standard, fist-pumping pictures, but did not forget the bike. With some sentimentality, I lined it up in the camera with a great view of the Rhine and the hills behind. I love it when something like that bike punches above its weight. They do say that the British love the underdog.

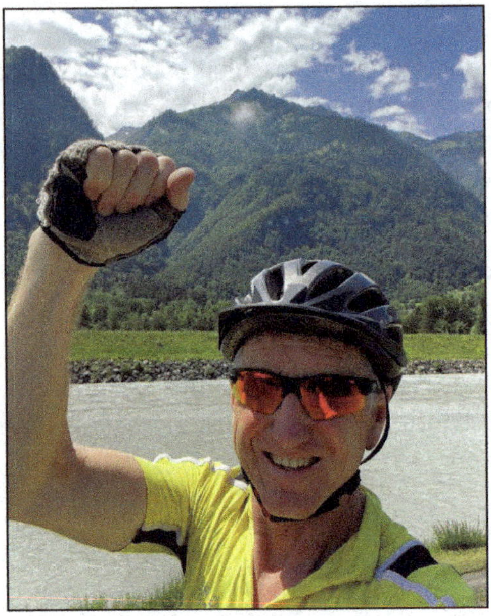

Too often, there is a temptation to over-prepare, with a new bike and all the gear, but there is something satisfying about sticking with what you have and maintaining it. Making do gives me a much more rewarding experience. It is not always the kit; it is the actual doing of stuff that matters. And my bike proved that in buckets.

I spent a few minutes lying in the grass on the verge, taking it all in: the warm wind – now that was a novelty – the increasingly tall mountains, the lush fields full of flowers, and the lazy cows chewing the cud. The river torrented along, busily carrying the melted mountain snow to the lowlands, and eventually out to the North Sea. I had got to know the River Rhine in all of its stretches, and it had been a good companion. Even though it was simply a marker to measure the journey's distance, travelling through centuries of history along this timeless river had been a delight.

I set off on the road to my stopover in Landquart and arrived in the early afternoon. It was a small town, and I had no intention of stopping just yet; it had been my best day by far, so I decided to add a bonus 10 miles, just to keep the fun going. I was in peak form and sped effortlessly toward Chur. There was a rail station at both Landquart and Chur, so I would get the train back, then the next day I would get the train again back to Chur and continue my journey.

There was nothing doing in Chur, so I headed back to the station and returned to Landquart. I finally found my accommodation behind a green door that was seemingly stuck onto a nondescript wall at the side of a filling station and mechanic's garage. I had to ring a number to summon the host, and she arrived from some flats across the way.

I had a top-floor, small room with a shared bathroom. There was no food available, but I managed to agree on boiled eggs for the morning. I was in luck and found that I was provided with a Nespresso machine. I took a shower, washed my kit, and headed for the balcony full of gnomes and model houses, with the occasional plastic animal. It had a wonderful view of the mountains, and a roaring, fast-flowing tributary was rushing past the end of the garden below.

I needed to head into the small town to get some food at some point. I could not find a lot of restaurants and I ended up, yet again, in a supermarket. I had the now-familiar offering of meat and cheese, plus a few mixed nuts – unimaginative, but this is what you must deal with on the road.

I needed to eat the correct macros, and as fresh as possible, but on occasions, this was difficult. That day, it was all about the journey and focusing on arrival in St Moritz on time. I had, however, managed to eat well most of the time, and had my fair share of the nutrient-dense foods that a real-food keto diet is all about; I had shown that it was possible to get by on a keto diet with more processed food while maintaining good blood glucose and low insulin volumes.

I trusted my food choices and did not take supplements. I knew a lot of people who did, though. My philosophy was that if I provided my body with nutrient-dense, fresh food, it would have enough minerals and vitamins to maintain health. However, I do take vitamin D in the winter for reasons that are obvious in Europe's northern climes.

I am so lucky that I hardly ever get ill since I have been on this optimised insulin lifestyle; I had had, perhaps, a cold every three years and, amazingly, only the occasional musculoskeletal injury or ache. From that perspective, this ride had confirmed the effectiveness of an optimised insulin strategy. Sure, there had been plenty of times when my muscles had been burning uphill, but I could honestly say I had had no morning aches and pains to work off. I was lucky – but I reckoned I had contributed to that run of luck.

I turned in early for bed and decided to go by my body clock. I used the same six units of Tresiba, and a couple for the meal. I had no long distances left to complete now, as I made my way to St Moritz. I could easily have done it tomorrow if I had wanted to, but I would arrive in St Moritz only when I needed to be there. In the meantime, I was determined to immerse myself in the wonderful and wild Alps.

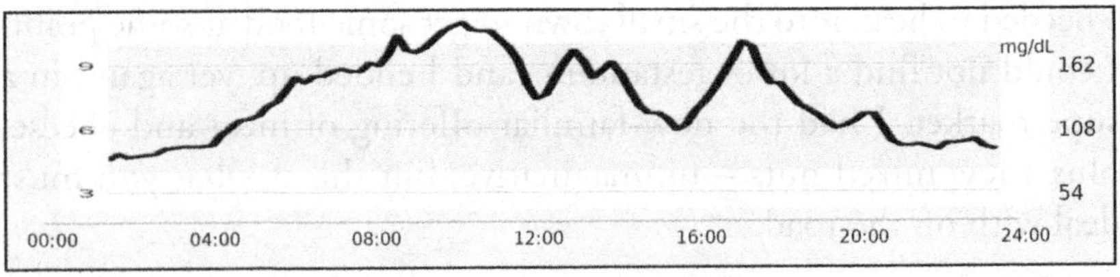

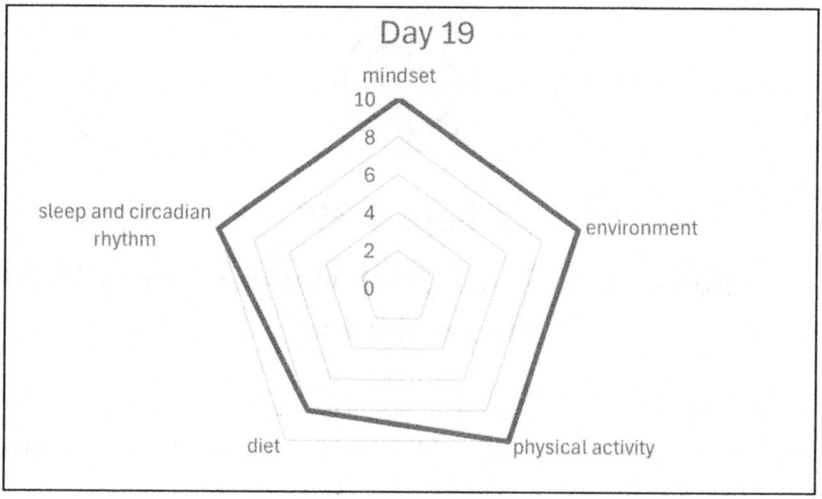
Day 19
mindset
10
8
6
4
2
0
environment
physical activity
diet
sleep and circadian rhythm

Chapter 39

The Retina and Dual-Fuel Metabolism: A View from the Eye

Some of the book's detailed chapters have been harder than others. Exploring biochemistry, metabolism and therapeutic nutrition over a three-week trip is a challenge. How can we explore the dynamic state of metabolism using a single example? One of the organs that does particularly well on multifuel is the eye.

Everyone with type 1 diabetes knows something about the eye. We get a lot of professional advice that the eye is vulnerable in type 1 diabetes, and every year the retinal screening tests become a stressful exercise, because only then can we tell if we are going to be okay or not. Being in control of glucose and having a good HbA1c helps, but the apprehension around any type of medical screening never fully goes away.

The retina is a good example of adaptability to metabolic demands, and combines many of the multifuelling concepts within its supporting structure, particularly the retinal pigment epithelium (RPE). This thin layer of cells supports the mechanics of vision and plays a central role in how the retina is fuelled. It is highly metabolic and can even be compared to a liver and a placenta rolled into one – an impressive claim! Have a go at this chapter and see what you remember.

Sensitivity to light is an ancient quality of lifeforms. It is thought to date back at least 600 million years, with primitive light-sensitive cells appearing in early multicellular organisms. These photosensitive structures likely helped early organisms align their internal clocks with the circadian cycle. The complex, camera-like eyes found in humans and many other species have evolved significantly from these specialised cells, but what is remarkable is that the fundamental process of sensing light has remained largely unchanged.

The anatomy and physiology of retinal photoreceptors, retinal circuitry and the camera-style eye show extremely close similarity across all jawed vertebrates. The human retina is made up of dense and specialised nerve tissue composed of rods and cones. It has very high energy demands. The retina is a sensory extension of the brain, and contains neurons sensitive to the wavelengths of visible light and non-visible light. Rods are very sensitive to light and dark but do not detect colour. Conversely, cones are responsible for colour vision and require about twice the energy of rods.

Both rods and cones get their energy from the RPE, which sits behind the retina and has a high-volume blood supply. The integrity of the RPE is crucial for retinal health. It helps clear out waste products from photoreceptors, recycles vitamin A, and supports the blood-retinal barrier (BRB), which controls the flow of nutrients, fluids and ions between the retina and the blood supply. The RPE, which has a black pigment, also absorbs excess light, protecting retinal cells from oxidative damage. Moreover, the RPE makes growth factors and helps maintain the structural integrity of the retina.

So, how do we see? A large protein (348 amino acids, compared with the 51 amino acids of insulin), called rhodopsin, or visual purple, sits across the cell membrane of a photoreceptor cell. It contains a vitamin A derivative called retinal (pronounced retin-al, with the emphasis on the last syllable), which is sensitive to light. When light photons hit rhodopsin, they trigger a change in the retinal molecule to produce a signal that registers the light. This process ultimately depends on ATP to reset and recycle rhodopsin. The photon reaction is immediate, and rhodopsin is rapidly recycled.

This signalling system, through a protein that crosses the full width of a cell membrane, is known as a transmembrane signalling system.

It is a common signalling method. For example, insulin activates transmembrane receptors, which then allow GLUT4 to transport glucose into the cell. Rhodopsin most strongly absorbs green-blue light but appears reddish-purple to our eyes, hence the term "visual purple".

Rods make up about 95% of the retina's photoreceptors and are extremely sensitive to low light, down to a single photon. Cones are present throughout the retina, though they are concentrated in the yellow spot, or fovea. They are sensitive to light but operate best in bright light, when the rods do not.

In the bright conditions of metropolitan life, we rely on the cones far more than the rods. Our dark-adaptation advantage of the rods, which enabled early humans to see better in the dark, is being superseded by bright-light conditions. This shift in light exposure may well have implications for our circadian rhythm.

The retina's energy demands can vary dramatically between light and dark exposure – up to tenfold – and they change within milliseconds. It is analogous to an aircraft landing wheel going from zero speed and no load, to 100 tonnes and 150 mph in a second. It is truly incredible engineering for both examples.

For the eye to perform this way, it needs a highly efficient and flexible energy supply. Photoreceptor cells in the retina contain one of the highest densities of mitochondria in the body. This gives us a clue about fuelling when we remember that mitochondria produce most of the energy for a cell. There are also pathways for glucose to rapidly enter cells through glucose transporters, particularly GLUT1 in the retina, which facilitates glucose entry from areas of higher to lower glucose concentration.

The RPE is also responsible for "eating" the tips of photoreceptor cells that are recycled daily in a process known as phagocytosis. Phagocytosis means "cell eating" and refers to the process by which cells engulf and digest particles and debris. It happens continuously in many tissues in a controlled way, and is not the same as autophagy. We have immune cells called phagocytes for this purpose. Phagocytes also destroy foreign bodies such as bacteria and viruses, serving both tissue maintenance and immune-protective roles.

The retinal neurone phagocytosis process peaks in the hours after light exposure and is regulated by the body's circadian rhythms. It is estimated that about 10% of photoreceptor tips are recycled each day. Now, here is the clever bit: photoreceptor outer segments are rich in lipids, and these discarded fatty acids become fuel for the mitochondria in RPE cells. Remarkably, up to 50% of these fatty acids may be converted to ketone bodies, another metabolic fuel with anti-inflammatory, anti-oxidative and hormone-like properties.

Who would have thought that the process of recycling tissue is operating in a circadian rhythm without fuss in our retinas? We think of autophagy as cell recycling that responds better to "stress" through timed eating. This photoreceptor recycling is automated and circadian, with the waste products used directly as mitochondrial fuel.

The retina has more surprises: when energy demand is high, there is a fast-recycling shortcut of the citric acid cycle in the eye. There are some apparent "back-door" steps in the citric acid cycle that bypass some of the slower-reacting steps to ramp up the energy supply. This mini citric acid cycle pathway produces energy more rapidly than the slower pyruvate-based citric acid pathway, meeting the high energy demands of cones.

Type 1 Diabetes and Eyesight

In diabetes, the retina is especially vulnerable due to prolonged exposure to high blood glucose. An intact RPE controls glucose delivery to photoreceptors via GLUT1 and GLUT3 transporters. If the RPE is damaged, the normally laminated layers of RPE and photoreceptors are disrupted, and GLUT transporters can no longer function efficiently at the RPE/neurone interface. The energy supply chain is broken, and glucose floods the rods and cones in an unregulated manner, creating a toxic situation.

One mechanism involves the accumulation of sorbitol inside retinal cells, which draws water in and damages the cells. The sorbitol pathway can become pathological in the retina. You may remember from a previous chapter that when glucose levels are high, glucose is converted into sorbitol. Sorbitol is then converted into fructose via sorbitol dehydrogenase.

Certain tissues, such as the kidneys, retina and Schwann cells (which produce myelin in peripheral nerves), lack sorbitol dehydrogenase. This means that excess sorbitol builds up, causing osmotic stress, which can contribute to kidney disease, diabetic retinopathy and peripheral neuropathy.

In diabetic retinopathy, blood vessels in the retina become leaky due to damage caused by elevated glucose levels. Insulin can contribute to the formation of new, abnormal vessels in proliferative diabetic retinopathy. Vascular endothelial growth factor (VEGF) drives new vessel formation and increases leakiness in existing ones. This causes haemorrhages and swelling.

In addition to ischaemia (reduced blood and oxygen supply to tissues), levels of VEGF can also be influenced by insulin, hyperglycaemia, and other metabolic factors. Insulin, along with the inflammatory effect of advanced glycation end products (AGEs), also contributes to the process of fibrosis of retinal tissue, which makes the retina prone to detachment.

This example of the retina hopefully ties together some threads from the preceding chapters, helping you to better understand biochemistry and metabolism. It is helpful to have at least some idea of how multifuelling and adaptation happen, how pathological processes can take hold, and, crucially, how to modify things when they do go wrong. There is always hope through knowledge.

The body is complex and awe-inspiring in the way it interacts with and survives in its intended environment. In my view, we need to celebrate our ancestral heritage and reduce the stress of modern inventions where we can, working with them to enhance our lifestyle while understanding their effects on our metabolic state.

As the French philosopher Voltaire is often quoted, "The art of medicine is to amuse the patient while nature cures the disease." With a nod to him, perhaps a modern twist is appropriate: "The science of medicine is to amuse the patient and the clinician, while nature cures the disease." Just do not try to distract yourself too much, and take time to follow the laws that sustain a healthy life!

Chapter 40

Total miles: 1,077

Day 20 – Chur to Sur, 37 miles

"I choose, I choose the mountain with all its stress and strain, because only by climbing can I rise above the plain."
– From "I Choose the Mountain" by Howard Simon

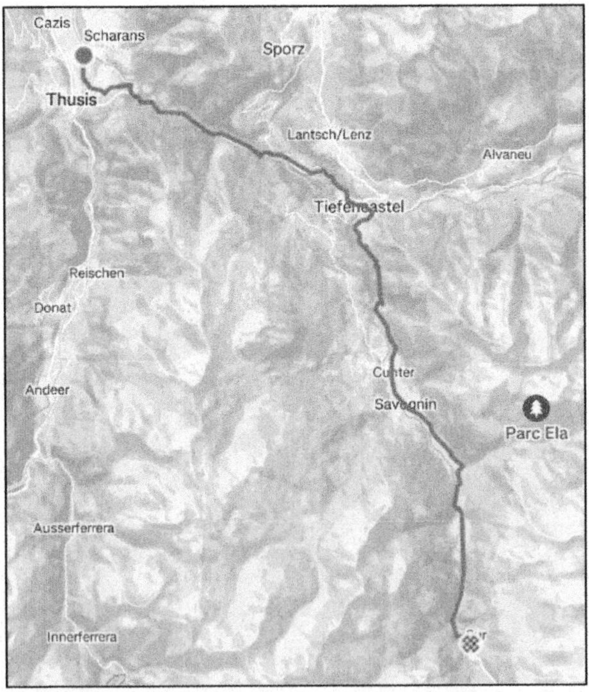

This morning, I began by catching the train back to Chur. I was up early and out on the patio with a coffee in the morning sun. I did my usual calibrations, dedicated to the end, and planned the route. I needed to choose which mountain pass to take.

I am in the Graubünden, or Grisons (same place, different language), area which is one of the largest cantons – a bit like the Swiss version of a U.S. state – in Switzerland. The name "Grau" referred to the Grey League of medieval times, when people wore grey cloaks. It is also where the Rhine begins its journey to the North Sea. There are two main mountain passes that cross from Tiefencastel, where I was headed for lunch, to St Moritz: the Albulapass to the east or the Julierpass to the west.

My first trip to the Keto Live conference, years ago, ended in Bergün, which is on the route to the Albulapass. It was a glorious summer, and my first time in this part of Switzerland. I motorcycled the Albulapass to St Moritz from the north, just as I was approaching it now, and looped back via the Julierpass from the south. I remember the drama and stark remoteness of it. At the time I crossed it, in June, the pass had been open for only a few days after the winter closure; there had still been snowdrifts at the roadside. The clouds were a solid blue-grey, and it was cold – yet both ends of the pass were basking in warm sunshine.

The Albulapass is slightly shorter than the Julierpass, but marginally higher – 2,312 metres above sea level – with one of the climbs reaching 12%, compared to the Julierpass at 10% and an elevation of 2,284 metres. What I remembered most about the Julierpass was that it was more developed and seemed to carry heavier traffic. I favoured the Albulapass, both for sentimental reasons and its remoteness.

I had been hoping to stay in Bergün and before reaching the Albulapass. This year, the Keto Live conference was being held in St Moritz for the first time. I called my good friend Josephine, the organiser of the conference; it was her vision to promote the use of ketogenic therapies in medicine that brought us together, and I have been proud to contribute to the conference ever since. She told me there was a big wedding in Bergün and no accommodation was available in the village or nearby.

Today, being Saturday, I was out of luck. There was just one room available, but it was outrageously priced and miles from the main route. So, the decision was made: the Julierpass it was. I checked some local cycling club websites. The full loop around both passes was a long ride, but these people did both in a day. This reassured me that one pass would be easily doable, even for a cyclist like me.

I was the only person dining that morning, and there was a lot of food laid out. Having negotiated some eggs the night before, the two I asked for were on the table, the shells dyed in red and blue. I also chose some cheese and cucumber. Then, the owner appeared, looked judgmentally at my plate, and asked if that was all I was having; I thought it was a generous plate of food.

She asked if I was having any of the Bircher, a Swiss hybrid of porridge and muesli in a creamy yoghurt base. I explained that I did not eat starchy foods and had mentioned this to her the day before. She looked wounded and proceeded to tell me it was full of nuts and seeds, and had no grains – especially for me. I could see banana pieces floating like icebergs in the mix; there were likely more carbs in that bowl than I had eaten in the whole fortnight. I really would rather have not, but I relented to my polite Britishness. I should have stood firm.

Not wanting to offend, I took a bowl and began spooning in the smallest amount I could, hiding some under yoghurt to try to bulk it out. I jettisoned some of the cheese and hurried to the patio. The woman came outside for a chat, and I slowly ate the Bircher with a "yes, thank you, it was lovely!" I was cross with myself for not holding out.

When she had gone, I gave some to the gnomes in the garden. It is more difficult to refuse when you only have a rudimentary vocabulary; it seemed that if I got my words wrong, I might be offending not just my host but the whole of Switzerland.

This lapse was going to mess up my glucose for half a day. Ten minutes of awkwardness had now created a few hours of juggling insulin and glucose. I agonised over what to do? I could not just ignore the carbs and rely on physical activity; I needed to manage the glucose surge. It would be perhaps an hour before I started riding properly, as I still had to reach the station and take the train.

I estimated I had consumed about 30g of carbs – a whole day's worth. With an insulin-to-carb ratio of 1:10 (perhaps even better), I would need around three units of insulin. The protein in the eggs and cheese could require another unit, but I would wait until after the train journey before doing that, as the protein spike would be delayed, if it happened at all.

I tentatively injected three units: once it is in, there is no getting it out. This is drilled into my training – when administering powerful drugs in an emergency, double-check and get it right. But this was nothing like the old days of carb-loading; back then, I might have eaten half that bowl and injected eight units of rapid insulin without a second thought. The idea of injecting that much in one go now fills me with dread.

I started the day with a short ride of a couple of minutes to the station. It was quiet, with only a few pigeons strutting on the platform for company. Watching them, I idly recalled that pigeons have a neck muscle linked to their feet, so that when they walk they are able to keep their centre of gravity in the right place to stop them falling over. It does make them a bit comical, though.

As departure time approached, the platform filled up. And finally, I was heading to Chur and facing the first significant climbs since day one. Once on my way, Google Maps added a flourish by diverting me from the main road onto a mountain track. It was grassy in parts and clearly little used. I had to walk some of the steeper sections, and other parts were a tough pedal through a pine forest that lined the valley walls.

I passed a few mountain bikers and, eventually, I reached the top, with a lovely view of the Rhine far below. From there, I could see the road I *should* have taken, complete with a cycle track beside it; the satnav had lured me onto a mountain bike route again! However, I did not mind; I had all day, the sun was shining, the views were fantastic, and it was downhill back to the main road. I felt fit, and even enjoyed the peace of the forest trails.

I hung around for a while and relaxed in the setting. This was forest bathing at its best. I checked my CGM. As expected, I had the steepest rise in glucose of the whole trip. It peaked at 14 mmol/L (252 mg/dL). I had been out for only a couple of hours, so a correction dose would be tricky. I needed to wait four or five hours, to be sure the previous insulin dose was out of my system; injecting now would be stacking insulin – overlapping doses before the previous one had worn off. Yet, clearly, I had underestimated the Bircher's carb load and needed more insulin. I was not planning to eat again soon, so I just had to monitor the action of what was already in. I did not want to go too low; physical activity makes me very insulin sensitive.

I finally opted for two units. I estimated that it would bring glucose down to about 9 mmol/L, plus the additional effect of riding and the previous dose. In fact, it plummeted to 4 mmol/L (72 mg/dL).

My ketones had not changed, staying around 1.5 mmol/L, so I had got away with the Bircher episode, but I noted my poor calculation of insulin dose. I was twice as insulin-sensitive as I had estimated, so that caught me out. Even for an experienced T1 like me, this condition poses daily challenges. For someone without type 1 diabetes, the same insulin would have been needed, but they would have secreted it at just the right time to keep glucose stable.

That is the life of a type 1: constant guesswork, planning, and unexpected results – especially with pens, which are likely to remain common for some time. Pumps might help finesse control, but they come with their own issues. I still believe an insulin optimisation strategy is the best philosophy for type 1 diabetes, however. For now, I am perfectly happy with my pens. I have done a good job managing things in a challenging metabolic environment, under prolonged physical stress; I have found that it is possible to maintain good control by understanding insulin and optimising its use.

It was late morning, and my satnav diversions were finally behind me. Ahead was the only road into the municipality of Thusis, and then it was on to the village of Tiefencastel and beyond. Between Thusis and Tiefencastel there was a steady climb into a tunnel which was over a kilometre long, narrow, and had no lighting. I was not happy about going in there. I double-checked Google Maps – yes, the cycle route was through this tunnel. I checked for alternatives; there were none without a massive detour, and I could not guarantee those mountain routes would be tunnel-free. I have done tunnels on a bike before, but this one bent around a corner and had the narrowest of kerbs, with a big drop to the road; I might buckle my wheel, or fall and be at risk of being hit by traffic. So far, traffic on this road had been light, which was a bonus, and being Saturday, thankfully, I did not anticipate large vehicles.

There was nothing for it – I had to set off. I lifted the bike onto the pavement and pedalled tentatively, ducking to accommodate the tunnel's slope. I was grateful I did not have panniers, otherwise it would have been very dangerous. My rear light was flashing and lit up the tunnel walls.

Then came a loud, hollow rush of tyres on tarmac mixed with engine noise; a car was behind me, somewhere. It seemed like forever before it passed. The tunnel held the sound, reverberating it all around. In the end, there were several cars on my tail, and I endured ten minutes of constant, loud, threatening noise, never quite sure when a vehicle would pass. Eventually, I rounded the bend and saw daylight. I dared not speed up for fear of falling, so I focused very hard and pedalled steadily until I was out.

Once back in the fresh air, I stopped immediately to rest and gather myself. That was the worst experience of the whole trip, bar none. I finished most of a water bottle; my mouth was dry. I hoped there would be no more long, narrow tunnels, and was not disappointed. The rest of the journey to Tiefencastel was a joy: lush meadows, wild flowers, chewing cattle. The green hills rose gently into mountains, although I could only occasionally see them as the treeline was high. There was snow on the higher peaks.

My long climb ended, and I freewheeled the last mile into Tiefencastel. There, I bought another litre of water at a filling station, and drank it while looking out over the distant valley and the next part of my route climbing up and over the crest. To the water, I added 20g of 90% dark chocolate – that was my fuel for the final part of the day's riding. My meagre food intake would not balance energy in versus energy out, but I could draw on fat reserves if needed.

I click-clacked across the garage forecourt and got back on the bike, heading down the rest of the hill to the turn for the mountain passes. Some road signs really stand out, and this was one of them. At the roundabout in town, the blue sign pointed me to St Moritz, Julierpass, Savognin, Albulapass and Davos. This was my first road sign to St Moritz, and it was exciting. I could not wait to head into the Alps and savour their stark beauty.

I rode on to Savognin, where well-kept, freshly cut hayfields were crossed by ski-resort chairlifts from Val Surses. It was all so pretty. There was a small stretch of valley floor before the final climb to Sur and my hotel just out of the town.

It was a small, family-run affair with goats and chickens in the yard. A couple of locals were enjoying a late-afternoon beer as I freewheeled into the parking area. The hosts were wonderful and took my bike to a safe spot, then I took the final shower of the trip and washed my cycling clothes one last time. In an almost final ritual, I hung them on the curtain rail and left the window open to help them dry.

I love the Alps and could easily have stayed here for days, walking the mountain trails. It was quiet and peaceful – this little hotel and a handful of houses were all that was here. I sipped a cold sparkling water while sitting on the warm stone wall outside. The evening was warm and dry, and I soaked up the sun. It was bliss. The road was quiet, but the occasional passing motorbike or cyclist added to the scene; there were even a few classic cars to complete the holiday feel.

A road sign at the T-junction pointed to a village called Alp Flix – surely one of the most discordant names I had seen. Thankfully, my accommodation was called "Hotel Edelweiss", which brought back the reassuring feeling that I was, indeed, in Switzerland. Dinner was a delicious pork steak with green salad and vegetables, served on the sunny terrace. Strava told me this had been my most significant climb since leaving Stroud, and I expected more tomorrow.

Glucose had been very good all day since the "Bircher episode". I used my usual six units of Tresiba and two of Novorapid, and had not thought much about glucose since the morning's correction – just the occasional glance at the CGM. There were no surprises. My dosing was good today. If anything, it was slightly too much, as glucose drifted down overnight and I woke at 3.8 mmol/L (68 mg/dL).

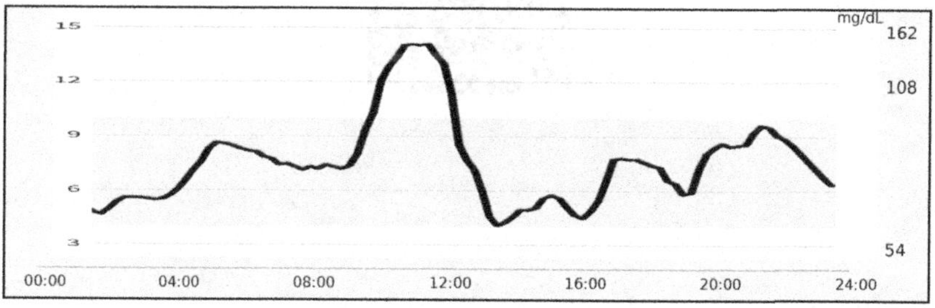

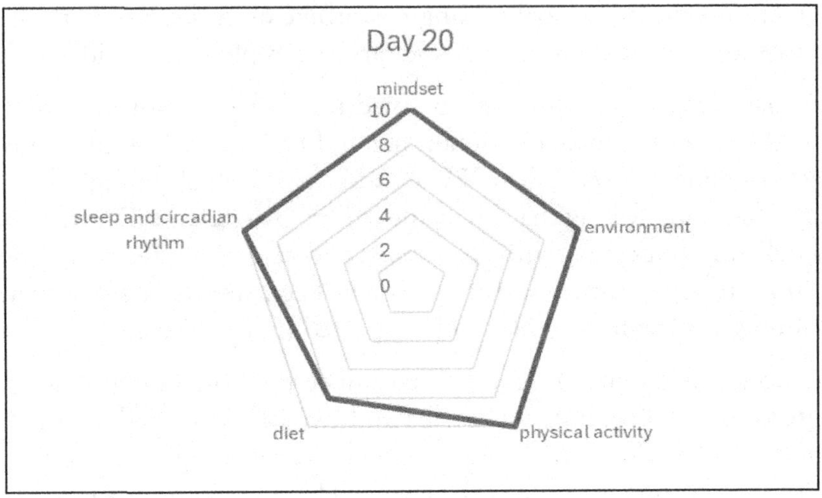
Day 20
mindset
10
8
6
4
2
0
environment
physical activity
diet
sleep and circadian rhythm

Chapter 41
Breathing

"If you know the art of deep breathing, you have the strength, wisdom and courage of ten tigers."
– Chinese adage

I have talked about the easy win of going outside, especially in the mornings, to give us a general improvement in our health. Another easy win is to understand breathing. Deep breathing can be practised regularly until it becomes a habit, and it can be very calming.

No one teaches us to breathe; it is considered an innate life skill that is naturally acquired. We can all breathe. But how we breathe is rarely something we think about.

Shallow breathing is very common, and we often move air mainly through the upper airways, with only enough reaching deeper into the lungs to keep us alive. Deep breathing can help us get more air in and out of the lungs, but breathing too deeply and too quickly can affect gas exchange and make us feel light-headed.

The lungs rely on two main anatomical structures for breathing. One is the rib cage, and the other is the diaphragm. Most people use a combination of the two, but the diaphragm is considered the more efficient and calming option.

The diaphragm is controlled by the phrenic nerve, which loosely translates to "of the mind", and originates in the cervical spinal cord. The vagus nerve, which as we know is the main nerve for many of the body's automatic functions, also plays an important role in the lungs by influencing heart rate, airway tone, and relaxation responses. The rib cage is moved by intercostal muscles, which are primarily controlled by spinal nerves. During heavy breathing, additional accessory muscles in the neck may also be used.

The breathing response can be strongly linked to stress. In humans, a feeling of non-specific alarm sometimes occurs before any conscious awareness of the stimulus. With that stimulus, we quickly prepare for avoidance. Our pulse rate increases, we might sweat, freeze physically, and our breathing might change – often with a short pause for breath-holding before becoming more rapid – as the brain prepares for an unclear threat. It is a sixth-sense fear that can override more rational responses, as it is mediated by the amygdala, a brain region involved in processing fear and threat. The amygdala is almond-shaped and derives its name from the Greek word for the same nut.

The amygdala prepares the body for an anticipated threat; it does not last long. When the amygdala is stimulated, blood pressure rises, muscles tense, and the heart rate increases. Breathing may briefly pause and then speed up as the brain prepares for a threat that may not even be real. The accessory muscles are used in this amygdala-driven response.

The rational brain then quickly assesses the threat and can override the amygdala if it decides there is no real danger. However, the amygdala response can be trained, much like Pavlov's experiment with dogs salivating at the sound of a bell; the same can be applied to amygdala-driven breathing.

The normal state of breathing is driven by the diaphragm and responds to immediate metabolic needs. Breathing changes when the body's needs change – for example, more oxygen during exercise. When breathing is driven by the amygdala, it often does not match the metabolic demand and can become unbalanced.

The trouble arises when the threat is non-physical and not imminent, such as anxiety about a future event or anger over something seen on social media. The body then operates on amygdala drive, preparing for action as if the threat were physical and close at hand.

If such responses become habitual, this preparation becomes chronic, with accessory-muscle breathing to support a higher breathing rate, elevated blood pressure and heart rate, and increased muscle tone. The breathing has been trained – just like Pavlov's dogs.

Under chronic stress, the higher breathing rate is often due to mouth breathing, because airway resistance is about 50% lower through the mouth than through the nose. It is also easier to speak and shout when breathing through the mouth, which might be useful in a survival situation.

However, just because mouth breathing is easier does not mean we should rely on it. It is the least healthy of the two options. The resistance of nasal breathing is not a disadvantage; in fact, it has benefits. The increased pressure needed to inhale through the nose makes the air denser, which helps inflate the alveoli – the gas-exchange sacs in the lungs. Inhaling against this resistance creates a slight vacuum, increasing oxygen transport by about 10–20%. This improves lung elasticity.

The natural human state is believed to be nose breathing. Mouth breathing is more of a chronic stress response. Of course, some people will have difficulty breathing through the nose due to obstruction or trauma, leading to enforced mouth breathing. But if imbalanced breathing becomes established, or if we subconsciously train ourselves into poor habits through Pavlovian signalling, we need to identify the issue and retrain our breathing.

Even airborne irritants or smells can trigger an amygdala response if a fear association has been established. Amygdala responses will almost certainly involve glucose-raising activity from the sympathetic nervous system, and a small rise in blood glucose may follow. This is possibly significant in type 1 diabetes.

Practising mindful, nasal breathing regularly is a good habit. Eventually, it becomes subconscious. There is plenty of information online about diaphragm breathing, and it is no accident that many Eastern relaxation practices place great emphasis on correct breathing techniques. As a way of contributing to a relaxed state of being, it is an easy, cost-free win.

How to Breathe With Your Diaphragm

Begin either sitting or standing, with your shoulders relaxed and arms loose at your sides. Keep your chest open without tensing your muscles. If possible, keep your head level and your spine upright but not rigid. Use a mirror at first, to observe your posture and movement.

Start by taking a deep breath in through your mouth. You will likely see your rib cage rise; this shows that you are using accessory muscles in your chest and shoulders. While common, it is not ideal for deep, efficient breathing. The goal is to engage your diaphragm, the main muscle responsible for healthy, relaxed breathing.

For your next breath, reset your posture by relaxing your upper body again. Now inhale through your nose and gently push your belly button outward. This outward movement shows that your diaphragm is descending, creating a vacuum that draws air deeply into the lungs. Then exhale through your nose, using only gentle effort.

You may notice that this feels more difficult at first – that is because the diaphragm has to be consciously engaged, which most of us are not used to doing. But with practice, it becomes easier, and you may even start to feel a calming effect during and after the exercise.

If you need to control your rib cage, you can place your hands on your head, but be aware that you might be overusing your arm muscles. When you get used to relaxing your ribs, return to a more natural posture, with your arms on your lap.

Over time, as you strengthen your awareness and control of the diaphragm, you may find that symptoms like acid reflux improve. That is because using the diaphragm properly supports not only breathing but also digestion and posture.

To visualise what is happening, think of the lungs as a slinky toy. If you lift the top, only the upper coils open while the lower ones stay compressed – similar to breathing only with your chest. But when you use the diaphragm correctly, you free up the lower portion of the lungs, which is actually the largest and most efficient area for gas exchange.

Chapter 42

Total miles: 1,095

Day 21 – Sur to St Moritz, 18 miles

"Long have I travelled, In storm, in the sun, in the rain,
And it is homeward singing,
Journey's at an end, journey's at an end."
– Journey's at an End, Clannad

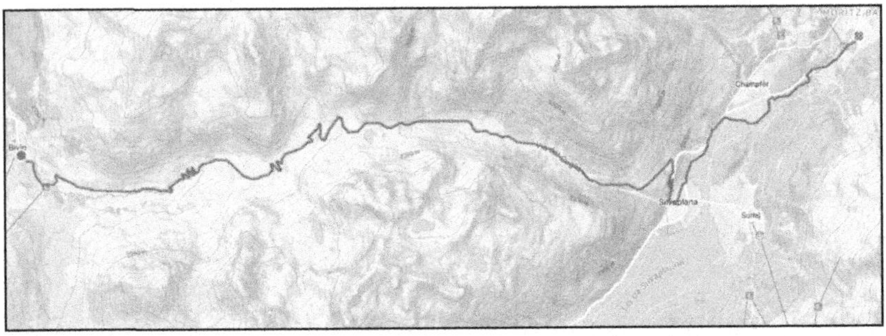

Well, this is it, my final day on the road – I would reach St Moritz on time after all! I woke up naturally at around 7 am. It was overcast and cool, but the forecast looked favourable. My clothes were still a little damp but would soon dry out; I would be climbing nonstop for at least a couple of hours, and my muscles would warm up quickly.

I left the kit hanging in the open window frame and decided I would put it on at the last minute. I had an hour to kill before breakfast and was not in a rush. I was meeting Josephine and her husband

Stephan at 1 pm, and today's ride was only 18 miles. It would easy, even with a mountain pass. That would bring my total to 1,095 miles, comfortably past the 1,000 I had aimed for.

I was about to cross the Julierpass and descend into the Engadin Valley, still within the canton of Grisons. Engadin is a high plain around 3,000 metres up. The word means "garden of the Inn", referring to the River Inn, which drains this high plain across to the northeast, through Innsbruck to the Danube – the longest river in Europe.

Last summer, I briefly stayed in the village of Maloja, on the road from St Moritz to Italy, and explored the Engadin. It is remarkably wide and dotted with glacial lakes. St Moritz lies at one end of the valley.

I checked the map. Very soon, I would be on the steady uphill climb to the summit of the Julierpass, which is named after Piz Julia, the 3,380-metre peak to my left as I ascend. Then, I would be on the long, winding descent to the village of Silvaplana, which is situated on the lake of the same name, just a few miles from St Moritz. Today's map showed many hairpin bends with lots of climbing – though eventually they would be downhill. I expected to reach the high point at the Surses ski resort, where the pass topped out at 2,240 metres.

I did a final calibration of my glucose and ketone meters. They were as expected: glucose was consistent across the three devices; the continuous ketone monitor under-read compared to the finger-prick device. I clipped on the heart-rate monitor, grateful it would be the last time. Worn around the chest, the strap is never quite comfortable and either slips or cuts off circulation. Yesterday, I spent 35% of the ride in heart-rate zone 4, which did not surprise me, given the climb; I was pleased I could still manage that effort at my age.

My glucose this morning was steady at 3.8 mmol/L and would likely rise with the stress hormone input from the climb and the effects of breakfast. I chose a couple of ham slices, some salami, a boiled egg, a thin wedge of cheese, and a black coffee – 309 calories, and 28g of protein for the journey ahead. I injected my usual six units of Tresiba for the last time. Tomorrow, I would return to taking eight as the conference began and I returned to a relatively sedentary lifestyle.

Should I cover the protein? If it were a sedentary day, like the Keto Live conference tomorrow, I would, but today, I chose not to inject a bolus dose of Novorapid. My glucose would likely peak at 9 mmol/L (162 mg/dL) with no bolus, but I did not want to chase a hypo up the mountain if I injected. A half-unit pen or a pump might have managed that peak more precisely, limiting glucose to around 6 mmol/L (108 mg/dL), but I was using pens, and had done well so far.

I was well into my routine and felt fit. My glucose was under control, and my insulin doses were minimal but also optimal. And I was in the middle of the Alps. I would have liked to stay longer, but that was for another time. I was expected in St Moritz that afternoon, and looking forward to meeting my friends again.

I saddled up and took the only road out of town. It was uphill from the start, and I took a while to warm up. It caught me out; I was panting after a few hundred metres and was not sure why. A check of glucose showed that it was okay, and the sudden feeling of exertion settled after a few minutes.

I spotted a cycle track at the next bend and decided to take it. I could see the road continue to snake up the mountain and it was busy with all kinds of traffic, so I took a meandering detour along a small track via a dammed alpine lake, Lai da Marmorera. It was worth it. I had to push the bike up the bank, but it was filled with wildflowers – mainly blue, white and yellow. I was not in a hurry today and I delayed the inevitable with a prolonged excursion into my "happy place".

Back on the main road, I climbed steadily to Surses, the ski resort, which marked about halfway. The snaky lines on the map were in two parts flanking a straight piece of road; I assumed these were the uphill and then the downhill hairpin bends of the pass. I stopped for a coffee at one of the ski-resort hotels, which was very quiet at this time of year, and was told by the barman that I still had another hour of climbing – I had completely misread the route! The hairpins were not, in fact, on both the ascent and descent; they were on the uphill.

There were posses of motorcyclists out that day, a few cyclists going the other way, and lots of campervans. People were clearly out for Sunday adventures, and it added to the atmosphere of anticipation. I could see where I needed to go by the slow, snaking procession of vehicles climbing ahead. That part was meant to be downhill, according to my previous reckoning. I made a note to be more careful next time – I mistook a ferry for a road earlier in the trip, I am a slow learner.

There was nothing for it but to dig in and pedal. But once into my rhythm, it was not overly difficult, just a hard slog. I followed the bends on the satnav, and this helped me manage the climb. Knowing when the end of the hairpin series was coming helped me relax into the ride. Before long, I was at the snowline, having taken only short breaks to soak in the scenery and capture the beauty on my camera. I loved it here. But I had to move on and get to the top.

It was a slow grind of persistence rather than a lung-buster, and the highest point of the Julierpass eventually appeared around a snowbank. Lots of people were taking photos at the top, and I did the same; I even persuaded someone to take my picture by the marker post. I got a bit of kudos for having cycled from England, but the pleasure was personal. I had done it!

But it is never over until it is over. I freewheeled downhill, the increasing warmth of the sun on the descent offsetting the wind. I smiled as I cruised at 40 mph on thin wheels, in shorts and a T-shirt. If I had been on my motorbike, I would have been dressed in full protective gear, but I did not mind; I felt in control, and even took off my cycling helmet to get the full wind-in-the-hair experience.

The long, winding downhill continued into Silvaplana. Then I took a left turn to the hotel. I could see the road stretching out ahead. The sun was out. Silvaplana lake was full of kitesurfers. By the time I coasted in, the village was hot. I knew the trip would end in just minutes and thought of dawdling, but had a deadline and was 15 minutes early – not bad for a 1,000-mile journey. In the end, I used up those 15 minutes by taking a detour on a gravel path through the woods. Then I joined the road and picked up the pace for the final stretch. I was in great shape, and soon rounded the corner to the hotel.

Josephine, Stephan, and some family and friends greeted me. It was lovely. After warm welcomes and hugs, Josephine asked, "How is your blood sugar?" I had to admit: "Josephine, I don't know. I haven't checked it since I left the hotel four hours ago."

It was true. I took a look; it was a perfect 4.8 mmol/L (86 mg/dL). I had to take a moment to absorb that sentence: I had not checked my glucose. That in itself is remarkable in type 1 diabetes, if you think about it. Yes, you can do anything you want with type 1 diabetes, but doing it with that degree of nonchalance? Well, that's doing it with style.

It was finally over. I had done what I set out to do: explore the practicality and safety of an insulin optimisation strategy. It required me to honour all the foundations of health and adapt my insulin to suit the conditions; in doing so, I felt liberated from the burden of type 1. Of course, it still demands respect – but I have bossed *it* these past three weeks.

It has been a joy.

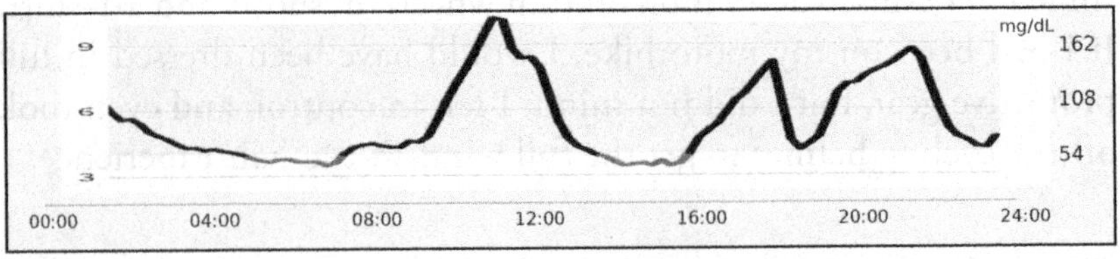

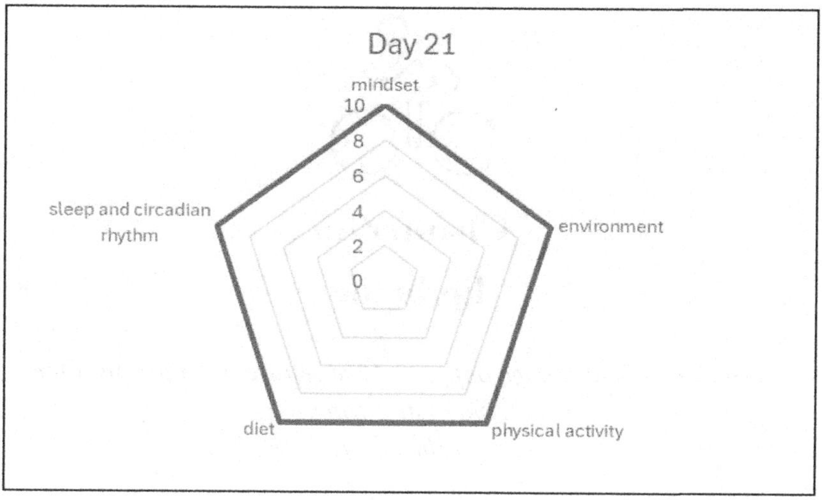
Day 21
mindset
10
8
6
4
2
0
environment
physical activity
diet
sleep and circadian rhythm

Chapter 43
Epilogue

"And that is how change happens. One gesture. One person. One moment at a time."
– Libba Bray

As I sit here one year later, writing down my thoughts on the journey, I savour the lovely memories of another adventure. Exactly one year ago, I was approaching Harwich, looking forward to crossing on the ferry to Hoek van Holland. I remember it well; I have an album of photos that jog the memory. I loved this trip more than I expected. There was something almost every day that challenged me to think and adapt.

I never imagined I would be dealing with an onboard insulin issue on Day One. That erratic trace of bouncing hypos did not look great coming from someone advocating for optimised insulin. It was not unexpected, but I had to consider how I would explain it. My type 1 is personal, and while some might fare better, others might struggle more.

It has been uncomfortable at times, opening up to my vulnerabilities and putting myself out there for potential criticism, but now you know who I am, and I expect you have identified with some of the diabetes challenges I have faced. I would bet many of you have stories far more dramatic than mine. And, of course, every person with type 1 diabetes would get different results and have different insulin requirements than I did. This book is not about comparisons; it is about information. Each of us is on a personal journey with type 1 diabetes.

I have tried to give you everything you need to understand type 1 diabetes, how complex it is, and how I approach managing it. If you have read this far, you will also understand my paradigm: to optimise insulin. I believe this is the key to smoothing out glucose control.

Glucose will follow insulin's lead – but, as I have said before, glucose is a symptom, not the cause, of type 1 diabetes. If we focus solely on controlling glucose, we miss the bigger picture. Our insulin gets out of control, and our other health markers suffer, too. The philosophy of "eat what you want and shoot as much insulin as you need" might suit some, but it is ultimately hedonistic.

Insulin is not a free ride; it is one of the central hormones in our metabolism. Overdo the insulin, and you increase inflammation. I do not want just my glucose in range, I want my insulin in range, too. We inject insulin in the wrong place, at the wrong time, in the wrong amount, and remarkably, it still works. If we optimise it, even within these limitations, we can not only smooth glucose but also bring inflammation markers like CRP, kidney function and lipid profiles into a healthier range. And when insulin is closer to a physiological level, the other hormones it interacts with are also more likely to function properly.

For me, simply counting carbs is a poor substitute for addressing the deeper foundations of health. If we manage those, we will feel more vital and we will know our insulin is working as it should; we will be as close to a non-diabetic state as possible. It might sound complex, but in practice it is not. I hope I have shown over the 21 days of my journey that it does not get in the way of living a free, full life.

My clinical colleagues would probably be gobsmacked, and may be horrified, that I barely ate or checked my blood glucose on the final day, but honestly, I just forgot; I was immersed in the cycling and the sights of the Alps. To have that kind of confidence with type 1 diabetes is a privilege. Equally, my clinical colleagues might recoil at my final thought…

Imagine we could bring back to life Banting and Best, McLeod and Collip – those early pioneers of insulin therapy for type 1 diabetes. The way they approached the condition then was to use the best available knowledge and technology. They discovered the root cause of type 1 diabetes and used insulin as the medicine to control glucose levels.

If we resurrected them and put them to work in the most state-of-the-art diabetes facility, they would fit right in, and with minimal training. Because, in spite of the technological advances, insulin is still injected into the skin, and we are still chasing glucose as the measure of control. Those four men would likely marvel at the advances in metabolic science and biochemistry; I think they would be shocked to find that, essentially, nothing has changed in type 1 diabetes management in a century. We are managing type 1 diabetes just like they did, with little regard for the incredible molecule, insulin, that saves our lives daily.

Now that we know better, I think we can do better. Let's hope that in the next hundred years, we will cure type 1 diabetes – but while we wait, let's embrace the current science and technology to make our lives easier, and hopefully free of complications. Let's optimise insulin for all foundations of health.

Technology is brilliant, and one day I would like to try a pump, to see if it is able to reduce my insulin volumes. If it can, I will likely stick with it, but if it does not, I might well stick with the convenience of pens. However, I will not stop living an optimised insulin lifestyle – it applies no matter how insulin is delivered.

I spoke to someone recently who has been optimising insulin for a year, and she told me that even if she got all her insulin function back, she would not change a thing regarding her lifestyle. She felt that good. I believe her; I would do the same. Because in exploring how to live our best life through the five foundations of health, we have also learned how the world around us affects type 1 diabetes, well beyond carbohydrates. We are trying to mimic the lifestyles of healthy people without diabetes.

Would I do the cycle trip again? Absolutely! Next time, though, I would take some friends, go at a more leisurely pace, and spend more time soaking it all in. I could do without the rain, almost losing my phone, my tech being soaked, getting spooked in tunnels, and discovering the difference between ferries and bridges. I would love to take cooking lessons next time, and sleep under canvas again; I missed my tent. Hopefully there will be time for all that… the world is big, and my time here is short. I need to keep moving toward new horizons – but another trip along the Rhine would be wonderful.

I am glad I did it. It has been a wonderful experience. Most of all, I hope you now understand your diabetes a little better, and maybe feel ready to set off on your own adventure, armed with the confidence and vitality that come from optimising your insulin.

Go well.

Acknowledgements

My sincere thanks to Professor Eric Westman for providing the foreword.

To Dr Suzanne Schneider for her guidance and gentle persuasion to continue when the task felt challenging. I am also grateful to Keto Live – especially Josephine and Stephan Barbarino – for your unwavering belief in me all these years and for choosing me as Scientist in Residence in Berghausen, providing a quiet, inspiring place to begin those difficult first chapters.

I would like to thank the following individuals for taking the time to read chapters of this book and for providing thoughtful peer review and feedback – whether as healthcare professionals, non-clinical specialists, or fellow people living with type 1 diabetes: Dr Suzanna Lake; Dr Eirin Wijne; Nick Chase; Dr Ian Collins; Dr Eric Smith; Nayiri Mississian; Chris Hill; Emma Clegg; Alice Dogruyol; Colin Gummer; Andy Wood; Dr Sarah Pugh; Dr Roshani Sanghani; Dr Garry Tan; John Cripps MD; Dr Alex Williams; Dr Zoe Harcombe; Dr Georgia Ede; and Professor Tim Noakes; Dr John Meadley, MBE; Fiona Meadley; and Thomas Meadley.

To my family: thank you for enduring years of keto evangelism – and for your sudden and impressive ability to become "busy" the moment the K-word appears in conversation. To my mum, first to read the draft, my greatest cheerleader. My fellow type 1 "ninjas" – Emma Porter, Dr Jon Furniss, Jane and Neil Hall-McLean, Dr Suzanne Schneider, and Ian Moseley – thank you for the early days when we were teaching, learning and supporting one another, and for the fun we had while doing it. Still good friends.

And to all those people who have encouraged and tolerated my enthusiasm along the way, too many to mention, including my close friends from a past life, with whom I shared so many memories.

Finally, thank you, Shirley McLellan and your team at Wellness Books, including medical editor Dr Said Qabbaah, for your support with the preparation and printing of this book.

Appendix

What to Consider Before Adopting Optimised Insulin Management

This chapter is rather complicated and is intended for clinicians; that's why there are so many references. However, the content is separated into the common complications and will help you understand the risks of a ketogenic diet with diabetic complications.

The vast majority of people will not have any need to worry about adopting a keto diet, but for anyone with complications that are advancing, it is strongly recommended that you read this. In most cases, when the person has type 1 diabetes without serious complications, the switch to a ketogenic diet can be fast or slow, depending on what the patient prefers. Usual symptoms during the change, like headaches, cramps or constipation, are usually easy to handle.

Adjusting insulin should be simple for most people. However, more care and close attention are needed for people with advanced complications. Even so, a ketogenic diet can be helpful in managing type 1 diabetes. Better glucose control and lower inflammation often bring medium- to long-term benefits. There are many reports of improved retinopathy and even recovery from neuropathy. Blood pressure usually falls, too.

The biggest challenges happen when patients with advanced complications try to begin a ketogenic lifestyle. Damaged tissue may seem to worsen before it improves, and some tissue may never recover. A slow and careful reduction of carbohydrates, along with a slow increase in fat and protein, is usually safest. There are no strict rules. A patient example appears later in the chapter on retinopathy.

A rough estimate for the transition is three to six months, based on what many clinicians have seen, but some patients may need more time. You should expect to watch the transition closely. In some cases, working with a whole team and sharing knowledge is the best way to help the patient.

Not all tissue damaged by diabetes can recover. While almost everyone agrees that good glucose control is important, years of high blood sugar and high insulin levels do cause harm. Patients with advanced disease will need lifelong monitoring. It is not guaranteed that damaged tissue will heal, which is why caution is needed when changing the body's fuel supply. Cells and the spaces around them can be harmed by sudden changes, especially when the micro-blood vessels are fragile. This means a fast switch to a ketogenic diet could cause further or permanent damage in these cases.

A Brief Overview of Diabetes Pathophysiology

More detail is available in specialist articles. For metabolic management, it is important to understand how damaging long-term high blood sugar can be.

One such article can be found at
www.ncbi.nlm.nih.gov/books/NBK560805/

The two strongest indicators of diabetes complications are the time since diagnosis and the level of chronic hyperglycaemia, usually measured by HbA1c (and also Time in Range). Higher HbA1c means a higher risk of complications.

Many metabolic pathways are affected by high blood sugar, and others are affected by high insulin levels caused by insulin doses (and the way insulin is given). High blood sugar activates alternate glucose pathways, including the polyol pathway. High insulin and high glucose trigger the creation of advanced glycation end products (AGEs), cytokines, and growth factors. These lead to abnormal cell signalling, injury to blood vessel lining, and oxidative stress.

Different tissues respond differently to high blood sugar partly because they have different levels of the enzyme sorbitol dehydrogenase. Tissues low in this enzyme – kidneys, retina, and peripheral nerves – are more at risk of swelling and stress (MB2). Other tissues may develop more AGEs, causing problems like reduced blood flow and more risk of tissue death.

Early-stage disease may be reversible with very tight glucose control. But this is not always true once serious tissue damage has occurred, so great caution is needed. It makes sense that improving blood sugar levels should help, but the safest speed for doing so is still debated. Most agree that slow progress toward normal blood sugar is safest.

Insulin Resistance

People using higher amounts of basal insulin usually have had type 1 diabetes for a long time and often have insulin resistance. These patients should be told that their need for basal insulin may fall over weeks or months as their insulin resistance decreases. They should watch carefully for low blood sugar caused by too much basal insulin.

Basal insulin usually lowers glucose slowly, so there is usually time to prevent and correct low blood sugar. Over time, the basal dose can be adjusted until it matches a ketogenic lifestyle.

Hypertension

High blood pressure often appears later in type 1 diabetes as insulin resistance and treatment-related high insulin levels develop. This is similar to type 2 diabetes appearing on top of type 1. Weight may rise, insulin doses may increase, and signs of fatty liver may appear.

A ketogenic or low-carb diet may reverse these problems. Patients should know that their blood pressure may fall, and if they take medication, they should know the symptoms of low blood pressure. The earliest sign is usually dizziness when standing up. Many patients have a home blood-pressure monitor; if not, encourage them to get one or borrow one for the first three months. Blood pressure often falls in the early months, and many patients can reduce or stop medication. In patients with advanced complications, this may not be possible.

Chronic high blood sugar and high insulin cause AGEs and amyloid deposits, leading to blood vessel problems. These changes may not be reversible. A gradual transition to a ketogenic diet may slow or stabilise the damage, but strong evidence is lacking.

Chronic Renal Failure

At this time, there is limited data on the effects of a ketogenic diet in people with chronic kidney disease (CKD). The role of dietary protein in CKD remains debated, and most published work comes from animal studies rather than human trials.

Further information is available from:
www.nejm.org/doi/full/10.1056/nejm198209093071104

One argument for limiting protein in kidney disease is that protein increases renal blood flow and glomerular pressure. This causes an early rise in the glomerular filtration rate (GFR), followed later by a gradual fall as the kidney becomes strained.

You can find article of interest here:
www.ncbi.nlm.nih.gov/pmc/articles/PMC5962279/

This paper discusses the complexity of protein choice in renal medicine and summarises multiple studies showing mixed findings. It is available from:
www.ncbi.nlm.nih.gov/pmc/articles/PMC4952055/

A "high-protein diet" is often defined as protein making up more than 20% of calories or more than 0.8 g/kg ideal body weight/day. You can find more information here:
www.ncbi.nlm.nih.gov/pmc/articles/PMC4258944/

Other sources define high protein as >1.2 g/kg/day:
www.ncbi.nlm.nih.gov/pmc/articles/PMC5962279/

People who eat less than 0.6 g/kg/day over time may develop protein malnutrition and muscle loss. Many ketogenic diets naturally fall between 0.8–1.5 g/kg/day, though some experts recommend around 1.5 g/kg/day depending on goals and health.

Ketogenic Diets and PKD

Important new evidence comes from research led by Thomas Weimbs and colleagues, who have studied ketogenic metabolism in Autosomal Dominant Polycystic Kidney Disease (ADPKD).

Animal Evidence

Early work in animal models showed that ketogenic diets – and even direct ketone treatment with β-hydroxybutyrate – reduced cyst growth and improved kidney structure. This is laid out in the following article:
www.pubmed.ncbi.nlm.nih.gov/31631001/

Human Retrospective Study

A large retrospective survey of 131 people with PKD who chose to follow ketogenic or time-restricted diets for six months found:

- A slight average increase in eGFR (from 58 to 61)
- Protein intake of 1.5–1.7 g/kg ideal body weight/day
- Those who achieved higher ketone levels had greater improvements in eGFR
- Only 14% had professional dietary advice

This suggests that ketone bodies themselves may have a direct positive effect on kidney health in PKD. For more information, see:
www.academic.oup.com/ckj/article/15/6/1079/6369511

Human Clinical Trial: KETO-ADPKD

A recent clinical trial (KETO-ADPKD tested ketogenic diets in PKD patients and found that the diet was:

- Safe and feasible
- Associated with improved GFR
- Associated with reduced body fat
- Not associated with harmful changes in kidney function markers

While the trial did not show a statistically significant reduction in kidney volume over the short study period, the overall results were encouraging. You can find further details here:
www.labs.mcdb.ucsb.edu/weimbs/thomas/sites/labs.mcdb.ucsb.edu.weimbs.thomas/files/biblio/files/2023cellreportsmedicine_0.pdf

Taken together, the Weimbs PKD studies suggest that nutritional ketosis may support kidney health, even in genetic kidney disorders, although larger and longer trials are needed.

Low-Carb Diets in Early CKD

Beyond PKD, another study of people with type 2 diabetes and early CKD who followed a low-carbohydrate diet for five years showed improved renal function.

Further information is available from:
www.journals.lww.com/co-endocrinology/Fulltext/2021/10000/Renal_function_in_patients_following_a_low.8.aspx

In contrast, high-protein diets were linked to faster GFR decline only in people who already had reduced kidney function, not in those with normal kidneys.

Follow this link:
www.journals.lww.com/co-endocrinology/Fulltext/2021/10000/Renal_function_in_patients_following_a_low.8.aspx

Real-World Impact of Poor Glycaemic Control

In type 1 diabetes, average HbA1c in England and Wales is about 70 mmol/mol, and 70% of people remain above 58 mmol/mol. Each year spent above 58 mmol/mol is associated with a loss of around 100 days of life, often due to kidney damage caused by long-term hyperglycaemia.

When a patient wants to begin a ketogenic diet, kidney function should be an important part of the discussion. Until more research exists, following current kidney guidelines is safest.

Ketogenic diets do not appear to harm people with early-stage CKD (Stages 1–2). Existing data do not show kidney decline due to keto in these stages.

Renal Stones

Children using a ketogenic diet for epilepsy have a higher chance of kidney stones:
www.ncbi.nlm.nih.gov/pmc/articles/PMC2852806/

In a two-year study of people with type 1 diabetes who used a ketogenic diet for an average of 2.6 years, there was no sign of kidney or liver damage:
www.pubmed.ncbi.nlm.nih.gov/29737587/

Because there is some association between keto diets and kidney stones in children with epilepsy, it is wise to be aware of this risk. Take a history of kidney stones or family risk. If none exists, stones are unlikely.

Kidney stones can be made of uric acid, calcium oxalate, or mixtures. Less common stones include struvite (from infection) and cystine (from genetic disease). Uric acid rises with meat, legumes, pulses, and fructose (mostly removed on a keto diet). Oxalates are common in plant-heavy diets such as those with spinach, kale, nuts or aubergine.

Chronic acidosis can reduce calcium absorption in the kidney and lead to high calcium in the urine. Some believe that a keto diet may make urine more acidic and raise uric-acid stone risk. However, a 1926 study showed that even with high urine ketones, blood pH did not change:
www.adc.bmj.com/content/archdischild/1/1/50.full.pdf

Athletes on keto diets also showed no change in blood acidity:
www.ncbi.nlm.nih.gov/pmc/articles/PMC5852812/

Dehydration is a common cause of kidney stones. Early in the keto transition, water loss can occur due to metabolic changes and lower insulin doses. Good hydration is important.

The exact cause of kidney stones in children on keto diets is not known.

Some sources suggest potassium citrate may prevent stones. There was no difference in serum citrate levels between stone-formers and others, but metabolic acidosis, low potassium, and starvation lower urine citrate. Nutritional ketosis is not starvation, but alkalising supplements may help. An article on this can be found here: www.pubmed.ncbi.nlm.nih.gov/19911682/.

Recommended potassium citrate dose: **15–30 mEq twice daily**, maximum **100 mEq/day**.

Chronic Renal Failure

Right now, there is not much data about how ketogenic diets affect people with chronic kidney disease (CKD). The role of protein in CKD is still debated. Most research comes from animal studies. Further information is available here:
www.nejm.org/doi/full/10.1056/nejm198209093071104

One argument about protein and kidney disease is that protein increases kidney blood flow and raises pressure inside the kidney filters. This increases the glomerular filtration rate (GFR) at first, but over time may lead to a drop in GFR:
www.ncbi.nlm.nih.gov/pmc/articles/PMC5962279/

GFR and protein in the urine (proteinuria) are key signs of kidney disease. The best diet for CKD remains unclear. The body's blood pH does not change much from diet, but urine pH changes depending on what the person eats. Protein quality and quantity matter. Diets high in meat contain amino acids like cysteine and methionine, which can lower urine pH.

This article below summarises the debates about protein and kidney problems: www.ncbi.nlm.nih.gov/pmc/articles/PMC4952055/

A "high-protein diet" is sometimes defined as protein making up more than 20% of calories, or more than **0.8 g/kg** ideal body weight per day:
www.ncbi.nlm.nih.gov/pmc/articles/PMC4258944/

Other sources say **1.2 g/kg/**day is high:
www.ncbi.nlm.nih.gov/pmc/articles/PMC5962279/

A person who is no longer growing (an adult) may be at higher risk of kidney problems with long-term high protein intake. Less than **0.6 g/kg/day** leads to protein malnutrition and muscle loss, which is a challenge in advanced kidney disease. Albumin in urine is also an important sign of kidney damage.

Protein from food or muscle breakdown becomes ammonia and then urea in the liver (and partly in the kidney). Because of this, protein intake must be considered when kidneys are failing. Many guidelines suggest **0.8–1.0 g/kg ideal body weight per day** for CKD.

For a 100 kg person, this means **80–100 g/day**. In real life, most people do not eat the same amount every day, so flexibility is needed. Many ketogenic diets naturally fall into this protein range. Some ketogenic experts recommend around **1.5 g/kg ideal body weight per day**, depending on goals and health.

A study by Strubl et al. looked at 131 people with polycystic kidney disease (PKD) who followed a ketogenic diet for six months. Their average GFR went from 58 to 61, even with protein intake of **1.5–1.7 g/kg/day**, and the diet was not plant-focused.

The results are outlined here:
www.academic.oup.com/ckj/article/15/6/1079/6369511

Only 14% had professional dietary advice. Those with higher ketone levels (BOHB) had greater rises in GFR. This suggests ketones themselves may help kidney health.

There is no sign that ketogenic diets harm kidneys in early CKD (stages 1–2). Another study looked at people with CKD and type 2 diabetes who followed a low-carb diet for five years. They showed **improved kidney function**. For more information, see:
www.journals.lww.com/co-endocrinology/Fulltext/2021/10000/Renal_function_in_patients_following_a_low.8.aspx

In contrast, high-protein diets led to faster decline in GFR in patients who already had low kidney function:

www.journals.lww.com/co-endocrinology/Fulltext/2021/10000/Renal_function_in_patients_following_a_low.8.aspx

For people with type 1 diabetes, average HbA1c in England and Wales is **70 mmol/mol**, and 70% are above **58 mmol/mol**. For every year spent above 58 mmol/mol, the person loses about **100 days of life**. Much of this loss is caused by kidney disease from chronic high blood sugar, not protein intake alone.

If a patient wants to start a ketogenic diet, kidney function should be part of the decision. Until more research exists, following current kidney guidelines is safest.

UK Guidelines

NICE CKD Guidelines:
www.nice.org.uk/guidance/ng203/chapter/Recommendations#classification-of-ckd-in-adults

Dietary Advice

- Give advice about potassium, phosphate, calories and salt based on CKD severity.
- If a dietary plan is chosen, give education and careful monitoring to avoid malnutrition.

Low-Protein Diets

- Do not offer diets below **0.6–0.8 g/kg/day** to adults with CKD.

Blood Pressure

- With ACR < 70 mg/mmol: aim for **<140/90 mmHg.**
- With ACR ≥ 70 mg/mmol: aim for **<130/80 mmHg.**

NICE guideline for Type 1 diabetes renal disease:
www.nice.org.uk/guidance/ng17 and
www.nice.org.uk/guidance/ng203

Diabetic Kidney Monitoring

People with Type 1 diabetes should bring a first-morning urine sample yearly to check albumin:creatinine ratio and have eGFR measured.

If albuminuria is found, discuss its meaning.

Target blood pressure is **<130/80 mmHg**.

Advise people with nephropathy to avoid high-protein diets.

Referral Criteria

Patients should be referred to specialists if they have:

- 5% five-year risk of needing kidney replacement
- ACR ≥ 70 mg/mmol unless due to diabetes
- ACR > 30 mg/mmol plus blood in urine
- Large drops in eGFR
- Poorly controlled hypertension
- Rare or genetic kidney diseases
- Suspected renal artery stenosis

A Diet for Renal Disease

One diet for people with stage 3–4 CKD comes from Santa Barbara Nutrients and PKD clinicians. It includes:

- ~50% plants
- Eggs, cream, fish, white meat, butter, cheese
- Plenty of healthy fats

Suggested supplements:

- L-carnitine
- B-complex
- Calcium citrate
- Vitamin D
- Occasional zinc

This is only one possible diet. It is discussed on the Diet Doctor podcast at 34:30 minutes:
www.youtube.com/watch?v=hNnFRbpyMd8

Gallstones (Cholelithiasis)

There are some reports of people getting gallbladder attacks when starting a ketogenic diet. Like kidney stones, gallstones have a genetic component. There is little evidence linking keto diets directly to gallstone formation. A study of 51 obese men found that "healthy diets" reduced gallstone risk:
www.pubmed.ncbi.nlm.nih.gov/3031240

Another study showed that calorie reduction lowered gallstone risk in obese male health workers:
www.ncbi.nlm.nih.gov/pmc/articles/PMC6280928/

Another study found that women with poor-quality diets had a higher risk of gallbladder disease:
www.ncbi.nlm.nih.gov/pmc/articles/PMC4438647/

A very low–calorie diet (500 calories/day) increased new gallstones by 25% over eight weeks:
www.pubmed.ncbi.nlm.nih.gov/2669662/

A small study of 32 people found no gallstones in the higher-fat group, but six cases in the very low-fat group. Further details here:
www.pubmed.ncbi.nlm.nih.gov/9665682/

Meaning for ketogenic dieting:

- Keep calorie intake normal; severe calorie restriction may increase stone risk.
- High-fat diets may actually protect the gallbladder by keeping bile flowing.
- People with a family history of gallstones should taper slowly into keto over 6–8 weeks.

There are no widespread reports of long-term keto causing gallbladder problems.

Diabetic Retinopathy

Rapid drops in blood sugar (over about four months) can worsen retinopathy in some cases. This has been seen in:

- Bariatric surgery
- Pancreas transplant
- Intensive insulin treatment

Further information is available from:
www.pubmed.ncbi.nlm.nih.gov/29217386/

A review showed that among patients aged 58.1 years with type 1 or type 2 diabetes:

- 34.6% had some retinopathy
- 6.96% had proliferative DR
- 6.81% had macular edema
- 10.2% had vision-threatening disease

Studies can be found at:
www.ncbi.nlm.nih.gov/pmc/articles/PMC3322721/

Retinopathy can appear at any HbA1c level because disease duration and insulin exposure also matter.

A 1% drop in HbA1c reduces retinopathy risk by 31%.

A 10 mmHg drop in systolic blood pressure reduces risk by 11%.

For more information, see:
www.emedicine.medscape.com/article/1225122-treatment?reg=1

Some people need laser treatment, vitrectomy, or anti-inflammatory injections.

Insulin resistance and high insulin levels may promote abnormal blood vessel growth by raising VEGF and IGF levels:
www.ncbi.nlm.nih.gov/pmc/articles/PMC5380736/#B22

About 10–20% of people may experience "early worsening" of DR in the first 3–6 months after sudden glucose improvement. This is more common with advanced DR:
www.ncbi.nlm.nih.gov/pmc/articles/PMC5380736/

This is a warning, but a slow ketogenic transition is different from sudden drops caused by surgery or rapid insulin changes.

There are also many reports of reversible retinopathy improvements on ketogenic diets.

Some insulins may stimulate angiogenesis (new vessel growth), including glargine, Lispro, Detemir and others: www.link.springer.com/article/10.1007/s00125-009-1415-7 (DOI: 10.1007/s00125-010-1687-y)

The patient must understand the risks. Reducing insulin doses and stabilising glucose with a ketogenic diet may help long-term.

Diabetic Neuropathy

Studies in mice have shown that a ketogenic diet can reduce diabetic neuropathy: www.ncbi.nlm.nih.gov/pmc/articles/PMC5994385/

There are many reports from people saying they feel improvements in nerve pain after switching to a keto diet, but at this time there is very little trial evidence in humans. Still, because beta-hydroxybutyrate (a ketone body) can support nerve health, it makes sense that a ketogenic diet may help stabilise or even improve neuropathy, as long as the nerve damage is not already permanent.

There are no formal guidelines about whether the start of a ketogenic diet needs to be slow or fast for people with neuropathy. Decisions should be based on the patient's health and the condition of other tissues affected by diabetes.

Autonomic Neuropathy

Many people with type 1 diabetes for more than 10 years develop some degree of autonomic neuropathy. Symptoms may range from mild to severe.

Common mild signs include:

- Dizziness on standing (postural hypotension)
- Fast heartbeat (sinus tachycardia)

More serious signs include:

- Digestive problems
- Diarrhoea
- Gastroparesis (the stomach empties slowly or unpredictably)

Gastroparesis can cause nausea and unstable blood glucose. "Brittle diabetes", where blood sugars swing rapidly and unpredictably, may have an autonomic component.

A low-carb diet may stress damaged nerves that already have a weak blood supply. There is very little evidence showing that keto diets make autonomic neuropathy worse, but a slow transition over about three months is probably safest. This allows the tissues to adjust slowly. Over time, people with gastroparesis may benefit from eating fewer carbohydrates, because carbs tend to cause large swings in glucose.

There are many reports of improvements in symptoms like dizziness, palpitations, joint pain and brain fog when people follow nutritional ketosis.

Contraindications

Below is a list of conditions that are often cited as reasons **not** to start a ketogenic diet:

- Acute pancreatitis
- Severe liver disease
- Pyruvate kinase deficiency
- Pyruvate carboxylase deficiency
- Porphyria
- Fatty acid oxidation defects
- Primary carnitine deficiencies
- Organic acidurias
- Defects in ketone metabolism
- Hypoglycaemia that is still under investigation

Primary Carnitine Deficiency (CDSP)

This condition prevents fatty acids from being transported into liver mitochondria. It is caused by a problem in the *SLC22A5* gene on chromosome 5. Patients may appear in infancy with high ammonia levels or in adulthood with high liver enzymes and episodes of low blood sugar without ketones. Treatment includes carnitine supplements, low-fat diet, and avoiding long fasting periods.

Medium-Chain Acyl-CoA Dehydrogenase (MCAD) Deficiency

MCAD deficiency occurs in about 1 in 10,000 White infants. It is usually detected early through newborn screening. MCAD is needed to break down medium-chain fats into acetyl-CoA inside mitochondria. Without treatment, patients may have seizures, coma, low blood sugar without ketones, or failure to thrive. Treatment is avoiding fasting and early detection.

Most of these metabolic diseases appear in infancy and often cause early death. It is extremely unlikely that a person with type 1 diabetes will also have one of these disorders.

Pyruvate Carboxylase Deficiency

This rare disorder affects about 1 in 250,000 births. Only Type C allows a person to reach adulthood. A high-carb diet is usually recommended, and keto diets can make the condition worse.

Pyruvate Kinase Deficiency

This is a rare form of haemolytic anaemia (red blood cell breakdown). It has dominant and recessive forms. It is very uncommon.

Porphyria

Porphyria is a group of rare metabolic disorders caused by problems in the body's ability to make haem, a key part of blood. The disorders fall into **acute porphyrias** and **cutaneous porphyrias**. Porphyria is usually inherited. Some people never develop symptoms.

Acute Intermittent Porphyria (AIP)

AIP is the most common acute form. It is caused by a partial lack of the enzyme hydroxymethylbilane synthase. Attacks affect the nervous system and can be life-threatening. Symptoms can include:

- Severe abdominal pain
- Muscle pain (especially in legs, chest, back)
- Sudden nerve problems, sometimes seizures
- Red or brown urine
- Fast heartbeat, palpitations, or high blood pressure
- Mental changes such as anxiety, confusion, or paranoia

Attacks usually last from days to weeks and improve slowly. Treatment must be started quickly. Glucose is often used in treatment because it blocks the build-up of harmful haem precursors. This is why porphyria symptoms may worsen if someone begins a ketogenic diet.

Testing for Porphyria

The main test is a **urine porphobilinogen (PBG) test**.

- It must be done early in the attack because PBG levels fall quickly.
- Urine samples must be kept in a dark container because porphyrins break down in light.

More testing is done in special laboratories. A useful resource is available from: http://porphyria.org.uk/

Porphyria Cutanea Tarda

This is the most common type. It causes:

- Skin sensitivity to sunlight
- Blisters
- Itching
- Excess hair in affected areas
- Red or brown urine

It may be triggered by:

- Oestrogens
- Smoking
- Alcohol
- Stress

Inherited Defects in Ketone Metabolism

Some genetic conditions affect ketone production or use. These include:

- Systemic primary carnitine deficiency
- Medium-chain acyl-CoA dehydrogenase deficiency

These conditions make ketogenic diets unsafe because the person cannot properly break down fat for fuel.

Inherited Disorders That Affect Ketone Use

Some rare inherited conditions make it dangerous for a person to enter ketosis because their body cannot properly break down or use fatty acids. These include:

Systemic Primary Carnitine Deficiency

People with this condition cannot move fatty acids into the mitochondria, where they are used for energy. This leads to:

- Low ketone levels
- Low blood sugar
- Liver problems
- Weakness or tiredness

Diagnosis is usually by genetic testing or by checking blood carnitine levels. Treatment includes giving carnitine supplements, lowering fat in the diet, and avoiding long periods without food.

Medium-Chain Acyl-CoA Dehydrogenase (MCAD) Deficiency

This is one of the most common fatty acid oxidation defects. It prevents the breakdown of medium-chain fats into acetyl-CoA. It is usually picked up by newborn screening.

People with MCAD deficiency can suffer:

- Seizures
- Fainting
- Coma
- Low blood sugar with few or no ketones
- Failure to thrive

Patients must avoid fasting because the body cannot switch to fat-burning safely.

These conditions are rare, and it is extremely unlikely that a person with type 1 diabetes will also have one of them. Still, clinicians should be aware of them.

Summary and Final Clinical Considerations

A ketogenic diet can offer major benefits for many people with type 1 diabetes, including:

- Lower and more stable blood glucose
- Reduced inflammation
- Lower insulin doses
- Possible improvement in neuropathy
- Possible stabilisation or even improvement of retinopathy
- Lower blood pressure
- Mild improvement in kidney markers in early CKD (based on limited data)

However, the **speed of transition matters** – especially in people with long-term or advanced complications.

Why a slow transition is safest:

- Sudden drops in blood sugar can stress fragile tissues.
- Microvascular damage may temporarily worsen.
- Retinopathy can flare (early worsening).
- Damaged nerves or kidneys may react poorly to abrupt metabolic changes.

A 3–6 month gradual taper of carbohydrates, with slow increases in fat and protein, is a reasonable guide. Many people may take longer.

People who need special caution:

- Those with advanced retinopathy
- Those with advanced neuropathy
- Those with chronic kidney disease (especially stage 3+)
- People with autonomic neuropathy
- People with genetic risks for gallstones or kidney stones
- Anyone with rare metabolic disorders (very unlikely in type 1 diabetes)

General Principles

1. Go slow.
2. Monitor closely.
3. Educate the patient clearly.
4. Adjust insulin carefully.
5. Use team-based care when needed.
6. Hydrate well, especially early on.
7. Review blood pressure, kidney function and eye assessments regularly.

For most people with type 1 diabetes without advanced complications, a ketogenic diet can be adopted safely and smoothly with good support.

For those with complications, the diet may still help – but only with a carefully controlled, slow transition, thoughtful monitoring, and attention to the patient's whole clinical picture.

References

Chapter 4. What Causes Type 1 diabetes?

1. New-Onset Type 1 Diabetes in Children During COVID-19
   Unsworth R, et al. *Diabetes Care.* 2020.

DOI: www.doi.org/10.2337/dc20-1551
Link: www.pubmed.ncbi.nlm.nih.gov/32816997/

Summary:
Multicentre UK study describing increased incidence and more severe presentation of type 1 diabetes in children during the COVID-19 pandemic.

Genetics (heritability / onset-related genetic liability)

2. Genetic Liability of Type 1 Diabetes and the Onset Age
   Hyttinen V, et al. *Diabetes.* 2003;52(4):1052–1058.

DOI: www.doi.org/10.2337/diabetes.52.4.1052
Link: www.pubmed.ncbi.nlm.nih.gov/12663480/

Summary:
Twin and family data demonstrating strong genetic contribution to type 1 diabetes risk, while highlighting the role of non-genetic factors in determining age of onset.

SNPs / risk loci (TEDDY-related)

3. Role of Type 1 Diabetes–Associated SNPs on Risk of Autoantibody Positivity in the TEDDY Study
   Törn C, et al. *Diabetes.* 2015.

DOI: www.doi.org/10.2337/db14-1497
Link: www.pubmed.ncbi.nlm.nih.gov/25422107/
PMC: www.pmc.ncbi.nlm.nih.gov/articles/PMC4407865/

Summary:
Analysis of non-HLA genetic variants showing how specific SNPs influence autoantibody development and progression toward clinical type 1 diabetes.

Delaying progression to clinical type 1 diabetes (immunotherapy)

4. An Anti-CD3 Antibody, Teplizumab, in Relatives at Risk for Type 1 Diabetes
Herold KC, et al. *New England Journal of Medicine.* 2019.
DOI: www.doi.org/10.1056/NEJMoa1902226
Link: www.nejm.org/doi/full/10.1056/NEJMoa1902226

Summary:
Landmark trial demonstrating that immune modulation with teplizumab can delay progression from autoimmunity to clinical type 1 diabetes.

Autoimmunity / antibody-related immunogenetics (PTPN axis)

5. Genetic Variations of PTPN2 and PTPN22: Role in the Pathogenesis of Type 1 Diabetes and Crohn's Disease
Sharp RC, et al. *Frontiers in Cellular and Infection Microbiology.* 2015.
DOI: www.doi.org/10.3389/fcimb.2015.00095
Link: www.frontiersin.org/articles/10.3389/fcimb.2015.00095/full

Summary:
Explores shared immune-regulatory pathways involving PTPN genes that link type 1 diabetes with other autoimmune diseases.

6. The Role for Protein Tyrosine Phosphatase Non-Receptor Type 22 in Regulating Intestinal Homeostasis
Spalinger MR, et al. *United European Gastroenterology Journal.* 2016.
DOI: www.doi.org/10.1177/2050640615600115
Link: www.pubmed.ncbi.nlm.nih.gov/27403297/

Summary:
Describes how PTPN22 variants influence gut immune regulation, supporting a gut–immune axis in autoimmune disease development.

Regional variation (autoantibody profiles / incidence differences)

7. Islet Autoantibody Profiles Associated with Higher Diabetes Risk in Lithuanian Compared with English Schoolchildren
   Long AE, et al. *Clinical & Experimental Immunology.* 2021.

DOI: www.doi.org/10.1111/cei.13524
Link: www.pmc.ncbi.nlm.nih.gov/articles/PMC7744493/

Summary:
Demonstrates geographic differences in autoantibody patterns, suggesting environmental modifiers of autoimmune risk beyond genetics.

Gut permeability ("leaky gut")

8. The Role for Gut Permeability in the Pathogenesis of Type 1 Diabetes
   Li X, et al. Pediatric *Diabetes.* 2015.

DOI: www.doi.org/10.1111/pedi.12305
Link: www.pubmed.ncbi.nlm.nih.gov/26269193/
PMC: www.pmc.ncbi.nlm.nih.gov/articles/PMC4638168/

Summary:
Reviews evidence linking increased intestinal permeability with immune activation and type 1 diabetes development.

9. Enteroviral Infections in the Pathogenesis of Type 1 Diabetes
   Richardson SJ, Morgan NG. *Current Opinion in Pharmacology.* 2018.

DOI: www.doi.org/10.1016/j.coph.2018.07.006
Link: www.pmc.ncbi.nlm.nih.gov/articles/PMC6294842/

Summary:
Examines viral triggers, particularly enteroviruses, as potential initiators or accelerators of autoimmune beta-cell destruction.

Diet: milk / cow's milk proteins

10. A1 Beta-Casein Milk Protein and Other Environmental Pre-Disposing Factors for Type 1 Diabetes

Chia JSJ, et al. *Nutrition & Diabetes.* 2017.
DOI: www.doi.org/10.1038/nutd.2017.16
Link: www.pubmed.ncbi.nlm.nih.gov/28504710/

Summary:
Reviews evidence linking A1 beta-casein exposure with immune responses relevant to type 1 diabetes risk.

11. Diet, Cow's Milk Protein Antibodies and the Risk of Type 1 Diabetes
Virtanen SM, et al. *Diabetologia.* 1994.
DOI: www.doi.org/10.1007/s001250050121
Link: www.pubmed.ncbi.nlm.nih.gov/8063039/

Summary:
Early study demonstrating associations between cow's milk protein antibodies and increased type 1 diabetes risk.

12. Increased Frequency of IgM Antibodies to Cow's Milk Proteins in Children with Newly Diagnosed Type 1 Diabetes
Saukkonen T, et al. *European Journal of Pediatrics.* 1996.
DOI: www.doi.org/10.1007/BF02282839
Link: www.pubmed.ncbi.nlm.nih.gov/8891559/

Summary:
Reports heightened immune reactivity to cow's milk proteins at diagnosis of type 1 diabetes.

Diet: gluten / coeliac overlap

13. Celiac Disease in Patients with Type 1 Diabetes
Uibo R, et al. Cellular & Molecular Immunology. 2011.
DOI: www.doi.org/10.1038/cmi.2010.66
Link: www.nature.com/articles/cmi201066

Summary:
Reviews the strong association between coeliac disease and type 1 diabetes, highlighting shared autoimmune mechanisms.

14. Association Between Maternal Gluten Intake and Type 1 Diabetes in Offspring
Antvorskov JC, et al. *BMJ.* 2018.
DOI: www.doi.org/10.1136/bmj.k3547
Link: www.pubmed.ncbi.nlm.nih.gov/30232082/
PMC: www.pmc.ncbi.nlm.nih.gov/articles/PMC6283375/

Summary:
Large cohort study linking higher maternal gluten intake during pregnancy with increased risk of type 1 diabetes in offspring.

Microbiome

15. Gut Microbiome in Type 1 Diabetes: A Comprehensive Review
Zheng P, et al. *Diabetes Metabolism Research and Reviews.* 2018.
DOI: www.doi.org/10.1002/dmrr.3043
Link: www.ncbi.nlm.nih.gov/pmc/articles/PMC6220847/

Summary:
Reviews alterations in gut microbiota composition preceding and accompanying type 1 diabetes development.

16. Toward Defining the Autoimmune Microbiome for Type 1 Diabetes
Giongo A, et al. *The ISME Journal.* 2011.
DOI: www.doi.org/10.1038/ismej.2010.92
Link: www.nature.com/articles/ismej201092

Summary:
Identifies early microbiome shifts that may contribute to immune dysregulation and autoimmunity.

Vitamin D

17. Intake of Vitamin D and Risk of Type 1 Diabetes: A Birth-Cohort Study
Hyppönen E, et al. The Lancet. 2001.
DOI: www.doi.org/10.1016/S0140-6736(01)06580-1
Link: www.pubmed.ncbi.nlm.nih.gov/11705562/

Summary:
Prospective cohort study showing reduced risk of type 1 diabetes with higher vitamin D intake in infancy.

Paleolithic ketogenic diet case report

18. A Child with Type 1 Diabetes Successfully Treated with the Paleolithic Ketogenic Diet
    Paleomedicina Group.

Link: www.paleomedicina.com/en/a-child-with-type-1-diabetes-mellitus-t1dm-successfully-treated-with-the-paleolithic-ketogenic-diet-a-19-months-insulin-freedom

Summary:
Case report describing prolonged insulin independence in a child with type 1 diabetes following a paleolithic ketogenic diet.

Chapter 11, Day 4: Hook of Holland to Wijk bij Duurstede.

1. The Rhine Cycle Route: Cycle touring EuroVelo 15 through six countries
   McGregor M. *Cicerone Cycle Touring Guides.* 2022.
   ISBN: 978-1786311092

Summary:
Guidebook describing the EuroVelo 15 Rhine Cycle Route across six countries, including navigation, terrain, and touring logistics.

2. Variability of insulin absorption and insulin action
   Heinemann L. *Diabetes Technology & Therapeutics.* 2002; 4(5):673–682.

DOI: www.doi.org/10.1089/152091502320798322

Summary:
Review describing variability in subcutaneous insulin absorption and its impact on glycaemic control.

3. Absorption of soluble insulin injected subcutaneously in diabetic patients
Lauritzen T, Pramming S, Gale EA. *BMJ.* 1983; 286(6366):123–126.
DOI: www.doi.org/10.1136/bmj.286.6366.123

Summary:
Clinical study demonstrating variability in insulin absorption following subcutaneous injection.

4. Worldwide injection technique questionnaire study
Frid AH, Hirsch LJ, Menchior AR, Morel DR, Strauss KW. *Mayo Clinic Proceedings.* 2016; 91(9):1224–1230.
DOI: www.doi.org/10.1016/j.mayocp.2016.06.012

Summary:
International study linking injection technique, lipohypertrophy, and insulin absorption variability.

5. Diabetic gastroparesis
Camilleri M. *New England Journal of Medicine.* 2007; 356(8):820–829.
DOI: www.doi.org/10.1056/NEJMra067348

Summary:
Review of diabetic gastroparesis, including pathophysiology, symptoms, and treatment approaches.

Chapter 12: Life force

1. Cifarelli V, Eichmann A. The intestinal lymphatic system: functions and metabolic implications. Cell Mol Gastroenterol Hepatol. 2019;8(4):619,33. Available from: www.cmghjournal.org/article/S2352,345X(18)30177,2/fulltext

2. Glucose transporters: physiological and pathological roles
Navale AM, Paranjape AD. *Biochemical and Biophysical Research Communications.* 2016.
DOI: www.doi.org/10.1016/j.bbrc.2015.12.007
Link: www.ncbi.nlm.nih.gov/pmc/articles/PMC5425736/

Summary:
Overview of glucose transporter families (GLUT proteins), their tissue distribution, and their role in metabolic disease.

3. The GLUT4 glucose transporter
Huang S. Cell Metabolism. 2007.
DOI: www.doi.org/10.1016/j.cmet.2007.03.006
Link: www.sciencedirect.com/science/article/pii/S1550413107000678

Summary:
Explains insulin-dependent glucose transport via GLUT4 in muscle and adipose tissue.

4. Glucose transporters in the 21st century
Thorens B. *American Journal of Physiology – Endocrinology and Metabolism.* 2010.
DOI: www.doi.org/10.1152/ajpendo.00712.2009
Link: www.journals.physiology.org/doi/full/10.1152/ajpendo.00712.2009

Summary:
Comprehensive review of glucose transporter biology and regulation across tissues.

Chapter 15. Metabolism in Action

1. Multi-Dimensional Roles of Ketone Bodies in Fuel Metabolism, Signalling, and Therapeutics
Puchalska P, Crawford PA. *Cell Metab.* 2017;25(2):262–284.
Link: www.ncbi.nlm.nih.gov/pmc/articles/PMC5313038/

Summary:
Comprehensive review of ketone bodies as metabolic fuels, signalling molecules, and therapeutic agents, including roles in mitochondrial function, inflammation regulation, and metabolic disease.

2. Ketone Bodies: From Enemy to Friend and Guardian Angel
   Kolb H, et al. *BMC Med.* 2021;19(1):25.
Link: www.bmcmedicine.biomedcentral.com/articles/10.1186/s12916-021-02185-0

Summary:
Discusses the evolving understanding of ketone bodies as protective metabolic substrates with roles in oxidative stress reduction, inflammation control, and metabolic adaptation.

3. Ketone Bodies in Exercise, Health and Disease: Metabolic and Signalling Roles
   Li Y, et al. *Metabolites.* 2025;15(3).
Link: www.sciencedirect.com/science/article/pii/S2950273X25000293

Summary:
Reviews the role of ketone bodies in exercise metabolism, cellular signalling, and disease states, highlighting their importance in metabolic flexibility and endurance physiology.

Chapter 17. Insulin actions

1. Pharmacokinetics and pharmacodynamics of insulin analogues
   Home PD. *Diabetes Obes Metab.* 2012.
DOI: www.doi.org/10.1111/j.1463-1326.2011.01451.x
Link: www.dom-pubs.onlinelibrary.wiley.com/doi/10.1111/j.1463-1326.2011.01451.x

Summary:
How insulin structure affects absorption, duration and predictability.

2. Critical nodes in insulin signalling pathways
Taniguchi CM, Emanuelli B, Kahn CR. *Nat Rev Mol Cell Biol.*
DOI: www.doi.org/10.1038/nrm3351
Link: www.nature.com/articles/nrm3351

Summary:
Core molecular pathways of insulin action and glucose transport.

3. Insulin resistance and vascular function
Muniyappa R, et al. *Hypertension.*
DOI: www.doi.org/10.1161/HYPERTENSIONAHA.118.11728
Link: www.ahajournals.org/doi/10.1161/HYPERTENSIONAHA.118.11728

Summary:
Insulin's interaction with blood vessels and cardiovascular regulation.

4. Pancreatic β-cell electrical activity and insulin secretion
Rorsman P, Ashcroft FM. *Physiol Rev.*
DOI: www.doi.org/10.1152/physrev.00008.2017
Link: www.ncbi.nlm.nih.gov/pmc/articles/PMC6471380/

Summary:
Mechanisms governing insulin release from β-cells.

5. Pancreatic extracts in diabetes mellitus
Banting FG, Best CH, Collip JB, Macleod JJR. *J Lab Clin Med.* 1922.
DOI: www.doi.org/10.1172/JCI100319
Link: www.ncbi.nlm.nih.gov/pmc/articles/PMC153065/

Summary:
Original discovery and therapeutic use of insulin.

6. The unit of insulin
Scott DA, Fisher AM. *Diabetes.* 1967.
DOI: www.doi.org/10.2337/diab.16.3.198
Link: www.diabetesjournals.org/diabetes/article/16/3/198/2858/The-Unit-of-Insulin

Summary:
Standardisation and biological definition of insulin units.

7. Mutant insulin genes and hyperinsulinaemia
Steiner DF, et al. *Diabetes.*
DOI: www.doi.org/10.2337/diab.36.1.70
Link: www.pubmed.ncbi.nlm.nih.gov/3552828/

Summary:
Genetic insulin mutations causing abnormal insulin production.

Chapter 19: Insulin Modulation, Nutrient Signalling, and Systemic Effects

1. Brain insulin signalling and metabolic regulation
Kullmann S, et al. *Frontiers in Endocrinology.*
DOI: www.doi.org/10.3389/fendo.2014.00161
Link: www.frontiersin.org/articles/10.3389/fendo.2014.00161/full

Summary:
Insulin signalling in the brain and its effects on appetite, cognition and energy regulation.

2. Anti-inflammatory effects of insulin
Dandona P, et al. *Journal of Clinical Medicine.*
DOI: www.doi.org/10.3390/jcm6020024
Link: www.ncbi.nlm.nih.gov/pmc/articles/PMC5380736/

Summary:
Insulin as an anti-inflammatory and oxidative-stress-modulating hormone.

3. Nutrient regulation of insulin secretion
Ashcroft FM, Rorsman P. *Handbook of Physiology.*
DOI: www.doi.org/10.1016/B978-008013395-9.50021-6
Link: www.sciencedirect.com/science/article/pii/B9780080133959500216

Summary:
How amino acids and free fatty acids stimulate insulin secretion.

4. Insulin signalling pathways
Taniguchi CM, Emanuelli B, Kahn CR. *Nature Reviews Molecular Cell Biology.*
DOI: www.doi.org/10.1038/nrm3351
Link: www.nature.com/articles/nrm3351

Summary:
Core molecular mechanisms of insulin receptor signalling.

5. Insulin resistance and vascular function
Muniyappa R, et al. *Hypertension.*
DOI: www.doi.org/10.1161/HYPERTENSIONAHA.118.11728
Link: www.ahajournals.org/doi/10.1161/HYPERTENSIONAHA.118.11728

Summary:
Links between insulin resistance, vascular biology and cardiometabolic risk.

Chapter 21: Insulin – as much as necessary, as little as possible

1. Sleep-dependent regulation of glucose metabolism
DOI: www.doi.org/10.1152/ajpendo.00628.2020
Link: www.journals.physiology.org/doi/full/10.1152/ajpendo.00628.2020

Summary:
Review of how sleep and circadian physiology influence glucose metabolism, insulin sensitivity and endocrine regulation.

2. Altered neuroendocrine sleep architecture in patients with type 1 diabetes
Jauch-Chara K, Schmid SM, Hallschmid M, Born J, Schultes B. *Diabetes Care.* 2008;31(6):1183–1188.
DOI: www.doi.org/10.2337/dc07-1986

Link: www.doi.org/10.2337/dc07-1986

Summary:
Demonstrates changes in sleep architecture and neuroendocrine hormone patterns in people with type 1 diabetes.

3. Circadian rhythm, metabolism, and endocrine signalling
DOI: www.doi.org/10.3390/ijms242115621
Link: www.mdpi.com/1422-0067/24/21/15621

Summary:
Review linking circadian biology, mitochondrial metabolism and endocrine signalling pathways.

4. Sleep disturbance and metabolic control in diabetes
DOI: www.doi.org/10.1046/j.1464-5491.2003.01029.x
Link: www.onlinelibrary.wiley.com/doi/10.1046/j.1464-5491.2003.01029.x

Summary:
Clinical research exploring associations between sleep disturbance and glucose regulation in diabetes.

Chapter 24: Inflammation

1. Inflammation, Metaflammation and Immunometabolic Disorders
   Hotamisligil GS. *Nature.* 2017;542:177–185.
Link: www.nature.com/articles/nature21363

Summary:
Describes the concept of metaflammation, the chronic low-grade inflammatory state associated with metabolic disease, linking immune signalling pathways with insulin resistance and metabolic dysfunction.

2. Muscle-Derived IL-6: A "Myokine" with Many Roles
Pedersen BK, Febbraio MA. *Physiol Rev.* 2008;88(4):1379–1406.

Link: www.journals.physiology.org/doi/full/10.1152/physrev.90100.2007

Summary:
Explains how skeletal muscle releases IL-6 during exercise, acting as a signalling molecule that influences metabolism, inflammation and energy regulation.

3. Advanced Glycation End-Products: A Review
   Singh R, Barden A, Mori T, Beilin L. *Diabetologia.* 2001;44(2):129–146.

Link: www.link.springer.com/article/10.1007/s001250051591

Summary:
Reviews the formation of advanced glycation end-products (AGEs) and their role in oxidative stress, inflammation, and long-term diabetic complications.

4. Clinical Application of C-Reactive Protein for Cardiovascular Disease Detection and Prevention
   Ridker PM. Circulation. 2003;107(3):363–369.

Link: www.ahajournals.org/doi/full/10.1161/01.CIR.0000053730.47739.3C

Summary:
Discusses C-reactive protein (CRP) as a biomarker of systemic inflammation and its relationship to cardiovascular risk and metabolic disease.

5. Beyond Weight Loss: A Review of the Therapeutic Uses of Very-Low-Carbohydrate (Ketogenic) Diets
   Paoli A, Rubini A, Volek JS, Grimaldi KA. *Eur J Clin Nutr.* 2013;67:789–796.

Link: www.nature.com/articles/ejcn2013116

Summary:
Reviews therapeutic effects of ketogenic diets, including improved metabolic markers and anti-inflammatory effects, partly mediated by β-hydroxybutyrate signalling.

Chapter 25: Physical Activity

1. Living with Type 1 Diabetes: Exercise and Sport
   NHS (UK).

Link: www.nhs.uk/conditions/type-1-diabetes/living-with-type-1-diabetes/exercise-and-sport/

Summary:
Guidance on safe physical activity for people with type 1 diabetes, including insulin adjustment and glucose monitoring.

2. Managing Your Diabetes: Exercise
   Diabetes UK.

Link: www.diabetes.org.uk/guide-to-diabetes/managing-your-diabetes/exercise

Summary:
Overview of exercise benefits and practical glucose-management advice for people living with diabetes.

3. Diabetes and Sport
   RunSweet (Ian Gallen).

Link: http://www.runsweet.com/diabetes-and-sport/

Summary:
Educational resource explaining glucose responses to exercise and insulin adjustment strategies.

4. Exercise management in type 1 diabetes: a consensus statement
   Riddell MC, et al. *Lancet Diabetes & Endocrinology*. 2017.

DOI: www.doi.org/10.1016/S2213-8587(17)30014-1
Link: www.pubmed.ncbi.nlm.nih.gov/28126459/

Summary:
International consensus guidelines describing physiological responses to aerobic and anaerobic exercise in type 1 diabetes.

5. Rethinking fat as a fuel for endurance exercise
   Volek JS, et al. *Metabolism Open*. 2021.

DOI: www.doi.org/10.1016/j.metop.2021.100117
Link: www.pubmed.ncbi.nlm.nih.gov/34337229/

Summary:
Review examining fat oxidation and metabolic adaptation in endurance athletes.

6. Metabolic characteristics of keto-adapted ultra-endurance athletes
Volek JS, et al. *Metabolism: Clinical and Experimental.* 2016.
DOI: www.doi.org/10.1016/j.metabol.2016.02.003
Link: www.pubmed.ncbi.nlm.nih.gov/26892521/

Summary:
Study demonstrating increased fat oxidation capacity in keto-adapted endurance athletes.

7. High-fat diets induce mitochondrial biogenesis and improve mitochondrial function in skeletal muscle
Volek JS, et al. *Journal of Physiology.* 2005.
DOI: www.doi.org/10.1113/jphysiol.2005.092064
Link: www.pubmed.ncbi.nlm.nih.gov/15774529/

Summary:
Experimental research showing dietary fat adaptation can enhance mitochondrial function in muscle.

8. What Is the Evidence That Dietary Macronutrient Composition Influences Exercise Performance? A Narrative Review
Noakes TD. *Nutrients.* 2021.
DOI: www.doi.org/10.3390/nu14050948
Link: www.pmc.ncbi.nlm.nih.gov/articles/PMC8875928/

Summary:
Review evaluating how macronutrient composition influences endurance performance.

9. Carbohydrate ingestion eliminates hypoglycaemia and improves endurance exercise performance in triathletes adapted to very-low- and high-carbohydrate diets
American Journal of Physiology – Cell Physiology. 2025.
DOI: www.doi.org/10.1152/ajpcell.00583.2024

Summary:
Study comparing endurance performance and hypoglycaemia risk in athletes adapted to different macronutrient diets.

10. Exercise metabolism and glucose regulation
Link: www.pubmed.ncbi.nlm.nih.gov/37057184/

Summary:
Review describing interactions between exercise physiology, insulin action and glucose metabolism.

Chapter 27: Foundations of health – Circadian Rhythms and Sleep

1. Herzog ED, Hermanstyne T, Smyllie NJ, Hastings MH. Regulating the Suprachiasmatic Nucleus (SCN) Circadian Clockwork: Interplay between Cell-Autonomous and Circuit-Level Mechanisms. *J Biol Rhythms.* 2017;32(3):171-189.
Link: www.pmc.ncbi.nlm.nih.gov/articles/PMC5204321/

Summary:
Detailed review of how SCN neurons and circuits generate and synchronize 24-hour rhythms that drive sleep-wake cycles and physiology in mammals. (PMC)

2. Reddy S. Physiology, Circadian Rhythm. *StatPearls.* 2023.
Link: www.ncbi.nlm.nih.gov/books/NBK519507/

Summary:
A concise overview of circadian rhythm physiology, including how light cues entrain the rhythm and how the circadian clock interacts with sleep-wake states. (NCBI)

3. Gentry NW. Human Circadian Variations. *Frontiers in Physiology.* 2021.
Link: www.pmc.ncbi.nlm.nih.gov/articles/PMC8363277/

Summary:
Review of human circadian rhythm biology, including chronotype variability and genetic/environmental influences on rhythm patterns. (PMC)

4. Huang W, Ramsey KM, Marcheva B, Bass J. Circadian rhythms, sleep, and metabolism. *J Clin Invest.* 2011;121(6):2133-2141.
Link: www.pmc.ncbi.nlm.nih.gov/articles/PMC3104765/

Summary:
Review linking molecular circadian mechanisms with sleep physiology and metabolic health, emphasizing clock-controlled feedback loops. (PMC)

5. Roenneberg T, et al. The Circadian Clock and Human Health. *Curr Biol.* 2016.
Link: www.doi.org/10.1016/j.cub.2016.07.051

Summary:
Epidemiological perspective on circadian timing systems and their influence on human behaviour, health and disease. (Cell)

6. StatPearls & Circadian Model (S & C Processes)
Okechukwu CE, et al. The Neurophysiologic Basis of the Human Sleep-Wake Cycle. *Egypt J Neurol Psychiatr Neurosurg.* 2022.
Link: www.doi.org/10.1186/s41983-022-00468-8

Summary:
Describes the **two-process model of sleep regulation**: Process S (homeostatic sleep pressure) and Process C (circadian component driven by the SCN). (Springer Link)

7. **Siffre cave study on circadian rhythms** (general science psychology description).
Siffre (Cave Study) found that lack of external cues extended his intrinsic sleep-wake cycle beyond 24 h.
Link: www.tutor2u.net/psychology/reference/biopsychology-biological-rhythms-circadian-rhythms

Summary:
Classic human experiment showing how circadian rhythms free-run without environmental cues such as light. (tutor2u.net)

8. Ingram KK, et al. Molecular insights into chronotype and time-of-day effects. *Sci Rep.* 2016.
Link: www.nature.com/articles/srep29392

Summary:
Demonstrates that genetic variations in clock gene phases are linked with behavioural chronotype differences in humans. (Nature)

Chapter 29: Our Environment

1. Effects of Forest Environment (Shinrin-yoku / Forest bathing) on Health Promotion and Disease Prevention – The Establishment of "Forest Medicine"
Li Q. *Environ Health Prev Med.* 2010;15(1):9–17.
DOI: 10.1007/s12199-009-0086-9
Link: www.pmc.ncbi.nlm.nih.gov/articles/PMC9665958/

Summary:
Describes the physiological and psychological health benefits of forest exposure, including reductions in stress hormones, improved immune function, and the development of "Forest Medicine" as a preventive health discipline.

2. View Through a Window May Influence Recovery from Surgery
Ulrich RS. *Science.* 1984;224(4647):420–421.
DOI: 10.1126/science.6143402
Link: www.science.org/doi/10.1126/science.6143402

Summary:
Demonstrates that exposure to natural scenery during hospital recovery is associated with improved clinical outcomes, including reduced analgesic use and shorter hospital stays.

3. Far Infrared Radiation (FIR): Its Biological Effects and Medical Applications
   Vatansever F, Hamblin MR. *Photonics Lasers Med.* 2012;1(4):255–266.

DOI: 10.1515/plm-2012-0034
Link: www.pmc.ncbi.nlm.nih.gov/articles/PMC3699878/

Summary:
Reviews the biological effects of far-infrared radiation, including improved circulation, reduced inflammation, and potential therapeutic applications in tissue healing.

4. Modulation of Mitochondrial Function with Near-Infrared Light Reduces Brain Injury in a Translational Model of Cardiac Arrest
   Wider JM, et al. *Crit Care.* 2023.

DOI: 10.1186/s13054-023-04745-7
Link: www.ccforum.biomedcentral.com/articles/10.1186/s13054-023-04745-7

Summary:
Shows that near-infrared photobiomodulation can improve mitochondrial function and reduce neurological injury after cardiac arrest in experimental models.

5. Melatonin and the Optics of the Human Body
   Zimmerman S, Reiter RJ. *Melatonin Research.*

DOI: 10.32794/mr11250016
Link: www.doi.org/10.32794/mr11250016

Summary:
Explores how light interacts with human tissues and discusses melatonin's photobiological and antioxidant roles within the body.

6. Melatonin and Mitochondrial Function
Journal of Photochemistry and Photobiology B. 2022.
DOI: 10.1016/j.jphotobiol.2022.112614
Link: www.sciencedirect.com/science/article/abs/pii/S1011134422002287

Summary:
Reviews melatonin's role in mitochondrial protection, oxidative stress regulation, and cellular energy metabolism.

7. Vitamin D Production After UVB Exposure: Environmental and Personal Determinants
Bogh MKB. *Scand J Clin Lab Invest Suppl.* 2012;243:24–31.
DOI: 10.3109/00365513.2012.681929
Link: www.tandfonline.com/doi/full/10.3109/00365513.2012.681929

Summary:
Examines how ultraviolet-B exposure, latitude, season and individual characteristics influence vitamin D synthesis in human skin.

8. Ultraviolet Radiation and Skin Physiology: Mechanisms and Systemic Effects
Wacker M, Holick MF. *J Aging Res.* 2018;2018:9276380.
DOI: 10.1155/2018/9276380
Link: www.onlinelibrary.wiley.com/doi/10.1155/2018/9276380

Summary:
Reviews the biological effects of ultraviolet radiation on the skin, including vitamin D synthesis, DNA damage, and immune modulation, highlighting both beneficial and harmful systemic consequences of UV exposure.

Chapter 31: Foundations of Health – Mindset

1. The glutamate/GABA–glutamine cycle: transport, neurotransmitter homeostasis, and ammonia transfer
Journal of Neurochemistry. 2006.

Link: www.doi.org/10.1111/j.1471-4159.2006.03913.x (Wiley Online Library)

Summary:
Authoritative review of the astrocyte–neuron glutamine shuttle that maintains synaptic pools of glutamate (excitatory) and GABA (inhibitory), covering key transporters, compartmentation, neurotransmitter recycling, and the coupling of this cycle to ammonia handling and metabolic homeostasis.

2. The selfish brain: competition for energy resources
   Neuroscience & Biobehavioral Reviews. 2004.
Link: www.doi.org/10.1016/j.neubiorev.2004.03.002 (PubMed)

Summary:
A conceptual review proposing the "selfish brain" theory: the brain actively prioritises its energy supply via neuroendocrine and autonomic mechanisms. Discusses HPA-axis/limbic involvement, energy allocation under stress, and implications for body-weight regulation and metabolic disease phenotypes.

3. Factors that affect quality of life in young adults with type 1 diabetes
   The Diabetes Educator. 2018.
Link: www.doi.org/10.1177/0145721718808733 (SAGE Journals)

Summary:
Observational study identifying key psychosocial correlates of quality of life in young adults with T1D, highlighting fear of hypoglycaemia, fear of complications, and diabetes self-efficacy as major contributors – useful targets for supportive interventions.

4. A longitudinal examination of hope and optimism and their role in type 1 diabetes in youths
   Journal of Pediatric Psychology. 2015.
Link: www.pmc.ncbi.nlm.nih.gov/articles/PMC4945775/

Summary:
Longitudinal analysis in paediatric T1D showing that hope (goal-directed thinking) and optimism relate to aspects of diabetes management and adjustment, supporting the clinical value of assessing hope and potentially using hope-focused approaches to improve self-management trajectories.

5. Depression and poor glycemic control: a meta-analytic review of the literature
   Diabetes Care. 2000.
Link: www.doi.org/10.2337/diacare.23.7.934 (PubMed)

Summary:
Classic meta-analysis demonstrating an association between depressive symptoms and worse glycaemic control, consolidating evidence that mood disturbance is clinically relevant for diabetes outcomes and warrants active detection and treatment.

6. Longitudinal changes in depression symptoms and glycemia in adults with type 1 diabetes
   Diabetes Care. 2019.
Link: www.diabetesjournals.org/care/article/42/7/1194/36239/ (Diabetes Journals)

Summary:
Long-term follow-up study tracking depression symptom patterns over years in adults with T1D and examining how shifts in depression status relate to glycaemia, strengthening the case for integrated psychological and metabolic care.

7. Helpful or harmful? The impact of the ketogenic diet on eating disorder outcomes in type 1 diabetes mellitus
   Expert Review of Endocrinology & Metabolism. 2022.
Link: www.doi.org/10.1080/17446651.2022.2089112 (tandfonline.com)

Summary:
Focused review weighing potential benefits and risks when ketogenic diets are used in T1D populations vulnerable to disordered eating. Discusses DKA risk, hypoglycaemia, dyslipidaemia, and the limited evidence base on how carbohydrate restriction interacts with eating disorder behaviours and motivations.

8. Eating disorders in adolescent females with and without type 1 diabetes: cross sectional study
BMJ. 2000.
Link: www.doi.org/10.1136/bmj.320.7249.1563 (BMJ)

Summary:
Cross-sectional study reporting that clinically significant and subthreshold eating disorders are more common in adolescent females with T1D than peers, and are associated with insulin omission for weight control and worse metabolic control – high relevance to screening and safeguarding.

9. Eating disorders and disordered eating in type 1 diabetes: prevalence, screening, and treatment options
Current Diabetes Reports. 2013.
Link: www.pmc.ncbi.nlm.nih.gov/articles/PMC4002640/ (PMC)

Summary:
Clinical review synthesising prevalence data for eating disorders/disordered eating in T1D and outlining practical approaches to screening, recognition, and management, including why insulin manipulation is uniquely dangerous in T1D and how multidisciplinary care is typically required.

10. A simple model to enhance hope: GRIN (Goals, Resources, Increments, Noticing)
Journal of Holistic Healthcare. 2019.
Link: www.bhma.org/wp-content/uploads/2019/06/GRIN-Unwins-JHH-16.2.pdf (bhma.org)

Summary:
Practical, consultation-friendly framework for strengthening patient hope and momentum for behaviour change using structured questions across Goals, Resources, small Increments, and Noticing progress – useful for lifestyle medicine and chronic disease support conversations.

11. Type 1 anxiety
    Resolute Keto (Gina Roberts). Web article.

Link: www.resoluteketo.com/type,1,anxiety/

Summary:
First-person/patient-advocate style piece discussing anxiety in the context of living with T1D, with emphasis on lived experience, coping strategies, and practical reflections relevant to self-management psychology.

12. *Fork in the Road: A Hopeful Guide to Food Freedom*
    Book (Independently published). 2021.

Link: www.amazon.co.uk/Fork-Road-Hopeful-Guide-Freedom/dp/B08XX4ZH3F

Summary:
Accessible, recovery-oriented guide framing carbohydrate/ultra-processed food dependence through a behavioural and psychological lens; focuses on recognising addictive patterns, building motivation, and implementing practical strategies for long-term "food freedom".

13. A Low Carbohydrate Diet in Type 1 Diabetes
    Nielsen JV. A low carbohydrate diet in type 1 diabetes. *Ups J Med Sci.* 2005;110(3):193–204.

Available from: www.ujms.net/index.php/ujms/article/view/6465

Summary:
This paper describes the use of a low-carbohydrate diet in individuals with type 1 diabetes, demonstrating improved glycaemic control with reduced glucose variability and lower insulin requirements. It highlights how carbohydrate restriction can stabilise blood glucose

levels and reduce the burden of hypoglycaemia, supporting a shift toward insulin optimisation rather than reactive glucose management.

Chapter 33: Hydration

1. The Neurobiology of Thirst and Hydration Control: Anticipatory Mechanisms and Homeostasis
   Nature Reviews Nephrology. 2017.

Link: www.nature.com/articles/nrneph.2017.149

Summary:
Review of the neural regulation of thirst and fluid balance, including hypothalamic sensing mechanisms, anticipatory drinking behaviour, and physiological homeostasis of body water.

2. Overhydration and Exercise: Misinterpretation of Hydration Guidelines and Performance
   Noakes TD, et al. *British Journal of Sports Medicine.* 2005.

Link: www.ncbi.nlm.nih.gov/pmc/articles/PMC1872071/

Summary:
Explores the risks of excessive fluid intake during endurance exercise, including exercise-associated hyponatraemia, and argues that thirst-guided drinking may be safer than fixed hydration schedules.

3. The Dangers of Overhydrating During a Race
   Runner's World.

Link: www.runnersworld.com/uk/nutrition/hydration/a774377/the-dangers-of-over-hydrating-during-a-race/

Summary:
Accessible explanation of overhydration during endurance events, highlighting the physiology of sodium dilution and the importance of balanced hydration strategies.

4. Let's Talk About Water: Cultural and Survival Aspects of Water Access in Maasailand
Adumu Impact.
Link: www.adumuimpact.org/lets-talk-about-water/

Summary:
Discussion of water access, cultural practices, and survival strategies in Maasai communities, illustrating how hydration practices are shaped by environment and tradition.

5. How Much Water Does a Human Produce per Day by Cellular Respiration?
Quora discussion thread.
Link: www.quora.com/How-much-water-does-a-human-produce-per-day-by-cell-respiration

Summary:
Informal discussion of metabolic water production from cellular respiration, typically estimated at roughly 250–350 ml per day in adults depending on metabolic rate.

6. Controversial Studies on "Water Memory" Including Jacques Benveniste's Research and Subsequent Trials
Nature; Homeopathy literature; multi-centre replication attempts.
Link: www.ncbi.nlm.nih.gov/pmc/articles/PMC1872071/

Summary:
Discussion of controversial claims that water may retain structural "memory" of dissolved substances, including early experimental reports and subsequent critical evaluation and replication attempts.

Chapter 35: Cholesterol and Lipids

1. Animal Studies on Dietary Cholesterol
Ference BA, et al. *Circulation.* 2020.
Link: www.ahajournals.org/doi/10.1161/CIR.0000000000000743

Summary:
Review of experimental and genetic evidence linking cholesterol metabolism, LDL exposure, and cardiovascular disease risk across animal and human studies.

2. The Seven Countries Study
   Keys A, et al. Seven Countries Study.
Link: www.sevencountriesstudy.com/

Summary:
Landmark epidemiological study examining relationships between dietary fat intake, cholesterol levels, and cardiovascular disease across multiple populations.

3. The Minnesota Coronary Experiment: Dietary Cholesterol Trial
   Ramsden CE, et al. *BMJ.* 2016;353:i1246.
Link: www.bmj.com/content/353/bmj.i1246

Summary:
Reanalysis of a randomised dietary intervention trial investigating replacement of saturated fat with vegetable oils and its effects on cholesterol levels and mortality.

4. Advances in Lipid Management and Ketogenic Diets
   JACC Advances. 2025.
Link: www.jacc.org/doi/epdf/10.1016/j.jacadv.2025.101686

Summary:
Discusses emerging evidence on lipid responses to ketogenic and low-carbohydrate diets, including variability in LDL changes and cardiometabolic risk markers.

5. Low-Carbohydrate Nutrition and Metabolic Outcomes
   PubMed entry.
Link: www.pubmed.ncbi.nlm.nih.gov/38276308/

Summary:
Study examining metabolic outcomes associated with low-carbohydrate dietary patterns, including insulin sensitivity, lipid markers and body composition.

6. NICE Guidelines: Lipid Modification for Cardiovascular Risk
National Institute for Health and Care Excellence (NICE).
Link: www.nice.org.uk/guidance/cg181

Summary:
Clinical guideline for lipid management and cardiovascular risk reduction, including statin therapy and risk-based treatment strategies.

7. Bile Acids and FXR: The New Biology of Cholesterol Homeostasis
Cell Metabolism.
Link: www.cell.com/cell-metabolism/fulltext/S1550-4131(13)00117-4

Summary:
Explains how bile acids function as signalling molecules regulating cholesterol metabolism through FXR pathways.

8. Challenging the LDL Hypothesis: A Review of Clinical Trials and Evidence
Diamond DM, et al. *Nutrition & Metabolism.* 2022.
Link: www.nutritionandmetabolism.biomedcentral.com/articles/10.1186/s12986-022-00687-7

Summary:
Review discussing alternative interpretations of LDL cholesterol, cardiovascular risk, and dietary fat evidence, including critiques of the traditional lipid hypothesis.

Chapter 37: Intermittent Fasting

1. Intermittent Fasting and Autophagy
   de Cabo R, Mattson MP. Effects of Intermittent Fasting on Health, Aging, and Disease. *New England Journal of Medicine.* 2019.
Link: www.pmc.ncbi.nlm.nih.gov/articles/PMC9441677

Summary:
Review article describing how intermittent fasting affects metabolic switching, insulin sensitivity, mitochondrial function, and autophagy, with implications for ageing and chronic disease.

2. Ketones, Glucose, and Insulin in People with Type 1 Diabetes (ZeroFive100)
   Lake I. *ZeroFive100.* Type1Keto.
Link: www.type1keto.com/zerofive100

Summary:
Practical exploration of glucose, ketones and insulin balance in people with type 1 diabetes using carbohydrate restriction and optimised insulin strategies.

Chapter 39: The Retina

1. The evolution of phototransduction and eyes
   Lamb TD, Arendt D, Collin SP. *Philosophical Transactions of the Royal Society B: Biological Sciences.* 2009.
Link: www.pmc.ncbi.nlm.nih.gov/articles/PMC2781866/

Summary:
Review of the evolutionary origins of eyes and phototransduction, explaining how light-detecting systems developed across species and how modern visual pathways emerged.

2. Why rods and cones?
   Lamb TD. *Eye.* 2016.
DOI: www.doi.org/10.1038/eye.2015.236

Link: www.nature.com/articles/eye2015236

Summary:
Explains the physiological differences between rod and cone photoreceptors and their complementary roles in night vision, colour vision, and visual sensitivity.

3. Fatty acid oxidation-dependent metabolism is required for the activation of neural stem cells in the adult brain
Knobloch M, Pilz GA, Ghesquière B, Kovacs WJ, Wegleiter T, Moore DL, Hruzova M, Zamboni N, Carmeliet P, Jessberger S. *Journal of Biological Chemistry.* 2014;289(30):20570–20582.
DOI: www.doi.org/10.1074/jbc.M114.565457

Summary:
Demonstrates that fatty-acid oxidation supports activation of adult neural stem cells, highlighting the importance of lipid metabolism in brain function and regeneration.

Chapter 41: Breathing

1. Interaction of Psychological and Emotional Variables with Breathing Dysfunction
Gilbert C. Interaction of psychological and emotional variables with breathing dysfunction. In: Courtney R, Cohen M, editors. *Recognizing and Treating Breathing Disorders: A Multidisciplinary Approach.* 2nd ed. Churchill Livingstone Elsevier; 2014.

Summary:
Explores how psychological stress, emotional state, and behavioural patterns influence breathing function and contribute to dysfunctional breathing syndromes, highlighting the importance of multidisciplinary treatment approaches.

About the Author

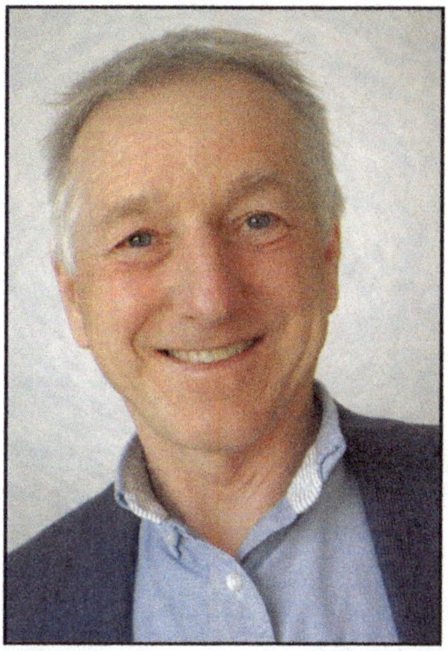

Dr Ian Lake, BSc (Cell Biology and Biochemistry), BM, MRCGP, is a UK-based medical doctor and long-term person living with type 1 diabetes (diagnosed in 1995). Over the past decade, he has conducted extensive independent research into insulin biology in type 1 diabetes, with a particular focus on how insulin function is influenced by lifestyle factors beyond diet. His work examines the effects of sleep, circadian rhythm, stress, physical activity, environmental cues, and behavioural patterns on insulin sensitivity and metabolic stability.

Dr Lake's research considers insulin not only as a glucose-lowering therapy but as a master metabolic hormone central to energy homeostasis, lipid metabolism and whole-body physiology. Through integrating clinical insight with lived experience, he has explored how aligning lifestyle with the body's natural metabolic rhythms can reduce glycaemic variability and total insulin requirements. His work supports the guiding principle of using "as much insulin as necessary, but as little as possible", a concept grounded in metabolic physiology and increasingly reflected in emerging scientific literature.

He is engaged in clinical education and public communication on the broader metabolic understanding of type 1 diabetes, promoting approaches that move beyond the limits of carb-focused management.

About the Author

Made in the USA
Monee, IL
12 September 2026

62976472R00223